A Text Book of

PHARMACEUTICAL BIOTECHNOLOGY

As Per PCI Regulations
Third Year B. Pharm.
Semester VI

Prof. Chandrakant Kokare
Professor and Head (Pharmaceutics)
Sinhgad Technical Education Society
Sinhgad Institute of Pharmacy
Narhe, Pune 411 041, India

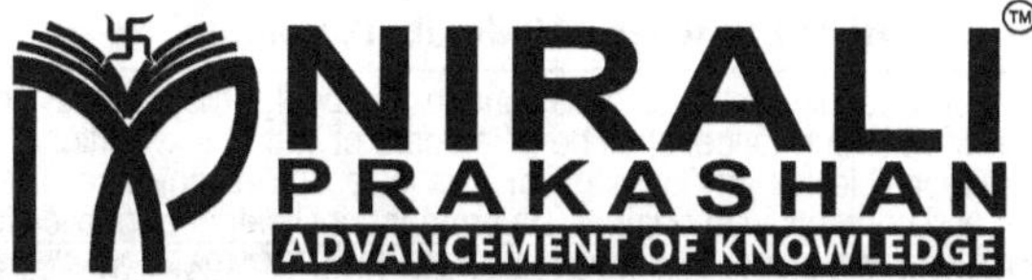

N4062

Pharmaceutical Biotechnology **ISBN 978-93-89686-34-0**

First Edition : **November, 2019**

Published By :

NIRALI PRAKASHAN

Abhyudaya Pragati, 1312, Shivaji Nagar

Off J.M. Road, Pune – 411005

Tel - (020) 25512336/37/39, Fax - (020) 25511379

Email : niralipune@pragationline.com

➢ DISTRIBUTION CENTRES

PUNE

Nirali Prakashan (For orders within Pune) : 119, Budhwar Peth, Jogeshwari Mandir Lane, Pune 411002, Maharashtra
Tel : (020) 2445 2044; Mobile : 9657703145
Email : niralilocal@pragationline.com

Nirali Prakashan (For orders outside Pune) : S. No. 28/27, Dhayari, Near Asian College Pune 411041
Tel : (020) 24690204; Mobile : 9657703143
Email : bookorder@pragationline.com

MUMBAI

Nirali Prakashan : 385, S.V.P. Road, Rasdhara Co-op. Hsg. Society Ltd.,
Girgaum, Mumbai 400004, Maharashtra; Mobile : 9320129587
Tel : (022) 2385 6339 / 2386 9976, Fax : (022) 2386 9976
Email : niralimumbai@pragationline.com

➢ DISTRIBUTION BRANCHES

JALGAON

Nirali Prakashan : 34, V. V. Golani Market, Navi Peth, Jalgaon 425001, Maharashtra,
Tel : (0257) 222 0395, Mob : 94234 91860; Email : niralijalgaon@pragationline.com

KOLHAPUR

Nirali Prakashan : New Mahadvar Road, Kedar Plaza, 1st Floor Opp. IDBI Bank, Kolhapur 416 012
Maharashtra. Mob : 9850046155; Email : niralikolhapur@pragationline.com

NAGPUR

Nirali Prakashan : Above Maratha Mandir, Shop No. 3, First Floor,
Rani Jhanshi Square, Sitabuldi, Nagpur 440012, Maharashtra
Tel : (0712) 254 7129; Email : niralinagpur@pragationline.com

DELHI

Nirali Prakashan : 4593/15, Basement, Agarwal Lane, Ansari Road, Daryaganj
Near Times of India Building, New Delhi 110002 Mob : 08505972553
Email : niralidelhi@pragationline.com

BENGALURU

Nirali Prakashan : Maitri Ground Floor, Jaya Apartments, No. 99, 6th Cross, 6th Main,
Malleswaram, Bengaluru 560003, Karnataka; Mob : 9449043034
Email: niralibangalore@pragationline.com

Other Branches : Hyderabad, Chennai

PREFACE OF FIRST EDITION

Pharmaceutical Biotechnology subject has been included in the syllabus of almost all colleges and universities both at under-graduate and post-graduate levels. This subject is related to development of new strains for pharmaceuticals, fermentation technology, recombinant technology, enzyme immobilization, developments of transgenic plants and animals, and production of new molecules by biotransformation.

This **'PHARMACEUTICAL BIOTECHNOLOGY** book has been written by considering the syllabus prescribed by **PHARMACY COUNCIL OF INDIA (PCI).** The book is designed for Third Year B. Pharm students (semester-VI). All the chapters in the present book are followed by objective type, short answer, long answer and multiple choice questions as per University examination pattern.

The book is a simple, handy, comprehensive and profusely illustrated digest on Pharmaceutical Biotechnology with special stress on the requirement of undergraduates. The basic principles and techniques of diverse biotechnological fields have been presented. The realization of the need and importance for students promoted me to write new book as per syllabus of PCI semester pattern. It is also hoped that it will serve as a useful resource for teachers of Pharmaceutical Biotechnology.

I express my sincere thanks to all my teachers, faculty members and students for their kind help, motivation and valuable guidance in writing this book. I express my deep sense of gratitude to my family for their love, support and motivation in academics and research. I am also thankful to team of Nirali Prakashan for their sustained efforts and keen interest in the publication of this book.

Readers are requested to write any shortcomings in this edition and give the valuable suggestions for the improvement of this book for the next edition.

November, 2019

Prof. Chandrakant Kokare

kokare71@rediffmail.com

■■■

SYLLABUS

Unit I **[10 Hours]**

(a) Brief Introduction to Biotechnology with reference to Pharmaceutical Sciences.
(b) Enzyme Biotechnology - Methods of Enzyme Immobilization and Applications.
(c) Biosensors - Working and applications of biosensors in Pharmaceutical Industries.
(d) Brief Introduction to Protein Engineering.
(e) Use of Microbes in Industry. Production of Enzymes - General Consideration - Amylase, Catalase, Peroxidase, Lipase, Protease, Penicillinase.
(f) Basic Principles of Genetic Engineering.

Unit II **[10 Hours]**

(a) Study of Cloning Vectors, Restriction Endonucleases and DNA Ligase.
(b) Recombinant DNA Technology, Application of Genetic Engineering in Medicine.
(c) Application of rDNA technology and Genetic Engineering in the Production of:
(i) Interferon (ii) Vaccines-hepatitis-B (iii) Hormones-Insulin.
(d) Brief introduction to PCR

Unit III **[10 Hours]**

Types of Immunity - Humoral Immunity, Cellular Immunity.
(a) Structure of Immunoglobulins.
(b) Structure and Function of MHC.
(c) Hypersensitivity Reactions, Immune Stimulation and Immune Suppressions.
(d) General Method of the preparation of Bacterial Vaccines, Toxoids, Viral Vaccine, Antitoxins, Serum-Immune Blood Derivatives and other Products Relative to Immunity.
(e) Storage conditions and Stability of Official Vaccines
(f) Hybridoma Technology - Production, Purification and Applications.
(g) Blood Products and Plasma Substituties.

Unit IV **[08 Hours]**

(a) Immuno Blotting Techniques - ELISA, Western blotting, Southern Blotting.
(b) Genetic Organization of Eukaryotes and Prokaryotes.
(c) Microbial Genetics including Transformation, Transduction, Conjugation, Plasmids and Transposons.
(d) Introduction to Microbial Biotransformation and Applications.
(e) Mutation: Types of Mutation/Mutants.

Unit V **[07 Hours]**

(a) Fermentation Methods and General Requirements, Study of Media, Equipments, Sterilization Methods, Aeration Process, Stirring.
(b) Large Scale Production Fermenter Design and its various Controls.
(c) Study of the Production of - Penicillins, Citric Acid, Vitamin B_{12}, Glutamic Acid, Griseofulvin.
(d) Blood Products: Collection, Processing and Storage of whole Human Blood, Dried Human Plasma, Plasma Substituties.

■■■

CONTENTS

SYLLABUS

Unit I **[10 Hours]**

(a) Brief Introduction to Biotechnology with reference to Pharmaceutical Sciences.
(b) Enzyme Biotechnology - Methods of Enzyme Immobilization and Applications.
(c) Biosensors - Working and applications of biosensors in Pharmaceutical Industries.
(d) Brief Introduction to Protein Engineering.
(e) Use of Microbes in Industry. Production of Enzymes - General Consideration - Amylase, Catalase, Peroxidase, Lipase, Protease, Penicillinase.
(f) Basic Principles of Genetic Engineering.

Unit II **[10 Hours]**

(a) Study of Cloning Vectors, Restriction Endonucleases and DNA Ligase.
(b) Recombinant DNA Technology, Application of Genetic Engineering in Medicine.
(c) Application of rDNA technology and Genetic Engineering in the Production of: (i) Interferon (ii) Vaccines-hepatitis-B (iii) Hormones-Insulin.
(d) Brief introduction to PCR

Unit III **[10 Hours]**

Types of Immunity - Humoral Immunity, Cellular Immunity.

(a) Structure of Immunoglobulins.
(b) Structure and Function of MHC.
(c) Hypersensitivity Reactions, Immune Stimulation and Immune Suppressions.
(d) General Method of the preparation of Bacterial Vaccines, Toxoids, Viral Vaccine, Antitoxins, Serum-Immune Blood Derivatives and other Products Relative to Immunity.
(e) Storage conditions and Stability of Official Vaccines
(f) Hybridoma Technology - Production, Purification and Applications.
(g) Blood Products and Plasma Substituties.

Unit IV **[08 Hours]**

(a) Immuno Blotting Techniques - ELISA, Western blotting, Southern Blotting.
(b) Genetic Organization of Eukaryotes and Prokaryotes.
(c) Microbial Genetics including Transformation, Transduction, Conjugation, Plasmids and Transposons.
(d) Introduction to Microbial Biotransformation and Applications.
(e) Mutation: Types of Mutation/Mutants.

Unit V **[07 Hours]**

(a) Fermentation Methods and General Requirements, Study of Media, Equipments, Sterilization Methods, Aeration Process, Stirring.
(b) Large Scale Production Fermenter Design and its various Controls.
(c) Study of the Production of - Penicillins, Citric Acid, Vitamin B_{12}, Glutamic Acid, Griseofulvin.
(d) Blood Products: Collection, Processing and Storage of whole Human Blood, Dried Human Plasma, Plasma Substituties.

■■■

CONTENTS

■■■

■■■

Chapter ... 1

INTRODUCTION TO BIOTECHNOLOGY

♦ LEARNING OBJECTIVES ♦

After completing this chapter, reader should be able to understand:

- *Introduction*
- *Milestones in Biotechnology*
- *Scope and applications in Pharmaceutical Sciences*

1.1 INTRODUCTION

Biotechnology has created many opportunities for the benefit of mankind and in the understanding of the fundamental life processes. The term biotechnology was introduced in 1917 by a Hungarian engineer, **Karl Ereky**. He used the term for large-scale production of pigs by using sugar beets as the source of food. According to Ereky, all types of work are biotechnology by which products are produced from raw materials using living organisms. Traditional Biotechnology that led to the development of processes for producing products like yogurt, vinegar, alcohol, wine and cheese. The modern biotechnology embraces all the genetic manipulations and the improvement made in the old or traditional biotechnological processes. Modern biotechnology has offered opportunities to produce more nutritious and better testing foods, higher crop yields and plants that are naturally protected from disease and insects.

Biotechnology is one of the world's fastest growing and most rapidly changing technology. During the end of 20th century biotechnology emerged as a new discipline of biology integrating with technology. Biotechnology is the application of scientific and engineering principles to the processing of materials by biological agents (microorganisms, plant and animal cell) to provide goods and services. The **Spinks Report** (1980) defined biotechnology as the application of biological organisms, system or processes to the manufacturing and service industries. Biotechnology can be represented as a mixture of various biological sciences for better services in the field of pharmaceuticals such as microbiology, biochemistry, biophysics, cell biology, genetics, molecular biology, engineering technology etc.

Biotechnology has given to humans several useful products by using microbes, plant, animals and their metabolic machinery. Recombinant DNA technology has made it possible to engineer microbes, plants and animals such that they have novel capabilities.

The basic areas and applied branches of biotechnology are shown in Fig. 1.1.

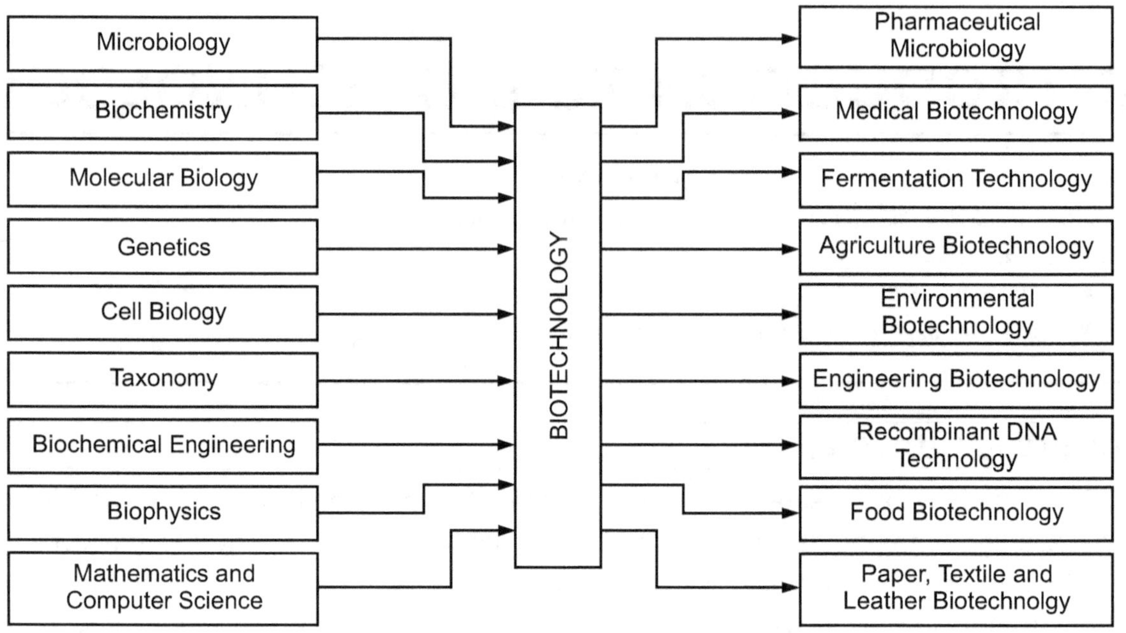

Fig. 1.1: Basic areas and applied branches of Biotechnology

A series of derived terms have been coined to identify several branches of biotechnology. **Bioinformatics** is an interdisciplinary field which addresses biological problems using computational techniques, and makes the rapid organization and analysis of biological data. The field may also be referred to as **computational biology,** and it is defined as, "conceptualizing biology in terms of molecules and then applying informatics techniques to understand and organize the information associated with these molecules." Bioinformatics plays a key role in various areas, such as genomics and proteomics, and forms a key component in the biotechnology, molecular biology and pharmaceutical sciences. **Blue biotechnology** is a term that has been used to describe the marine and aquatic applications of biotechnology. **Green biotechnology** is biotechnology applied to agricultural processes. The designing of transgenic plants to grow under specific environments in the presence or absence of chemicals is the example of green biotechnology. **Red biotechnology** is applied to medical processes. The designing of organisms to produce new active molecules such as antibiotics, and the engineering of genetic cures through genetic manipulation are the examples of red biotechnology. **White biotechnology**, also known as industrial biotechnology, is biotechnology applied to industrial processes. The designing of an organism to produce active chemicals which are useful for industry such as enzymes and proteins are the examples of white biotechnology. The investment and economic output of all of these types of applied biotechnologies is termed as **bioeconomy**.

1.2 MILESTONES IN BIOTECHNOLOGY

In the late 19th century, many discoveries and developments were made to gene birth of molecular biology by biochemists, geneticists and cell biologists. The term biotechnology was described in a bulletin of the Bureau of Biotechnology published in 1920. The articles in this bulletin described the different roles of microbes in leather industry, pest control and fermentations. The historical developments in biotechnology are summarized in Table 1.1.

Table 1.1: Historical development in biotechnology

Development	Year
Pasteur proposes that microbes that cause fermentation.	1857
Discovery of genetic basis of heredity by **Gregor Mendel**.	1860
Fleming discovers chromation, i.e. chromosomes.	1879
The first cancer causing virus is discovered by Rous.	1911
Microbes are used to treat sewage for the first time in Manchester, England.	1914
Development of fermentations process for acetone and n-butanol by **Chain Weizmann**.	1916
Discovery of penicillin by **Alexander Fleming**.	1929
Discovery of streptomycin by **Selman Waksman**.	1943
DNA is proven to carry genetic information.	1944
Elucidation of double helical structure of DNA by **Francis Crick** and **James Walson**.	1953
Mechanism of DNA replication was studied in *E. coli* by **Meseleson** and **Stahl**.	1958
Determination of genetic code by **Nirenberg** and **Mathaei**.	1961
DNA transformation into *E. coli*.	1970
Discovery of restriction enzymes.	1971
Preparation of monoclonal antibodies using hybridoma cells by **Cesar Milstein** and **George Kohler**.	1975
Sequencing of DNA by **Sanger** and **Coulson**.	1975
Genetically engineered microorganisms can be patented (US Supreme Court).	1980
Development of Gene Bank.	1982
Discovery of PCR.	1985
Development of human genome project.	1990
Complete sequencing of yeast genome.	1996
Dolly (sheep), first cloned animal.	1998
Maintenance of human stem cells in culture.	1998
Human genome, the first mammalian genome sequenced.	2001

The concept of molecular biology, microbiology, and biotechnology has changed the scenario of pharmaceutical developments. The advancements in recombinant (rDNA) and monoclonal antibody technology have led to developments of new drug molecules. Products developed from the basis of genetic engineering are recombinant soluble CD_4, tissue plasminogen, erythropoietin, colony stimulating factors etc. Different types of diagnostic kits are developed by using monoclonal antibodies. The most developing field in pharmaceutical biotechnology is the production of therapeutically active proteins and peptides. These drugs have been extensively utilized in replacement therapies where the patient is unable to produce the required protein (e.g. insulin). Many drugs and vaccines are developed by using basic concepts of biotechnology. Genomics, pharmacogenomics, proteomics, gene therapy, gene cloning and tissue engineering are the present focus of biotechnology.

Some major advancements in the field of pharmaceuticals in the last few decades have come forth as a result of extensive research and development in biotechnology. Human Insulin (Humulin) is the first pharmaceutical product derived from DNA technology which was discovered by Genetech and Eli Lilly and Company in 1882 and this product has been approved by US FDA. Recent advances in genetics, immune system, recombinant DNA, hybridomas and monoclonal antibiotics have led to a rapid increase in the number of biotechnological products (Table 1.2) for human use. In 1988, only five proteins from genetically engineered cells had been approved as drugs by the United States Food and Drug Administration (FDA), but this number would skyrocket to over 125 by the end of the 1990s. There was tremendous progress in agricultural field since the market introduction of the genetically engineered Flavr Savr tomato in 1994. Ernst and Young reported that in 1998, 30% of the U.S. soybean crop was expected to be from genetically engineered seeds.

Table 1.2: Important biotechnology drugs and vaccines

Generic name	Product name	Name of company	Year of discovery
Human insulin	Humulin	Eli Lilly	1982
Sometrem	Protropin	Genetech	1985
Digoxin Immune Fab	Digibind	Burroughs Wellcome	1986
Interferon-α - 2a	Roferon-A	Hoffmann – La- Roche	1986
Interferon-α - 2b	Intron-A	Schering- Plough	1986
Hepatitis-B-vaccine	Recombivax HB	Merk	1986
Somatotropin	Humatrope	Eli Lilly	1987
Heamophilus-B-conjugate Vaccine	Hib. Titer	Praxis Biologics	1988
Hepatitis-B-vaccine	Engerix-B	SmithKline Beecham	1989
Interferon-y-Ib	Actimmune	Genetech	1990
Sargramostim	Leukin	Immunex	1991

1.3 SCOPE AND APPLICATIONS IN PHARMACEUTICAL SCIENCES

Biotechnology is the applied science and has made many advances in different fields. Pharmaceutical biotechnology is based on the production of antibiotics, vaccines, therapeutic proteins, hormones, vitamins and other pharmaceuticals. It also includes targeted drug delivery system, standardization of chemotherapeutic agents, production control using biosensors, enzyme immobilization, gene cloning technology, monoclonal antibodies etc. Fields of medical biotechnology, agriculture biotechnology, environmental biotechnology and marine biotechnology are linked with pharmaceutical biotechnology. Major developments are taken place in the field of pharmaceuticals in the last few decades because of extensive research and advancement in the field of biotechnology, biochemistry, organic chemistry, pharmacology and new drug delivery systems.

Recombinant DNA technology: The recombinant DNA technology is appreciated as a milestone in development of pharmaceutical biotechnology. Different products are prepared by genetic engineering such as human insulin, erythropoietins, tumour necrosis factors, monoclonal antibodies, clotting factor, tissue plasminogen activator, interleukins, interferons, antitrypsin etc. The production of human insulin by recombinant DNA techniques was an early goal for the pharmaceutical industry. This technique has been used to produce number of natural proteins, vaccines and enzymes. Various diagnostic kits have been developed such as tumour kits, pregnancy testing, ovarian cancer detecting test, immunoradiometric assay kits etc.

Gene therapy: Inserting a missing gene or replacing a defective one in human cells is an important outcome of gene therapy. This technique uses a harmless virus to carry the missing a new gene into the appropriate chromosome. Gene therapy has been used to treat patients with adenosine deaminase (ADA) deficiency, a cause of severe combined immunodeficiency disease (SICD), in which cells of immune system are missing or inactive. Spliceosome-mediated RNA trans-splicing (SMaRT) is a new technology for gene therapy that exploits the expressed genetic differences between normal and diseased cells. This technology may be applied to a wide range of diseases that involve the expression of unique or mutated genes. Cystic fibrosis, duchenne muscular dystrophy (DMD), spinal muscular atropy (SMA) diseases are easily treated by SMaRT gene therapy.

Molecular markers: The last decade has seen great advances in the development of molecular biological reagents, robotics, arraying techniques, assay detection technologies and faster computers. This has made it possible to embrace comprehensive monitoring of complex biomolecular events at reasonable costs. The use of microarrays and other technologies has provided the ability to monitor the expression of essentially the whole genome in the form of individual mRNA levels for a wide variety of situations and settings. This has opened the door to use of molecular profiling or multi-variant biomarker strategies for every step in the drug discovery and development process. The use of large complex sets of genomic biomarkers, generally in the form of microarrays used to monitor the expression of large set of genes. It is used in the identification and validation of drug targets. Polymerase chain reaction (PCR), is also being used to more quickly and accurately identify the presence of infections such as AIDS, Chlamydias and other microbial diseases.

Criminal forensic: DNA fingerprinting is the process of cross matching two strands of DNA. In criminal investigations, DNA from samples of hair, body fluids or skin at a crime scene is compared with those obtained from the suspects. It uses highly developed technologies with scientific evidence to investigate criminal cases involving robbery, kidnapping, rape, murder or identification of any missing relatives in any calamity. It has become one of the most powerful and widely known applications of biotechnology today.

Monoclonal antibody: Antibodies are glycoproteins that can be made to specifically target the immunizing agent. They are very useful for *in-vitro* and *in-vivo* diagnostic applications. They are also being used to detect allergies, anaemias and heart diseases. Monoclonal antibody diagnostic kits are available for drug assays, blood typing and infectious diseases such as hepatitis, gonorrhoea, syphilis, streptococcal infections, AIDS etc. The most important utilization of the hybridoma technology is the target oriented therapy so as to attain cell specific delivery of drugs for cancer, HIV etc.

Genetically engineered vaccine: The first genetically engineered vaccine was approved in US in 1986 for hepatitis B. Genetic engineering allows large scale production of the protein components of a virus. Many vaccines are under development for production of humans against influenza, rabies, hepatitis, herpes simplex, poliomyelitis etc.

Plant tissue culture: Plant tissue culture is the technique of growing plant cells, tissues and organs in an artificially prepared medium under aseptic conditions. This technique has many applications for production of secondary metabolites. Many natural products are prepared by plant tissue culture such as vincristine, vinblastine, opium alkaloids, digitalis glycosides etc. Plant cells are also used in the process of biotransformation. It has potential for bioconversion of steroids, alkaloids, tannins etc. The method of immobilized plant cells has been found very effective for the production of secondary metabolites. Animal cell culture deals with the study of organs, tissues or individual cells *in-vitro*. Antibodies, enzymes, hormones, cytokines etc. are produced by animal cell culture techniques.

Genetically engineering plants: Genetically engineering plants are also poised to produce vaccines. A few hundred acres of genetically engineered banana plantation can provide enough vaccine to immunize 120 million children every year that need to be protected against common diseases. *Bacillus thuringiensis* produce proteins that kill certain insects such as lepidopterans (tobacco budworm, armyworm), coleopterans (beetles) and dipterans (flies, mosquitoes). *B. thuringiensis* forms protein crystals during a particular phase of their growth. These crystals contain a toxic insecticidal protein. The Bt toxin protein exist as inactive protoxins but once an insect ingest the inactive toxin, it is converted into an active form of toxin due to the alkaline pH of the gut which solubilise the crystals. The activated toxin binds to the surface of midgut epithelial cells and create pores that cause cell swelling and eventually cause death of the insect. Bt toxin gene has been cloned from the bacteria and been expressed in plants to provide resistance to insects without the need for insecticides

Genetically engineered animals: One of the future sources of cheap protein-drugs in the coming years, would be genetically engineered animals who would secrete these drugs in their milk. They will be available at a cost of three or more times lower than the current cost. Animals that have had their DNA manipulated to possess and express an extra (foreign) gene are known as transgenic animals. Transgenic rats, rabbits, pigs, sheep, cows and fish have been produced, although over 95 per cent of all existing transgenic animals are mice. Transgenic animals can be specifically designed to allow the study of how genes are regulated, and how they affect the normal functions of the body. Many transgenic animals are designed to increase our understanding of how genes contribute to the development of disease. These are specially made to serve as models for human diseases such as cancer, cystic fibrosis, rheumatoid arthritis and Alzheimer's so that investigation of new treatments for diseases is made possible. Transgenic animals that produce useful biological products can be created by the introduction of the portion of DNA which codes for a particular product such as human protein (α_1-antitrypsin) used to treat emphysema. In 1997, the first transgenic cow, **Rosie,** produced human protein-enriched milk. The milk contained the human alpha-lactalbumin and was nutritionally a more balanced product for human babies than natural cow-milk. Transgenic mice are being developed for use in testing the safety of vaccines before they are used on humans. Transgenic mice are being used to test the safety of the polio vaccine. Transgenic animals are made that carry genes which make them more sensitive to toxic substances than non-transgenic animals. Toxicity testing in such animals will allow to obtain results in less time.

Pharmacogenomics: Pharmacogenomics is the study of how the genetic inheritance of an individual affects his/her body's response to drugs. The term is derived from the root of the word "pharmacology" and the word "genomics". The vision of pharmacogenomics is to be able to design and produce drugs that are adapted to each person's genetic makeup. Using pharmacogenomics, pharmaceutical companies can create drugs based on the proteins, enzymes and RNA molecules that are associated with specific genes and diseases. These tailor-made drugs not only to maximize therapeutic effects but also to decrease damage to nearby healthy cells. The discovery of potential therapies will be made easier using genome targets. Genes have been associated with numerous diseases and disorders. With modern biotechnology, these genes can be used as targets for the development of effective new therapies, which could significantly shorten the drug discovery process.

Bioinformatics: Bioinformatics is an emerging interdisciplinary area of science and technology encompassing a systematic development and application of IT solutions to handle biological information by addressing biological data collection and warehousing, data mining, database searches, analyses and interpretation, modeling and product design. Being an interface between modern biology and informatics it involves discovery, development and implementation of computational algorithms and software tools that facilitate an understanding of the biological processes with the goal to serve primarily agriculture and healthcare sectors with several spinoffs. In the pharmaceutical sector, it can be used to reduce the time and cost involved in drug discovery process particularly for third world diseases, to custom design drugs and to develop personalized medicine. Computer-aided drug design (CADD) is a specialized discipline that uses computational methods to simulate drug-receptor interactions. CADD methods are heavily dependent on bioinformatics tools, applications and databases.

Human Genome Project (HGP): The Human Genome Project (HGP) is an attempt to map completely the entire spectrum of genetic materials that can be found in all human beings. It is used to determine the complete sequence of the DNA from a typical human cell and it provides information and resources to understand some of the critical differences that make us individuals and that often contribute to diseases. Technology and resources promoted by the Human Genome Project are starting to have profound impacts on biomedical research and promise to revolutionize the wider spectrum of biological research and clinical medicine. It is expected that the development in biotechnology will lead to a new scientific revolution that could change the lives and future of the people.

QUESTIONS

(A) Objective Type Questions:

1. Define: (i) Biotechnology, (ii) Recombinant DNA technology.
2. What is gene therapy?
3. Why insecticidal protein present in *B. thuringiensis* does not kill bacteria?
4. What is the most common application of PCR?

(B) Short Answer Questions:

1. Explain in short different branches of biotechnology.
2. What are the various approaches to treat DNA deficiency disease?
3. Write advantages and disadvantages of genetically modified crops.
4. How can biotechnology be useful in agriculture? Explain with examples.

(C) Long Answer Questions:

1. Write in short 'historical developments' in biotechnology.
2. Explain in detail importance of Biotechnology with reference to Pharmaceutical Sciences.

(D) Multiple Choice Questions:

1. The double helical structure of DNA is discovered by _____.
   (a) Crick and Walson (b) Meselesson and Stahl
   (c) Milstein and Kohler (d) Sanger and Coulson
2. Which one of the following is the first rDNA product?
   (a) Interleukins (b) Leptin
   (c) Tissue of plasminogen activator (d) Insulin
3. The enzyme not used in genetic engineering
   (a) Ligase (b) Polymerase
   (c) Phosphatase (d) Lipase
4. Fermentation technique was introduced by _____
   (a) Paul Ehrlich (b) Louis Pasteur
   (c) Robert Koch (d) A. Fleming
5. Pencillin was discovered by _____
   (a) Paul Ehrlich (b) Louis Pasteur
   (c) Milstein and Kohler (d) A. Fleming
6. Who is said to be founder of modern genetics?
   (a) Charles Darwin (b) Gregor Mendel
   (c) Robert Koch (d) August Weismann

■■■

Chapter ... 2

ENZYME BIOTECHNOLOGY

♦ LEARNING OBJECTIVES ♦

After completing this chapter, reader should be able to understand:

- *Introduction*
- *Enzyme Immobilization*
  - *Methods of Immobilization*
  - *Applications of Immobilization*
- *Production of Enzymes*
  - *Amylase*
  - *Catalase*
  - *Peroxidase*
  - *Lipase*
  - *Protease*
  - *Penicillinase*

2.1 INTRODUCTION

Enzyme technology is the technology associated with the use of enzymes as tools in industry, pharmaceuticals, agriculture or medicine. Enzymes are soluble, amorphous, colloidal, proteineous, bioactive organic catalyst produced by living cells. They are proteins, composed of one polypeptide (amino acid chain) or more associated polypeptide chains. The catalytic activity of enzymes depend on the L-α-amino acid sequence and peptide bonds constituting the protein molecule. Primary, secondary, tertiary and quaternary structures of enzyme proteins are necessary for their catalytic activity. Enzymes are called holoenzyme composed of protein (apoenzyme), non-protein (coenzyme) and metal. Protein part of enzyme is attached to non-protein part by covalent or non-covalent bond. When coenzyme is attached to apoenzyme tightly and permanently then it is called as prosthetic group. Enzymes have molecular weights ranging from about 12,000 to over one million.

Enzymes are mainly classified as extracellular enzymes (exoenzyme) and intracellular enzymes (endoenzyme). Exoenzymes are secreted outside the cell such as cellulose, polyglucturonase, pectinmethylesterase etc. Endoenzymes are secreted within the cell such as invertase, uric oxidase, asparaginase etc. Endoenzymes are isolated by breaking the cells by means of a homogenizer or a bead mill and extracting them through the biochemical processes.

Table 2.1: Sources and applications of enzymes

Source	Name of enzyme	Source of enzyme	Applications
Plant	Proteases	Pineapple, papaya	Inflammation gastritis
	Amylolytic	Wheat, potatoes, beans, soybeans	Production of glucose syrup
	α or β Amylase	Seeds	Paper, textile industries
Animal	Lipase	Pancreatic gland	Food and oil industry
	Chymotrypsin (protease)	Bovine pancreas	Inflammation
	Plasmin (protease)	Plasminogen	Thrombotic disorders
	Pepsin	Animal intestine	Digestion
	Glucose oxidase	Liver	Digestive aid
	Urokinase (protease)	Human urine	Thromboembolic diseases
	Hyaluronidase	Animal *testes*	Local anesthesia
Bacteria	α-Amylase	*Bacillus* spp.	Paper, textile, baking industries
	β-Amylase	*Bacillus cereus*	
	Streptokinase	*Streptococcus* spp.	Thromboembolic diseases
	Urokinase (protease)	*Bacillus fastidiosus*	Thromboembolic diseases
	Proteinase	*Escherichia coli, Bacillus subtilis*	Genetics, rDNA technology
	Penicillin acylase	*Bacillus megaterium*	Production of semi-synthetic penicillin
	Glucose isomerase	*Bacillus coagulans, Streptomyces* sp.,	Preparation of fructose
	Dextran sucrase	*Leuconostoc mesenteroides*	Production of dextran
Fungi	α-Amylase, proteinase	*Aspergillus oryzae*	Paper, textile and baking industries
	Catalase, lactase, amyloglucosidase	*Aspergillus niger*	Cytotoxic agent
	Cellulase	*Trichoderma reesi, Penicillium funiculsosum*	Polymer degradation in detergents
	Dextranase	*Penicillium* sp.	Dental plaque
	Glucoamylase	*Aspergillus niger, Rhizopus* sp.	Production of maltose syrup
	Invertase	*Saccharomyces* sp.	Sugar industry
	Lactase	*Aspergillus niger, Kluveromyces fragilis*	Milk and ice-cream industry
	Lipase	*Candida lipoytica Rhizopus delemar*	Food industry

Enzymes are mainly obtained from living cells from plants, animals and microorganisms (Table 2.1). Mitochondria, granular microsome, lysosome and ribosome are major sources for enzymes in plant and animal cells. Animal gland is source for hydrolyzing enzymes used as digestive aids. The pancreas is source of trypsinogen (23%) and chymotrypsinogen (10 to 14%). Pancreatin contains several enzymes such as amylase, protease etc. The selection of the sources for enzyme is dependent on specificity, activation, inhibition, pH, thermostability, availability and cost. The extraction of enzymes from plant and animal sources are simple as compared to microbial sources. Microbial sources are capable of producing a wide variety of enzymes from bacteria and fungi. The enzyme concentration in these cells is dependent on environmental conditions and genetic manipulations. Microbial cells require short fermentation times, inexpensive media and simple screening procedures.

2.2 ENZYME IMMOBILIZATION

Enzyme immobilization is a process in which 'enzymes are physically confined, or localized in a certain defined region of space with retention of their catalytic activities' and which can be used repeatedly and continuously. It is the process wherein an enzyme or cell makes use of safe carrier phase for stealth and safe homing. The use of enzymes in industrial applications is limited because most of the enzymes are relatively unstable and high cost of isolation, purification and recovery of active enzymes from the reaction mixtures after the completion of catalytic process. Hence, enzymes must be immobilized on the surface of some solid support or it can convert a continuous flow of substrate to product without being lost. The first commercial application of immobilized enzyme technology was realised in 1969 in Japan with the use of *Aspergillus oryzae* amino acylase for the industrial production of L-amino acids. The advantage of immobilized enzymes are as follows.

- The immobilization process can lead to increased activity and stability of the enzyme molecules.
- They are physically confined during a continuous catalytic process.
- Immobilized enzymes are easily recovered from the reaction mixture and reused. Hence, process is more economic.
- They can be operated continuously and can be readily controlled.
- Enzyme immobilization process avoids the contamination in products and increases enzyme: substrate ratio.
- The products can be easily separated.

Methods of enzyme immobilization:

Enzyme immobilization methods are classified as surface immobilization and within surface immobilization (Fig. 2.1). These methods depend upon physical relationship of the catalyst to the matrix (carrier).

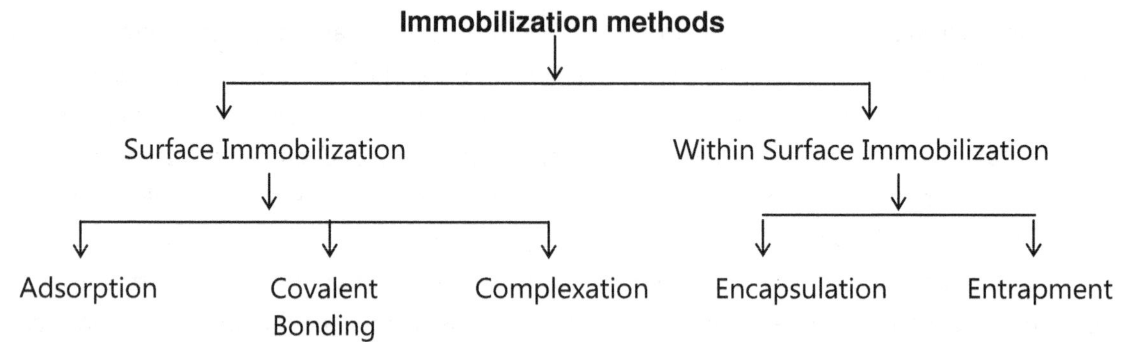

Fig. 2.1: Methods of enzyme immobilization

The major components of an immobilized enzyme are the enzyme, the matrix and the mode of interaction of the enzyme with the carrier. The selected matrix must enhance the operational stability of the immobilized enzyme purification. The carriers used for enzyme immobilization are porous or non-porous materials with organic (natural or synthetic) or inorganic nature. An ideal carrier matrix should be inert, cost effective, stable, high regidity, regenerability, large surface area, more permeability, suitable shape and highly resistance to microbial attack.

Adsorption: Adsorption is the most economical and simple method to immobilize enzymes by adsorbing them on to charged or neutral surfaces of inert substrate. Various kinds of supports are used for adsorption such as aluminium oxide, charcoal, starch, modified sepharose, cellulose derivatives, glass and ion exchange resins. The adsorption of an enzyme is dependent on the experimental variables such as pH, ionic strength, temperature, nature of solvent and concentration of enzyme and adsorbent. The surface of the support involves weak binding forces between protein and adsorbent such as hydrogen bonds, Van der Waals forces and ionic or hydrophobic interactions (Fig. 2.2).

The process of adsorption of an enzyme is performed by mixing the enzyme and polymer support in a stirred reactor or by percolating the enzyme through a packed bed, tube or membrane. The quantity of enzyme adsorbed to a solid support is dependent on the enzyme concentration exposed to the unit surface of carrier during the immobilization process. Time and temperature are important parameters in adsorption of enzymes with porous carrier. The disadvantage of adsorption is that the binding forces between the enzyme and the support are weak. Hence, adsorbed enzymes are liable to desorption during the utilization. The desorption of the protein is dependent on changes in temperature, pH and ionic strength. The various enzymes that may be immobilized by adsorption on respective carrier matrix are given in Table 2.2.

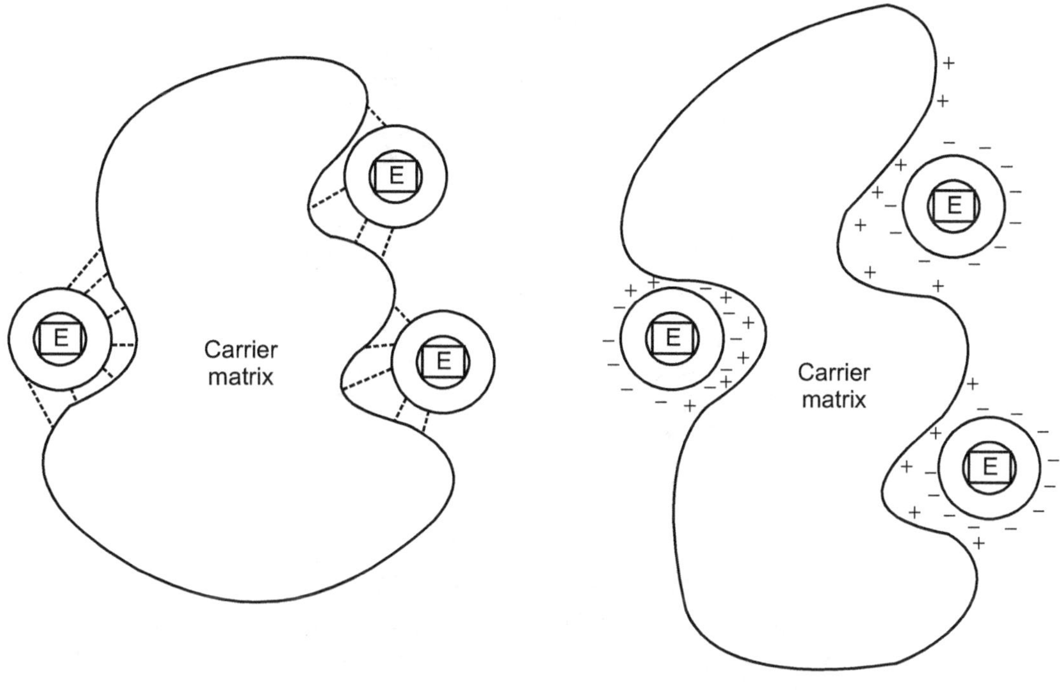

(a) Van der Waals forces (b) Hydrogen bonding

Fig. 2.2: Enzyme immobilization by adsorption

Table 2.2: Enzymes immobilized by adsorption

Enzymes	Carrier matrix
α - Amylase	Calcium phosphate
Catalase	Charcoal
Invertase	Charcoal, DEAE – sephadex
Subtilisin	Cellulose
Aminoglycosidase	Agarose gel, DEAE – sephadex
Glucose oxidase	Cellophane

Covalent bonding: Covalent bond is formed between the chemical groups of enzyme and chemical groups on surface of carrier (Fig. 2.3). Covalent bonding has an advantage of an attachment not reversed by pH, ionic strength or substrate. The active site of an enzyme may be blocked through the chemical reaction and the enzyme rendered inactive. Adsorption of enzymes to the carrier matrices is quite easy and convenient by covalent bonding.

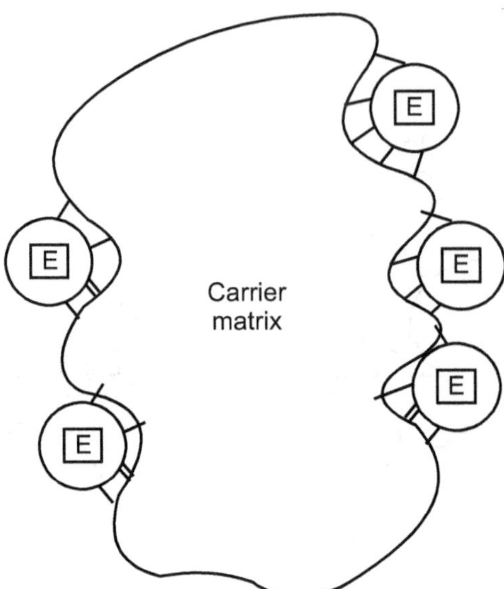

Fig. 2.3: Covalent bonding

The formation of covalent bond usually takes place particularly with the side chains of amino acids present in the enzyme. The various groups are sulphide, sulphahydril, oxide, amino, carboxyl, hydroxyl, ammonium, imino, amide, methylthiol, guanidyl, imidazole and phenol ring. Different methods of covalent bonding are classified as follows.

(i) Diazotation: This reaction involves bonding between the amino group of the support e.g. aminobenzyl cellulose, amino derivatives of polystyrene, aminosilanised porous glass and a tyrosyl or histidyl group of the enzyme. The amino functional moiety containing support material is converted to the corresponding diazonium chloride salt by treating with a mixture of sodium nitrate and diluted hydrochloric acid (Fig. 2.4).

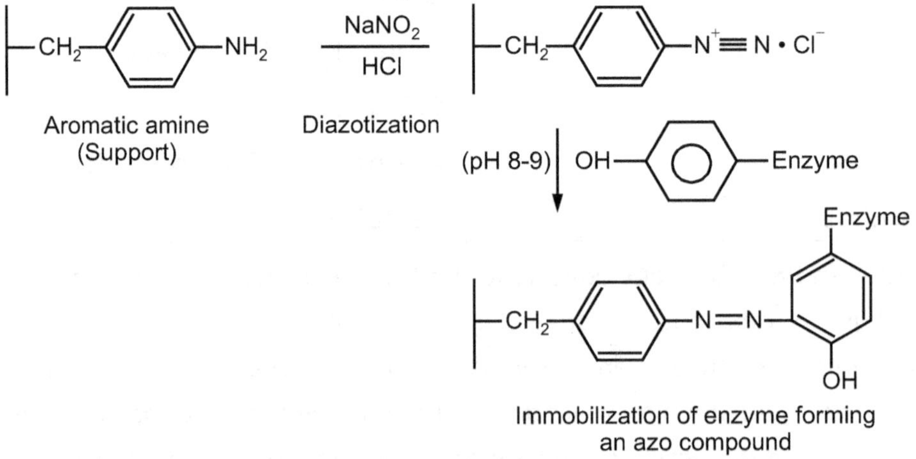

$$\vdash CH_2-C_6H_4-NH_2 \xrightarrow[HCl]{NaNO_2} \vdash CH_2-C_6H_4-\overset{+}{N}\equiv N\cdot Cl^-$$

Aromatic amine (Support) — Diazotization

$$\xrightarrow[(pH\ 8\text{-}9)]{OH-C_6H_4-Enzyme} \vdash CH_2-C_6H_4-N=N-C_6H_3(OH)-Enzyme$$

Immobilization of enzyme forming an azo compound

Fig. 2.4: Immobilization of enzyme forming an azo compound

(ii) Formation of peptide bond: The reaction occurs between the amino or carboxyl groups of the support and the carboxyl or amino groups of the enzymes. Acyl azide derivatives react with the enzyme protein involving predominantly the primary amino groups of enzyme to form the peptide bond (Fig. 2.5).

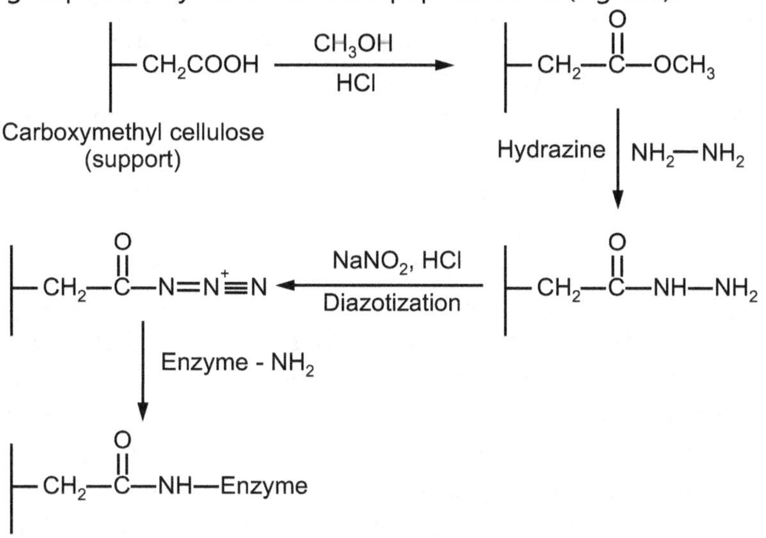

Fig. 2.5: Immobilization of enzyme using CMC support by peptide bond formation

(iii) Group activation: In this method, cyanogen bromide (Fig. 2.6) is applied to a support containing glycol groups e.g. cellulose, sephadex, sepharose etc.

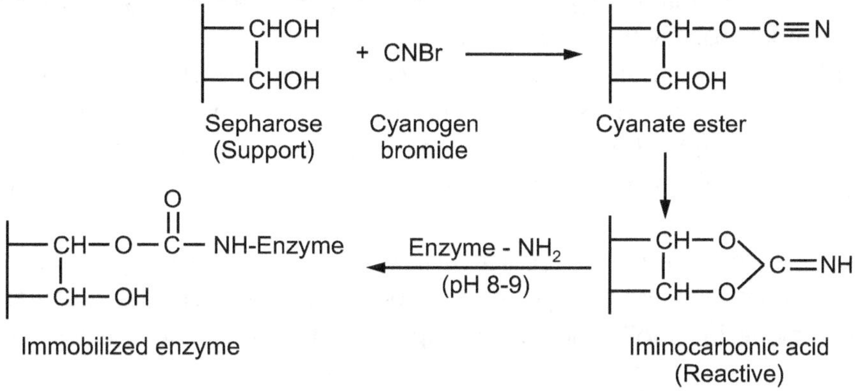

Fig. 2.6: Immobilization of enzyme by cyanogen bromide activation

(iv) Polyfunctional reagents: In this method, a bifunctional or a multifunctional reagent such as glutaraldehyde (Fig. 2.7) is used to create bonding between the amino group of the support and the amino groups of the enzyme. Some of enzymes immobilized by covalent bonding are given in Table 2.3.

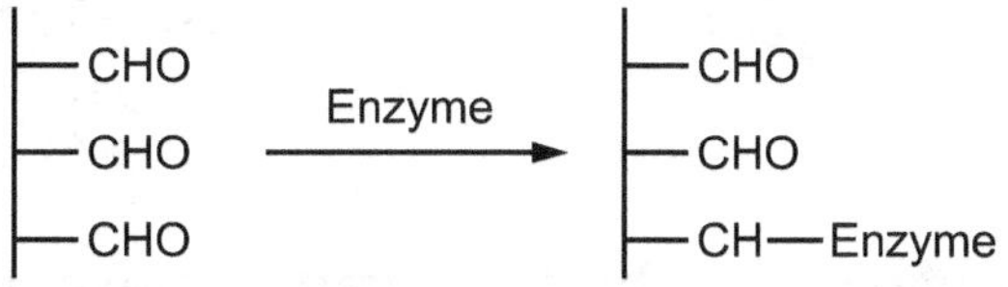

Fig. 2.7: Immobilization of enzyme by activation of bifunctional agent

Table 2.3: Enzymes immobilized by covalent bonding

Enzyme	Carrier matrix	Binding agent/Reaction
α-Amylase	DEAE – cellulose (cellulose – 2-(diethylamino) ethyl ether)	Direct coupling
Amyloglucosidase	DEAE – cellulose	Cyanuric chloride
Cellulose	Polyurethane	Isocyanate
Glucose isomerase	Polyurethane	Isocyanate
Glucose oxidase	Porous glass	Isothiocyanate
Pectinase	Polyurethane	Isothiocyanate
Pronase	Carbodiimide activation	CM-sephadex

Complexation or chelation: This method is based on the chelating properties of the transition metals, which can be employed to couple enzymes. Immobilized enzymes are prepared using transition metal compounds (e.g. titanium, zirconium metal salts) for the activation of the surface of organic carriers or using the corresponding hydrous metal oxides. The metals like Co (II), Cu (II), Mn (II), tin (II) (IV), Zn (II), chromium (II), zirchonium (IV) are converted into metal oxides and in the presence of enzyme it gives metal oxide enzyme. The interaction of the transition metal compounds with biopolymers are occur as follows.

Titanium metal + chloride ion = octahedral co-ordination = ligand + cellulose = glycosidic linkage = titanium chloride – cellulose.

Cellulose contains vicinal diol groups which are not involved in glycosidic linkage hence available for free chelation by transition metals.

Encapsulation: Enzymes are immobilized within microcapsules prepared from organic polymers. The membrane encloses the enzyme and remain semipermeable to the substrate and the products. The method of encapsulation is cheap and simple. It provides large surface area to enzyme to contact with the substrate and several enzymes can be immobilized in single step.

Encapsulation technique is not applicable for high molecular weight substrates. During the process of immobilization, enzymes may be inactivated or may be leaked through microcapsule. Enzyme immobilization by encapsulation and microenapsulation is shown in Fig. 2.8.

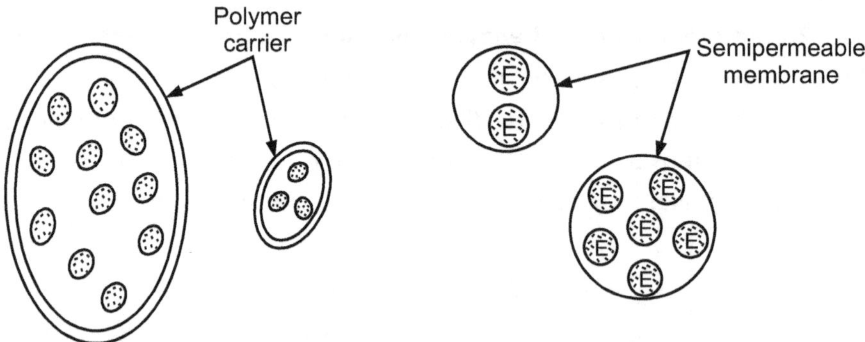

(a) Encapsulation **(b) Microencapsulation or membrane confinement**

Fig. 2.8: Enzyme immobilization techniques

derivatives react with the enzyme protein involving predominantly the primary amino groups of enzyme to form the peptide bond (Fig. 2.5).

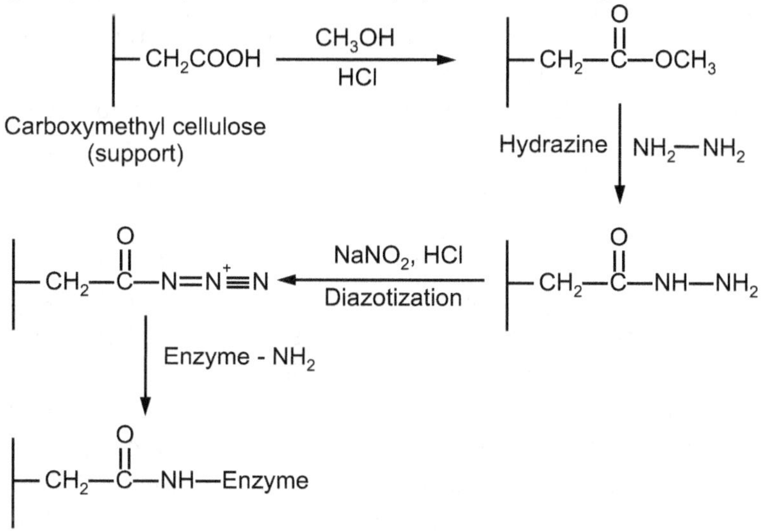

$$\text{—}CH_2COOH \xrightarrow[HCl]{CH_3OH} \text{—}CH_2\text{—}\overset{O}{\overset{||}{C}}\text{—}OCH_3$$

Carboxymethyl cellulose (support)

Hydrazine $NH_2\text{—}NH_2$

$$\text{—}CH_2\text{—}\overset{O}{\overset{||}{C}}\text{—}N{=}\overset{+}{N}{\equiv}N \xleftarrow[\text{Diazotization}]{NaNO_2,\ HCl} \text{—}CH_2\text{—}\overset{O}{\overset{||}{C}}\text{—}NH\text{—}NH_2$$

Enzyme - NH_2

$$\text{—}CH_2\text{—}\overset{O}{\overset{||}{C}}\text{—}NH\text{—}Enzyme$$

Fig. 2.5: Immobilization of enzyme using CMC support by peptide bond formation

(iii) Group activation: In this method, cyanogen bromide (Fig. 2.6) is applied to a support containing glycol groups e.g. cellulose, sephadex, sepharose etc.

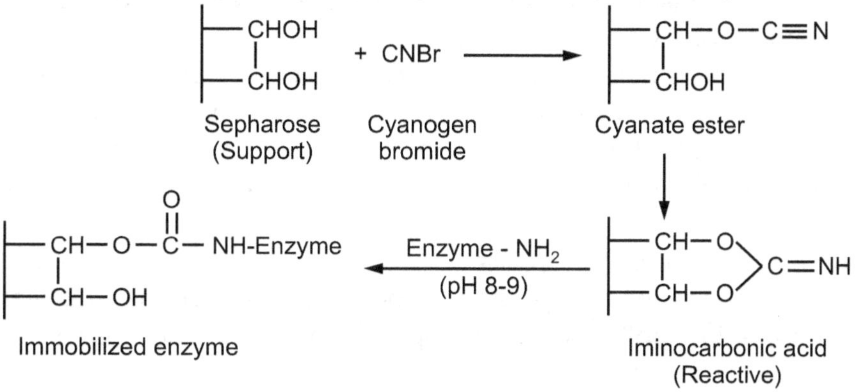

$$\begin{matrix}\text{—}CHOH \\ | \\ \text{—}CHOH\end{matrix} + CNBr \longrightarrow \begin{matrix}\text{—}CH\text{—}O\text{—}C{\equiv}N \\ | \\ \text{—}CHOH\end{matrix}$$

Sepharose (Support) Cyanogen bromide Cyanate ester

$$\begin{matrix}\text{—}CH\text{—}O\text{—}\overset{O}{\overset{||}{C}}\text{—}NH\text{-}Enzyme \\ | \\ \text{—}CH\text{—}OH\end{matrix} \xleftarrow[(pH\ 8\text{-}9)]{Enzyme\ \text{-}\ NH_2} \begin{matrix}\text{—}CH\text{—}O \\ | \\ \text{—}CH\text{—}O\end{matrix}\!\!>C{=}NH$$

Immobilized enzyme Iminocarbonic acid (Reactive)

Fig. 2.6: Immobilization of enzyme by cyanogen bromide activation

(iv) Polyfunctional reagents: In this method, a bifunctional or a multifunctional reagent such as glutaraldehyde (Fig. 2.7) is used to create bonding between the amino group of the support and the amino groups of the enzyme. Some of enzymes immobilized by covalent bonding are given in Table 2.3.

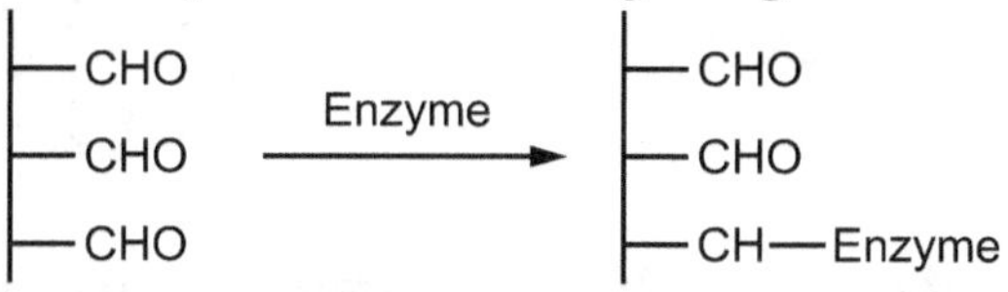

$$\begin{matrix}\text{—}CHO \\ \text{—}CHO \\ \text{—}CHO\end{matrix} \xrightarrow{Enzyme} \begin{matrix}\text{—}CHO \\ \text{—}CHO \\ \text{—}CH\text{—}Enzyme\end{matrix}$$

Fig. 2.7: Immobilization of enzyme by activation of bifunctional agent

Table 2.3: Enzymes immobilized by covalent bonding

Enzyme	Carrier matrix	Binding agent/Reaction
α-Amylase	DEAE – cellulose (cellulose – 2-(diethylamino) ethyl ether)	Direct coupling
Amyloglucosidase	DEAE – cellulose	Cyanuric chloride
Cellulose	Polyurethane	Isocyanate
Glucose isomerase	Polyurethane	Isocyanate
Glucose oxidase	Porous glass	Isothiocyanate
Pectinase	Polyurethane	Isothiocyanate
Pronase	Carbodiimide activation	CM-sephadex

Complexation or chelation: This method is based on the chelating properties of the transition metals, which can be employed to couple enzymes. Immobilized enzymes are prepared using transition metal compounds (e.g. titanium, zirconium metal salts) for the activation of the surface of organic carriers or using the corresponding hydrous metal oxides. The metals like Co (II), Cu (II), Mn (II), tin (II) (IV), Zn (II), chromium (II), zirchonium (IV) are converted into metal oxides and in the presence of enzyme it gives metal oxide enzyme. The interaction of the transition metal compounds with biopolymers are occur as follows.

Titanium metal + chloride ion = octahedral co-ordination = ligand + cellulose = glycosidic linkage = titanium chloride – cellulose.

Cellulose contains vicinal diol groups which are not involved in glycosidic linkage hence available for free chelation by transition metals.

Encapsulation: Enzymes are immobilized within microcapsules prepared from organic polymers. The membrane encloses the enzyme and remain semipermeable to the substrate and the products. The method of encapsulation is cheap and simple. It provides large surface area to enzyme to contact with the substrate and several enzymes can be immobilized in single step.

Encapsulation technique is not applicable for high molecular weight substrates. During the process of immobilization, enzymes may be inactivated or may be leaked through microcapsule. Enzyme immobilization by encapsulation and microenapsulation is shown in Fig. 2.8.

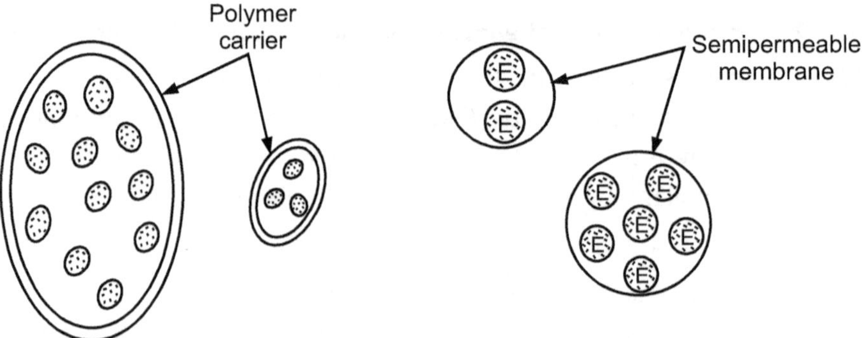

(a) Encapsulation **(b) Microencapsulation or membrane confinement**

Fig. 2.8: Enzyme immobilization techniques

The methods used for microencapsulation of enzymes are classified as (i) Phase separation method, (ii) Interfacial polymerization method, (iii) Liquid drying method and (iv) Liquid-surfactant-membrane method.

Many enzymes are microencapsulated by the process of phase separation method, which is based on coacervation. Aqueous enzyme solution is first emulsified in a organic solvent (water insoluble) containing the polymer and then to the organic phase containing aqueous microdroplets. Another organic solvent is slowly added in which the polymer is insoluble. The polymer is concentrated and membranes are formed around the microdroplets of the aqueous enzyme solution. Interfacial polymerization method is also similar to the phase separation method. In interfacial polymerization method, aqueous solution of the enzyme and a hydrophilic monomer are emulsified in a water immiscible organic solvent. In this emulsion, the hydrophilic monomer is added with stirring. These two monomers polymerize at the interface between the aqueous and organic solvent phases in the emulsion and forms a semipermeable membrane of the copolymer in which the enzyme in the aqueous phase is enclosed.

In liquid-drying method, the enzyme solution is emulsified in an organic solvent with a boiling point lower than that of water containing the membrane forming polymers and using an oil-soluble surfactant. The emulsion containing aqueous enzyme microdroplets is then dispersed in an aqueous medium with protective colloidal substances and secondary emulsion is formed. The final microencapsulated enzyme is obtained by removing the organic solvent. In liquid-surfactant-membrane method, the enzyme emulsion is prepared in two steps. First, the aqueous enzyme solution is emulsified in the organic phase at high shear stresses. The stability of the microdroplets is attained by adding suitable surfactants to the organic phase. In the second step, the stable emulsion is injected into the outer continuous aqueous phase.

Entrapment: Immobilization of enzyme molecules can be performed by the physical entrapping of the enzyme inside a polymer matrix, gel or fibres (Fig. 2.9). Entrapment is based on coupling enzymes to the lattice of a polymer matrix or enclosing them in semipermeable membrane. It prevents the release of proteins while allowing the diffusion of substrates and products.

Gels can be formed by polymerization in which covalent bonds are formed by use of prepolymers with very little change in covalent bonds. Enzymes are dispersed or dissolved into an aqueous buffer containing acrylamide and bis acrylate as a cross linker. Pore size and mechanical strength of gel is dependent on concentration of acrylamide.

In the process of inclusion in fibres, the mixture containing the polymer and the enzyme is extruded to have the enzyme trapped in fibre format. Penicillin acylase is immobilized by entrapment in the micro cavities of synthetic fibres.

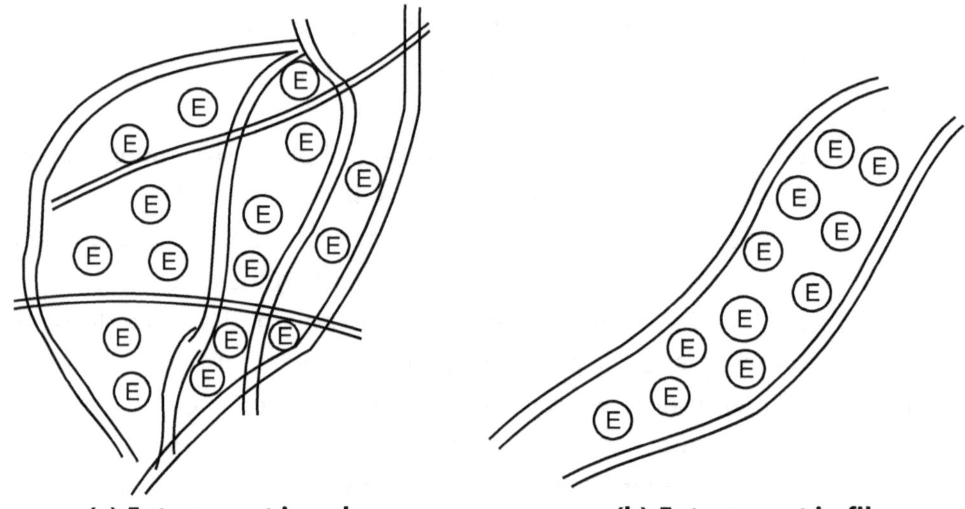

(a) Entrapment in gels **(b) Entrapment in fibres**

Fig. 2.9: Enzyme immobilization by entrapment

Applications of immobilization:

Immobilized enzymes and cells are commonly used in industrial processes, analytical techniques, secondary metabolic production, drug targeting, designing of bioreactors, bio-environmental modification etc. In 1969, Tanabe Seiyaku Co. were the first developed immobilized aminoacylase for the continuous production of L-amino acids from acyl-DL-amino acids. Immobilized enzymes have wide applications in the following areas.

Industrial processes: Immobilized biocatalysts are used for production of antibiotics, steroids and amino acids in pharmaceutical industries. Immobilized penicillin acylase has been used in the production of semisynthetic penicillin's through deacylation of penicillin G to 6-amino penicillianic acid (6-APA) using macroreticular ion exchange resin as supports. Cephalosporin amidase obtained from different microorganisms can be immobilized by various methods and are used for production of various cephalosporin derivatives. Macrolide antibiotic tylosin and the nucleoside peptide antibiotic nikkomycin are produced using living cells of *Streptomyces* spp. immobilized with calcium alginate.

Microbial cells containing systems of cofactors are immobilized and employed for large-scale steroid transformations. The synthesis of hydrocortisone and prednisolone from cortexolone is obtained by immobilizing the biocatalyst by entrapment with polyacrylamide. (Fig. 2.10)

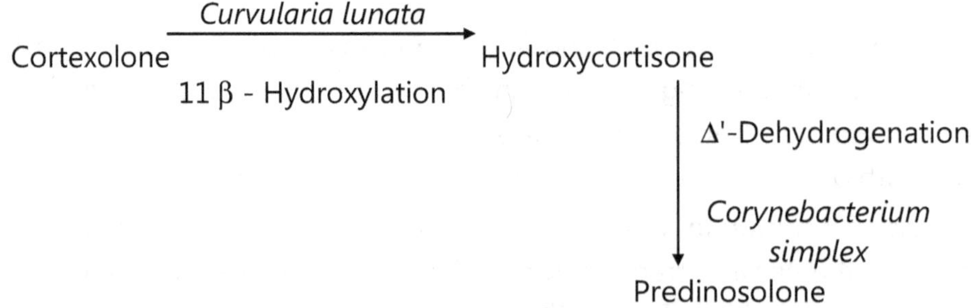

Fig. 2.10: Production of predinosolone from cortexolone

Sugar and sugar syrups prepared by enzyme technology has received much attention from food industry. Fructose manufactured by using glucoamylase and glucose isomerase is being produced on a large scale to replace sucrose as a sweetening agent. Aminoacylase is used for the continuous optical resolution of DL-amino acids and is isolated from *Aspergillus oryzae*. Enzyme is obtained by ionic binding of DEAE-sephedex covalent binding to iodoacetyl cellulose and entrapment of polyacrylamide gel. DL-Acylamino acid is asymmetrically hydrolyzed by enzyme aminoacylase and it produces L-amino acid and unhydrolyzed D-acylamino acid. L-alanine is produced from L-aspartic acid by using *Pseudomonas dacunhae* cells (L-aspartate 4-decarboxylase) which are immobilized with k-carrageenam. Immobilized biocatalysts used for chemical transformations in the pharmaceutical industries are shown in Table 2.4.

Table 2.4: Immobilized biocatalysts used for chemical transformations

Compounds	Microbial cells	Enzyme	Matrix for Immobilization
1. Antibiotics			
Ampicillin	*Bacillus megaterium*	Penicillin amidase	DEAE-cellulose
Penicillin G	*Penicillium chrysogenum*	Multi-enzymes	Polyacrylamide, calcium alginate
Cephalexin	*Achromobater* sp.	Cephalosporin amidase	DEAE-cellulose
Bacitracin	*Bacillus* sp.	Multi-enzymes	Polyacrylamide
Tylosin	*Streptomyces* sp.	Multi-enzymes	Calcium alginate
2. Steroids			
Prednisolone	*Arthrobacter simplex*	Complete cell	Photo-crosslinkable resin, calcium alginate
Hydrocortisone	*Curvularia lunata*	Complete cell	Photo-crosslinkable resin, polyacrylamide
3. Amino Acids			
L-Alanine	*Pseudomonas dacunhae*	L-aspartate 4-decarboxylase	Carrageenan
L-Arginine	*Serratia marcescens*	Multi-enzymes	Carrageenan
L-Glutamic acid	*Brevibacterium flavum*	Multi-enzymes	Collagen
D-α-Phenylglycine	*Bacillus* sp.	Hydantoinase	Polyacrylamide
L-Tryptophan	*Escherichia coli.*	Tryptophan synthase β-tyrosinase	Polyacrylamide
L-Tyrosine	*Erwinia herbicola*		Collagen and glutaraldehyde

contd. ...

4. Organic Acids			
Acetic acid	*Acetobacter aceti*	Multi-enzymes	Porous ceramic
Citric acid	*Aspergillus niger*	Multi-enzymes	Calcium alginate
Gluconic acid	*Aspergillus niger*	Glucose oxidase	Calcium alginate
Lactic acid	*Lactobacillus casei*	Multi-enzymes	Polyacrylamide
2-Ketogluconic acid	*Serratia marcescens*	Multi-enzymes	Collagen
L-Malic acid	*Brevibacterium flavum*	Fumarase	Carrageenan

Analytical applications: Enzymes are commonly used in medical diagnosis, industrial monitoring programs and analysis of specific reactions. Determination of organic and inorganic compounds in biologicals fluids is important in clinical analysis. Most of analysis of these compounds are performed by enzyme catalyzed reactions. Enzyme electrodes or biosensors are probes capable of generating an electrical potential as a result of a reaction catalysed by an immobilized enzyme. The first enzyme electrode to be reported was the glucose-sensitive electrode (Fig. 2.11). The enzyme glucose oxidase was immobilized in a polyacrylamide gel around a platinum oxygen electrode. When a solution of glucose is brought into contact with electrode, glucose and oxygen diffuses into an enzyme layer and are converted into gluconolactone and hydrogen peroxide lowering the oxygen concentration. The principle involved is the removal of oxygen from solution at a rate dependent upon the concentration of glucose present. The response of biosensor is measured in terms of substrate used or product form. Different biosensors are used for estimation of compounds (Table 2.5) such as glucose, lactic acid, alcohol, glutamic acid, vitamin B_1, nicotinic acid, urea, penicillin, nystatin etc. are easily analysed by using enzyme electrodes.

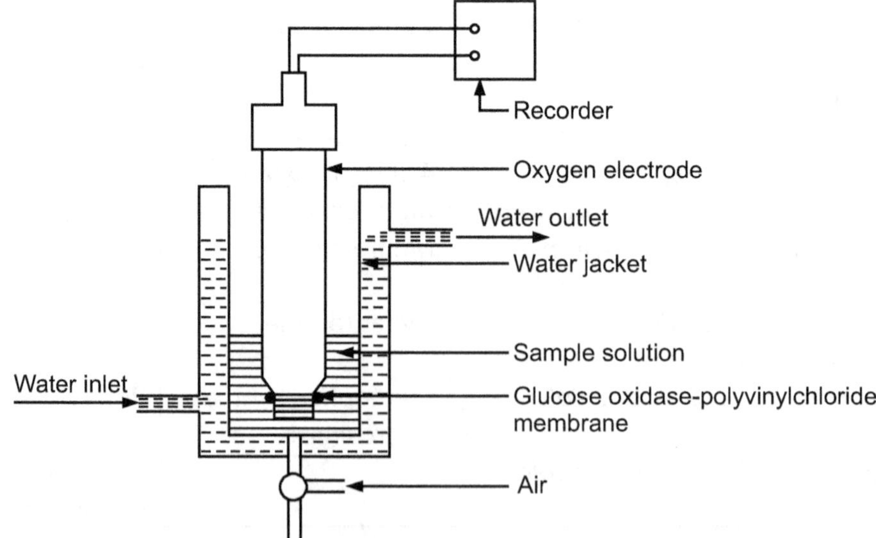

Fig. 2.11: Enzyme electrode for determination of glucose

Biosensors are composed of a bifunctional material and a transducer and it is applied to analytical fields, clinical analysis and food industry. Microbial sensors have been developed and applied to the measurement of biological compounds. Microbial sensors are based on either the change the respiration or the amount of produced metabolites as the result of assimilation of substrates by microorganisms.

Table 2.5: Electrochemical devices used for estimation of compounds

Electrochemical Devices	Sensor	Enzyme	Immobilization
1. Oxygen electrode	Glucose	Glucose oxidase	Covalent
	Ethanol	Alcohol oxidase	Crosslinked
	Uric acid	Uricase	Crosslinked
	Inosine	Nucleoside phosphorylase	Covalent
	Monoamine	Monoamine oxidase	Entrapment
	L-Alginine	Alginine decarboxylase	Crosslinked
2. Ammonia gas electrode	L-Amino acid	L-Amino acid oxidase	Covalent
	L-Asparagine	Asparaginase	Entrapment
	Urea	Urease	Crosslinked
	Nitrite	Nitrite reductase	Crosslinked
	L-Methionine	Methionine ammonia lyase	Crosslinked
3. CO_2 gas electrode	L-Tyrosine	L-Tyrosine decarboxylase	Adsorption
4. pH electrode	Penicillin	Penicillinase	Entrapment
	Neutral lipid	Lipase	Covalent
5. Platinum electrode	Cholesterol	Cholesterol esterase	Covalent
	Phospholipid	Phospholipase	Covalent

Immunoadsorption techniques: Enzyme-linked immunosorbent assay (ELISA) is widely used for detection of antigens and antibodies. This technique involves immobilization of antigen or antibody on to a microtiter plate. The excess antigen or antibody used for coating is washed off. The counter antibody linked with an enzyme is added and allowed to react with the immobilized antigen or antibody. A substrate specific for the enzyme is then added and colour produced is used for detection of antigen and antibody.

Protein A and G are generally immobilized on agarose or sephadex and used as affinity chromatography medium a typical immobilized protein complex or conjugation. The matrix based on an immobilized mannan binding protein support is most effective for purifying mouse IgM from ascites. Mannan binding protein is usually immobilized on agarose bead and used in affinity chromatography. Radioallergosorbent (Rast) test is based on absorption of IgE antibody by immobilized antigens and subsequently the degree of binding is determined.

Therapeutic applications: Preparation of immobilized enzymes such as streptokinase, urokinase, fibrinolysis in microgranules of sephadex can be effectively used for the treatment of thromboses and thromboemboli of any vessels. Urea-urease modulated system suggests the interesting possibility of using immobilized enzymes to alter local pH and consequently to change the pH sensitive polymer erosion rates. Enzymes, adsorbents or other material can be incorporated together with target enzyme into the artificial cells. The simple artificial organs are designed and constructed using the principle of artificial cells e.g. artificial liver, artificial kidney, blood detoxifier etc. Artificial cells containing multienzyme systems are used for the sequential conversion of substrates into products. Immobilized enzymes are also recommended in replacement therapy needed in hereditary enzyme-deficiency conditions.

2.3 PRODUCTION OF ENZYMES

Enzymes used in industry are isolated from microorganisms, plants and animals. Enzymes are commercially produced by semisolid culture method and submerged culture. In semisolid culture method, enzyme producing culture is grown on the surface of a suitable semisolid substrate supplemented with specific nutrients. Now-a-days submerged culture methods are widely used in the production of enzymes. The fermentation equipment used is the same as in the manufacture of antibiotics. Microbial enzymes produced by fermentation include amylases, proteases, catalase, penicillinase, streptokinase etc.

In general, the techniques used for microbial production of enzymes are described in following steps:

- Isolation and selection of microbial strains.
- Formulation of medium.
- Fermentation.
- Extraction and purification of enzymes.

The flowchart for enzyme production by microbial cell is given in Fig. 2.12.

Isolation and selection of microbial strains: The most important criteria for selecting the microbes are:

1. To produce high amount of enzyme,
2. Less fermentation time,
3. Simple isolation and separation (extracellular),
4. Non-pathogenic cell and
5. Utilization of low cost culture medium.

Best suitable microbial culture is selected based on all optimized parameters. Strain improvement techniques are used for optimization of enzyme production by appropriate methods such as mutagens or UV rays.

Formulation of medium: The culture medium should contain all the nutrients to support adequate growth of microorganisms that will result in maximum enzyme production.

All ingredients of the medium should be easily available at low cost and with high nutritional value. The production media must contain sources of carbon, nitrogen, energy, minerals, macronutrients, micronutrients, growth factors, etc. Commonly used substrates for the media are soybean meal, potato starch, molasses, starch hydrolysate, corn steep liquor, wheat or rice bran, cereal meal, casein, yeast extract, etc. the pH of medium should be adjusted to show optimal microbial growth and enzyme production.

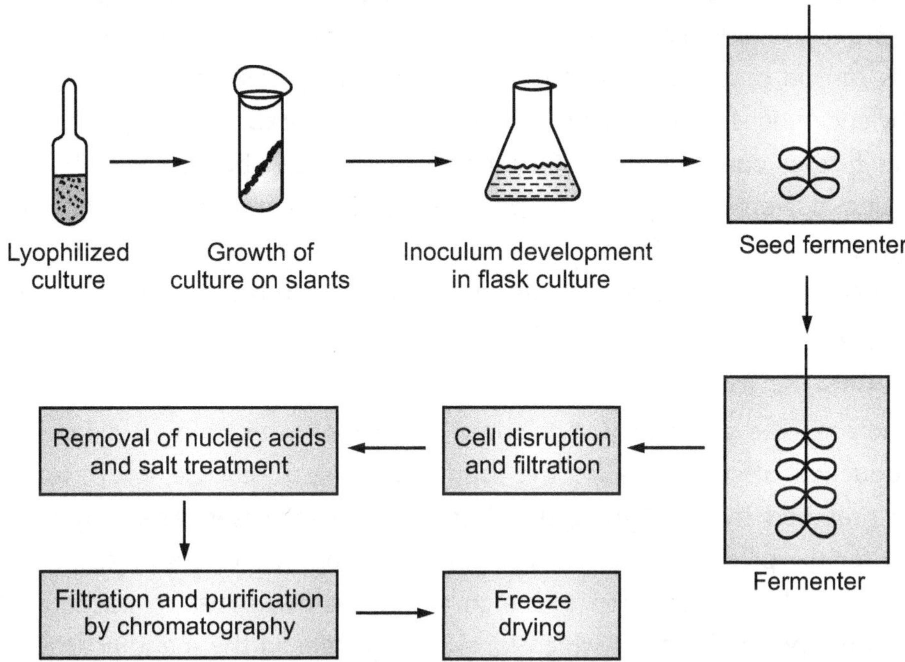

Fig. 2.12: Flowchart for production of enzymes by microorganisms

Fermentation: Submerged culture technique is commonly used for industrial production of enzymes. In some cases, solid-substrate culture as well as deep bed cultivation techniques are also used for enzyme production. Medium is sterilized batch wise or continuous sterilization method. Submerged culture method is most widely used because of less chances of infection and more yield. Surface culture technique is a traditional method but still in use for production of fungal enzymes such as amylase, protease, cellulases and pectinases.

Mechanically stirred bioreactors of capacities 20,000 to 1,00,000 liters are used for production of enzymes by submerged techniques. The duration of fermentation is around 2 to 7 days. Growth conditions such as pH, temperature and oxygen are maintained in optimal level. A small amount of oil is added to control the foam in the fermentation. Most of the enzymes are extracellular and produced at the end of exponential phase.

Solid-substrate culture method is mainly used for isolation of enzymes from fungi. Drum process and tray process are commonly used in solid-substrate culture. The substrate is spread in the form of thin layer and the culture is inoculated.

The trays are incubated in an air-conditioned room upto 1 to 7 days.

Extraction and purification of enzymes: The desired enzyme produced may be extracted into the culture medium based on extracellular or intracellular nature of isolate. The physical, chemical and enzymatic methods are used to break the cells and release the intracellular enzymes. Recovery of an extracellular enzyme is much simpler than intracellular enzyme. Fungal broth is directly filtered or centrifuged after pH adjustment. Bacterial broth is first treated with calcium salts to precipitate calcium phosphate which help in separation of bacterial cells and colloids. Filtration or centrifugation can be used to remove cell debris. Nucleic acids can be precipitated and removed by adding polycations such as polyamines and polyethyleneimine. Isolated enzymes can be precipitated by using salts and organic solvents, and further concentration of desired enzymes can be achieved by liquid-liquid extraction using polyethylene glycol or polyamines. Chromatographic techniques such as ion-exchange, size exclusion, affinity, hydrophobic interaction and dye ligand are commonly used for separation and purification of enzymes. The concentrated form of the enzyme can be obtained by vacuum drying or spray drying.

2.3.1 Amylases

Amylolytic enzymes are widely distributed in bacteria and fungi. Amylases are mainly used for production of sweetners for the food industry e.g. glucose syrup, fructose syrup. Dextrins are prepared by the hydrolysis of starch with amylases. The amylases are used commercially for the preparation of sizing agents and removal of starch sizing from woven cloth. It is also used in preparation of starch sizing pastes for use in paper coatings and liquefaction of heavy starch pastes which form during steps in the manufacture of corn and chocolate syrups. These amylases can be employed as a replacement for malt for starch hydrolysis in the brewing industry. Amylases are characterized by their ability to hydrolyze 1, 4 glucosidic linkages in polysaccharides e.g. starch, glucogen etc. They are mainly classified as α-amylases and β-amylases.

α-Amylases, 1, 4-α-glucanglucanohydrolyases are endoenzymes, responsible for affecting the cleavage of the substrate strategically positioned in the interior of the molecule. They attack all the linkages between glucose units in the starch molecule. A large number of bacterial species are used for production of α-amylases such as *Bacillus subtilis, B. cereus, B. licheniformis, B. amyloliquefaciens, Lactobacillus* sp., *Pseudomonas saccharophila, Arthrobacter* sp., *Escherichia* sp., *Thermononospora* sp. etc. Selected strains of *Bacillus subtilis* are mainly preferred for industrial scale production of amylase. Fungal α-amylases for commercial purposes are derived from *Aspergillus oryzae*. Different species of *Aspergillus, Candida, Cephalosporium, Penicillium* and *Rhizopus* are used for production of highly specific α-amylase. Bacterial α-amylase is produced only by submerged culture method. The media employed are generally based on the use of natural raw materials including certain growth factors such as trace elements, vitamins and amino acids. A careful balance of carbohydrate and nitrogen ingredients of the medium is most important. It is necessary to maintain the pH near neutrality and incubation temperature 30 to 40°C of the fermentation medium for 3 to 5 days. After fermentation, culture is filtered or centrifuged to separate the cells. Amylase can be precipitated from aqueous solution by the addition of cold acetone, ethanol, isopropanol or ammonium sulfate. It is purified by dialysis and chromatographic techniques. Fungal α-amylase was originally and is still produced in significant amounts in solid substrate culture.

The β-amylases, α-1, 4-glycanmalthodrolases hydrolyze starch and other amyloses by splitting off maltose molecules until the action is blocked by the occurrence of either 1, 3 linkages or branch points. The residual molecule is then called a limit dextrin. β-Amylases are mainly belong to plant origin however, certain specific microorganisms produce this enzyme such as *Bacillus polymyxa, Bacillus cereus, Streptomyces* sp., *Pseudomonas* sp. and *Rhizopus* species.

2.3.2 Catalase

Catalase is a common enzyme found in nearly all living organisms exposed to oxygen. Catalase is present in different sources such as microorganisms, plants and animals. It is a tetramer of four polypeptide chains, each over 500 amino acids long.

Catalases are antioxidant enzymes present in all aerobic organisms and it catalyze the conversion of hydrogen peroxide to water and molecular oxygen.

$$2H_2O_2 \xrightarrow{\text{Catalase}} 2H_2O + O_2$$

This prevents conversion to hydroxyl radical and other more toxic reactive oxygen species (ROS). Hydrogen peroxide is produced as a by-product of aerobic respiration. Hence, catalase enzyme act as an antioxidant and protects the cell against oxidative stress. Catalases can be classified into three categories on the basis of structure and sequence such as mono-functional or typical catalase, catalase-peroxidase and pseudo-catalase or Mn-catalase.

Different strains are used for production of catalase enzyme such as *A. niger, S. cerevisiae, Penicillium variable, Thermoascus aurantiacus, Bacillius subtilis, Staphylococcus,* etc. This enzyme is located in the cytoplasm or in peroxisomes. The extracellular liberation of an enzyme is more advantageous for extraction and isolation. The commercial source of catalase is extracellular production by different microorganisms, mainly fungal strains.

This enzyme is used in several industrial applications such as food or textile processing to remove hydrogen peroxide which is used for sterilization or bleaching. This enzyme is used to remove hydrogen peroxided from milk prior to cheese production. It is used in contact lens hygiene to decompose the hydrogen peroxide which is used as disinfectant. Catalase enzyme also used in paper, pharmaceutical industry and in the field of bioremediation.

2.3.3 Peroxidase

Peroxidases are also an oxidoreductase class of enzyme, which catalyze oxidoreduction reactions. Many peroxidases contain an iron-porphyrin derivative (heme) in their active site and they can catalyze oxidation of a wide variety of organic compounds using hydrogen peroxide.

$$AH_2 + H_2O_2 \xrightarrow{\text{Peroxidase}} A + 2H_2O$$

Peroxidase includes a group of specific enzymes such as NAD peroxidase, fatty acid peroxidases and glutathione peroxidase. It is isolated from different sources of plants, animals and microbes (Table 2.6).

Table 2.6: Different sources of peroxidases

Sources	Examples
Plant sources	Horseradish *(Armoracia rusticana)*, papaya *(Carica papaya), bare (Acorus calamus)*, banana *(Musa paradisiaca)*.
Bacterial strains	*Bacillus subtilis, Escherichia coli, Pseudomonas species.*
Fungal strains	*Penicillium geastrovirus, Thanatephorus* species, *Auricularia* species, *Pleurotus ostreatus, Candida tropicalis, Debaryomyces polymorphus.*

Peroxidases are primarily intracellular enzymes but many cells produce extracellular enzymes, which are involved in the degradation of complex organic compounds. Peroxidases are useful in a number of industrial and analytical bioprocesses, due to high reduction potential. It is used for reduction of water pollution by bioremediation of phenol and chlorinated phenolic compounds in waste water. It degrades synthetic dyes such as azo, remazol blue, anthraquinine, etc. by using lignin and manganese peroxidase. Peroxidases are also used in the degradation of wood compounds in paper industry by lignin and cellulose hydrolysis. It is also used in the construction of biosensors for determination of hydrogen peroxide and phenolic compounds.

2.3.4 Protease

Complex mixtures of true proteinases and peptidases are usually called proteases. Microbial proteases can be divided into three groups based upon the pH range in which their activity is higher, namely acid, neutral or alkaline proteases. Proteolytic enzymes are produced by various bacteria such as *Bacillus, Pseudomonas, Clostridium, Proteus* and *Serratia* species and fungi such as *Aspergillus niger, Aspergillus oryzae, Aspergillus flavus, Penicillium roquefortii* and *Mucor pusillus*. However, the enzymes associated with these microorganisms are actually mixtures of proteinases and peptidases. Proteinases are excreted to the fermentation medium during growth while the peptidases are liberated only on autolysis of the cells.

Proteases are used on a large scale in detergent, food and leather industries. The enzymes cause adequate alterations in the hides to provide a finer grain and texture, greater pliability and better general quality. Proteases also find usage in the textile industry to afford proteinaceous sizing. In the silk industry, proteases help in the liberation of the silk fibres from the naturally occurring proteinaceous material wherein they are actually imbedded. Proteases are also employed as a meat tenderizer e.g. papain. Proteases are used in brewing industry, film industry, waste-disposal management and manufacture of protein hydrolyzates. They are the active ingredient in spot-remover preparations for removing food spots in the dry-cleaning industry. Industrial production of microbial proteases is carried out by cultivation of the microorganisms in the submerged fermentation for the bacteria. However, fungi usually give higher yields when cultured on solid media. Most of the microorganisms excrete more than one kind of protease. The type of proteolytic enzyme formed may depend on the composition of the medium.

2.3.5 Penicillinase

Penicillinase is a bacterial extracellular enzyme produced from *Bacillus* species, *Staphylococcus* species and members of the coliform group of bacteria. The enzyme penicillinase inactivates penicillin by the process of hydrolysis and converts to penicilloic acid (Fig. 2.13).

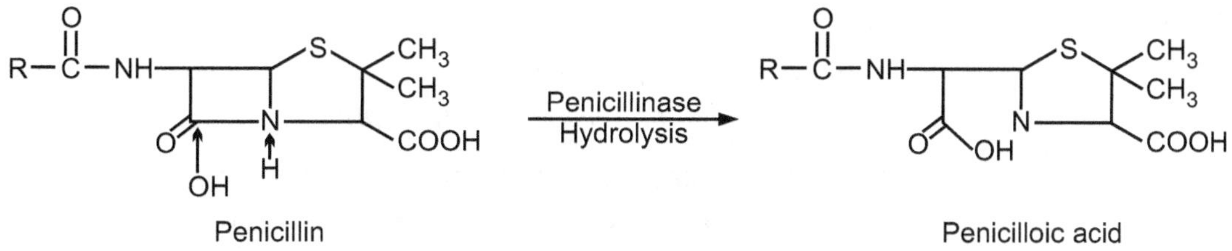

Fig. 2.13: Hydrolysis of penicillin by penicillinase

The enzyme penicillin amidase is normally produced by fungal species such as *Penicillium, Aspergillus* and *Mucor*. Penicillinase is divided into two major classes based on their activity such as penicillin amidase or penicillin acylase and β-lactamase or penicillinase. The enzyme penicillin amidase is specific on attacking the acyl group attached to the basic nucleus i.e. 6-amino-penicillanic acid. This enzyme is more specific with penicillin 'V' and 'K'. The enzyme β-lactamase acts on the basic nucleus itself. It breaks the β-lactam bond and produce penicilloic acid. This enzyme is more specific with penicillin G and penicillin X.

2.3.6 Lipase

Lipases are glycerol ester hydrolases that split fats into diglycerides or monoglycerides and fatty acids. A triglyceride is hydrolysed by lipase to form glycerol and fatty acids (Fig. 2.14). Lipases are also used to catalyze the trans-esterification reaction using alcohol together with fats, oils and free fatty acids to produce alkyl esters.

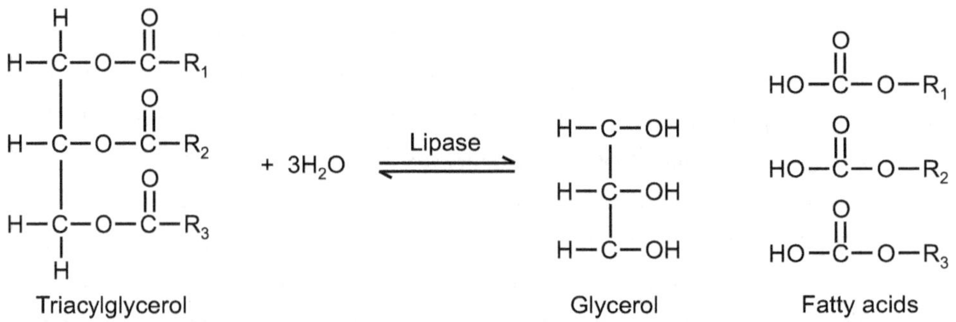

$$\text{Triacylglycerol} + 3H_2O \xrightleftharpoons{\text{Lipase}} \text{Glycerol} + \text{Fatty acids}$$

Triacylglycerol: $H-C(H)(-O-C(=O)-R_1)-C(H)(-O-C(=O)-R_2)-C(H)(H)(-O-C(=O)-R_3)$

Glycerol: $H-C-OH$, $H-C-OH$, $H-C-OH$

Fatty acids: $HO-C(=O)-O-R_1$, $HO-C(=O)-O-R_2$, $HO-C(=O)-O-R_3$

Fig. 2.14: Hydrolysis of triglyceride by lipase

Lipases are produced by animals, plants and microorganisms. The most common animal lipase is produced from pancreatic gland. Papaya latex, oat seed and castor seed can be source of plant lipase. Microorganisms (Table 2.7) are most important source of lipases compare to the plants and animals. The lipases produced for commercial use mainly isolated from fungi and bacteria. Screening of lipase produces on agar plate is performed by using tributyrin as a substrate and clear zones around the colonies indicate the cell produce lipase enzyme.

Table 2.7: Lipase producing microorganisms

Microbes	Species
Bacteria	*Acinetobacter radioresistens, Bacillus cereus, Photobacterium lipolyticum, Pseudomonas aeruginosa, Bacillus coagulans, Pseudomonas fragi, Achromobacter lipolyticum, Aeromonas hydrophila.*
Fungi	*Aspergillus oryzae, Candida antarctica, Candida rugosa, Penicillum roqueforti, Penicillium chrysogenum, Geotrichum candidum, Rhizopus delemar.*

Microbial lipases are generally extracellular nature and these can be produced by submerged fermentation or solid state fermentation. Submerged fermentation requires large space, complex media and also needs different equipments and control systems. Solid state fermentation is an another alternative method for enzyme production due to use of residues and by-products of agro-industries as nutrient sources. These components are high value and low-cost substrates which are mainly responsible to reduce the cost of enzyme production. Immobilization of microbial cells producing lipases increase the extent of reaction and facilitate downstream processing. Lipase production is influenced by the type and concentration of carbon and nitrogen sources, growth, temperature, pH and dissolved oxygen concentration.

Lipases are mainly used in the processing of fats and oils, detergents, food processing, synthesis of fine chemicals and pharmaceuticals, paper industry and production of cosmetics. Lipases mainly modify the properties of lipids by altering the location of fatty acid chains in the glycerol and replace some fatty acids with new ones. It synthesis esters of short chain fatty acids and alcohols which are known flavour and fragrance compounds. Lipases are also used to remove fat from meat and fish products to produce lean meat.

Lipases are commonly used as biocatalyst in cosmetic industry for production of personal care products. It plays a main role in production of speciality lipids and digestive aids. Lipases modify monoglycerides for use as emulsifiers in pharmaceuticals.

QUESTIONS

(A) Objective Type Questions:

1. What is enzyme technology? Explain.
2. Write advantages and disadvantages of immobilization of enzymes using entrapment.
3. Write different properties of enzymes.
4. Explain the roles of the following:
   (i) Penicillinase
   (ii) Protease
   (iii) Peroxidase

(B) Short Answer Questions:

1. Explain in short methods used for microencapsulation of enzymes.
2. Explain the production and applications of Lipase.
3. Write notes on:
   (a) Catalase
   (b) Amylase

(C) Long Answer Questions:

1. Explain in short different applications of enzyme immobilization.
2. Explain in detail methods for enzyme immobilization.
3. Explain in short general method for production of enzymes.

(D) Multiple Choice Questions:

1. The synthesis of hydrocortisone and prednisolone from cortexolone is obtained by immobilizing the biocatalyst by entrapment with ________
   (a) Starch (b) Acacia
   (c) Calcium alginate (d) Polyacrylamide
2. ________ is the method of covalent bonding.
   (a) Adsorption (b) Diazotation
   (c) Phase separation (d) Polymerization

3. ________ precipitation method, enzymes are recovered from fermentation broth.
   (a) Ammonium chloride (b) Ammonium oxalase
   (c) Ammonium nitrate (c) Ammonium sulfate
4. ________ enzyme is used for saccharification of starch.
   (a) Amylase (b) Invertase
   (c) Protease (d) Xylanase
5. ________ are glycerol ester hydrolases that split fats into monoglycerides and fatty acids.
   (a) Amylases (b) Lipases
   (c) Peroxidases (d) Catalases
6. Enzymes are recovered from fermentation broth by using ________ as a protein precipitants.
   (a) Ammonium chloride (b) Sodium chloride
   (c) Ammonium sulfate (d) Sodium nitrate

■■■

Chapter ... 3

BIOSENSORS

♦ LEARNING OBJECTIVES ♦

After completing this chapter, reader should be able to understand:

- *Introduction*
- *Types of biosensors:*
  - *Amperometric biosensor*
  - *Potentiometric biosensor*
  - *Conductimetric biosensor*
  - *Thermometric or Calorimetric biosensor*
  - *Optical biosensor*
  - *Piezoelectric or Acoustic biosensor*
  - *Whole Cell biosensor*
- *Applications of Biosensors*

3.1 INTRODUCTION

A biosensor is an analytical device consisting of an immobilized layer of biological component (e.g. nucleic acid, hormone, antibody, enzyme, whole cell, tissue) in the intimate contact with the transducer i.e. sensor. A transducer is a physical component which analyses the biological signals and converts into an electrical signal which is measurable. Biosensors are analytical devices that convert a biological response into an electrical signal. Biosensors are functionally composed of three main components. The first part of biosensor is biological element. Biological element is responsible for detecting the analyte (drug, glucose, urea, pesticide etc.) and generating a response signal. The signal generated by the biological element is then transformed into a detectable response by the second component called as transducer. The third component of the biosensor is the detector which amplifies and processes the signals which are displayed an electronic display system. The various steps in signal processing of a biosensor is shown in Fig. 3.1.

The biological recognition components are enzymes, microbial cells, plant or animal cells, tissues, immune binding or receptor proteins. It is important and beneficial to use immobilized biocatalyst as it provides reusability, long half-life and ensures same catalytic activity in a series of analyses. The desired biological material (enzyme) is immobilized by conventional methods such as adsorption, entrapment, microencapsulation, covalent or cross binding. This immobilized biological component is in intimate contact with the transducer.

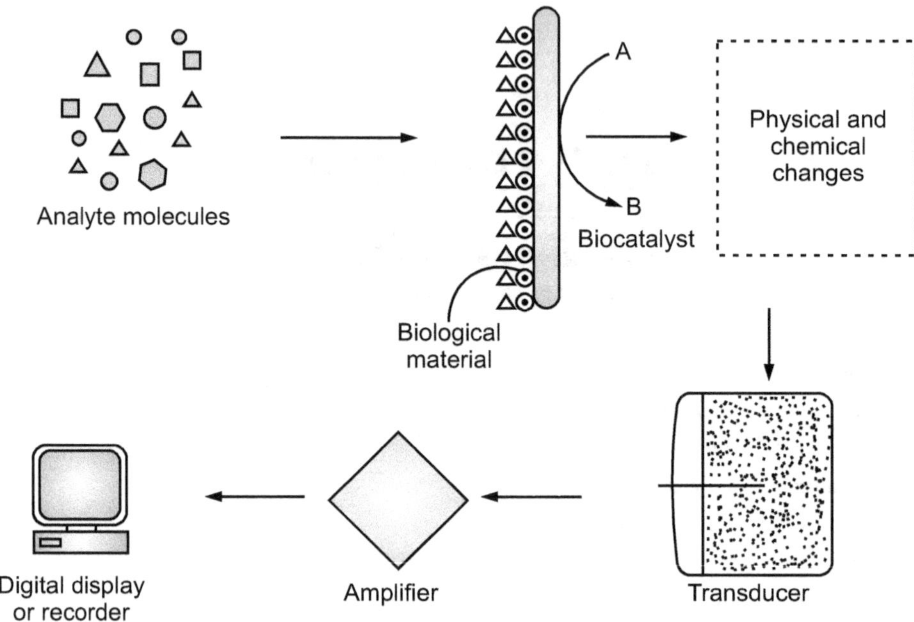

Fig. 3.1: General principle and components of biosensors

The system is responsible for the detection of the analyte and subsequent response in same measurable parameters. Transducer is the main part of biosensor which makes use of a physical change accompanying the reaction. The detection systems used in biosensing are electrochemical detection, photometric detection, thermal and mass detection, fluorescence, signal processing and instrumentation based detection system. The analyte binds to the biological component to form bound analyte which in turn produces the electronic response that can be measured. The analyte is converted to a product which may be associated with the release of heat, oxygen, electrons, hydrogen ions or the product of ammonium ions. The product passes through another membrane to the transducer. The transducer converts product into an electric signal which is amplified. Processor is used to process the signal by subtracting the base line signal which is taken by an electrode without a biocatalyst and converts the resultant signal to digital output.

3.2 TYPES OF BIOSENSORS

Biosensors are classified as enzyme-based, tissue-based, immunosensors, DNA biosensors and thermal and piezoelectric biosensors. Enzyme biosensors are prepared by immobilization methods such as ionic bonding, covalent bonding or van der Waals forces. The commonly used enzymes are peroxidases, aminoxidases, polyphenoloxidases, oxidoreductases etc. Bacterial biosensors directly utilize a chain of bacterial enzyme reactions to achieve detection of one or more species. Organelle-based sensors are prepared by using membranes, chloroplasts, mitochondria, microsomes etc. Immunosensors are prepared on the fact that antibodies have high affinity towards their respective antigens, i.e. antigen-antibody specific reaction properties. Labelled antigens or antibodies may be used in biosensors based on enzyme linked immunoassary (ELISA) principles. The DNA biosensors are based on the property that single-strand nucleic acid molecule is able to recognize and bind to its complementary strand in a sample.

Biosensors can be classified according to the mode of physicochemical transduction or the type of biorecognition element. Based on the transducer, biosensors can be classified as electrochemical, optical (measure the absorbed or emitted light), thermal and piezoelectric (detect stress) biosensors. Electrochemical biosensors can be further classified as amperometric biosensors (measure the electrical current), potentiometric biosensors (measure electrical voltage) and conductometric biosensors (measure electrical conductance).

3.2.1 Amperometric Biosensor

These biosenors are based on the movement of electrons as a result of enzyme-catalysed redox reactions. The amperometric biosensors contain either enzyme-electrode or chemically modified electrodes. A redox reaction catalyzed by an enzymes is directly coupled to an electrode where enzyme is presented with the oxidizable substrate. The electrons are transferred from the substrate to the electrode via enzyme and redox mediator (Fig. 3.2). The magnitude of the current is proportional to the substrate concentration. The most common amperometric biosensor is glucose biosensor which is based on a Clark oxygen electrode. In this case, the platinum cathode is held next to an oxygen permeable membrane on which glucose oxidase enzyme is immobilized. This membrane is also permeable to substrate glucose.

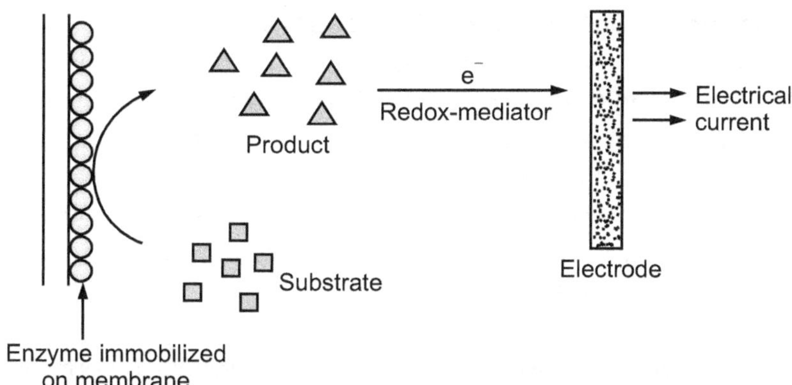

Fig. 3.2: Working of amperometric biosensors

3.2.2 Potentiometric Biosensor

In potentiometric biosensor, changes in ionic concentrations are measured by use of ion-selective electrodes (pH electrode). These biosensors consist of a membrane containing immobilized enzyme and surrounding the probe from a pH meter. The potential difference obtained between the potentiometric electrode (Fig. 3.3) and the reference electrode can be measured. It is proportional to the concentration of the substrate. The major limitation of these biosensors are the sensitivity of enzymes to pH, ammonia, carbon dioxide or other analytes. Ion-selective field effect transistors (ISFET) can be used for miniaturization of potentiometric biosensors. The intramyocardial pH is monitored by an ISFET biosensor during human open-heart surgery.

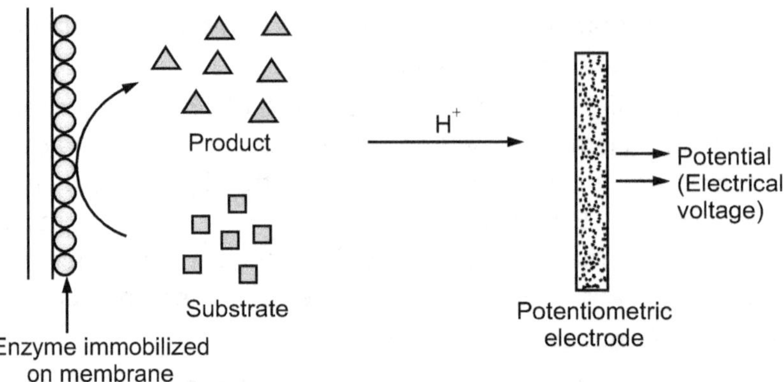

Fig. 3.3: Principle of potentiometric biosensor

3.2.3 Conductimetric Biosensors

The changes in the ionic species is transferred or altered into electrical conductivity in conductimetric biosensors. Conductivity measurement is based on the biocatalytic reaction of the sample on an electrode. The conductimetric transducer consists of reference electrode and working electrode. Both electrodes are coated with a nata de coco membrane and enzyme is immobilized only on working electrode. The reaction produces ions which results in the change of conductivity. Urea biosensor utilizing immobilized urease is a example of conductimetric biosensors.

3.2.4 Thermometric or Calorimetric Biosensors

Many enzyme catalyzed reactions are exothermic (production of heat), which may be used as a basis for measuring the rate of reaction. These changes are determined by thermal biosensors or calorimetric biosensors. In this method, substrate enters into the enzyme packed bed reactor and then it converted to a product by generating heat. The difference in the temperature between the substrate and product is measured by thermistors (thermal biosensors) calorimetric microsensors have been used for detection of cholesterol in blood serum based on production of heat by enzymatic reaction.

3.2.5 Optical Biosensors

Optical biosensors are the devices that utilize the principle of optical measurements i.e. fluorescence, absorbance, chemiluminescence, internal reflection spectroscopy; etc. These involve determining changes in light absorption between the reactants and products of a reaction or measuring the light output. Optical biosensors primarily involve enzyme and antibodies as the transducing elements. It allow a safe non-electrical remote sensing of materials and these biosensors usually do not require reference sensors. The most common application of this biosensor is estimation of blood glucose for monitoring of diabetes.

Fibre optic lactate biosensor is one of important example of optical biosensors. The principle of this biosensor is based on the measurement of changes in molecular oxygen concentration. This reaction is catalysed by the enzyme lactate monooxygenase.

$$O_2 + \text{Lactate} \xrightarrow[\text{monooxygenase}]{\text{Lactate}} CO_2 + \text{Acetate} + H_2O$$

Oxygen has quenching (reducing) effect on the fluorescence and hence, the amount of fluorescence generated by the dyed film is dependent on the oxygen. Lactate present in the reaction mixture utilize oxygen and proportionate decrease in the reducing effect of oxygen. This results, increase in the fluorescent output which can be measured. Optical fibre sensing devices are used for measuring pH, pCO_2 and pO_2 in critical care and surgical monitoring.

3.2.6 Piezoelectric or Acoustic Biosensor

Piezoelectric biosensors are based on the principle of sound vibrations (acoustics). Piezoelectric crystals with positive and negative changes vibrate with characteristics frequencies. The optimal resonant frequency for acoustic wave transmission is dependent on the physical dimensions and properties of the piezoelectric crystals. Adsorption of molecules on the crystal surface alters the resonance frequencies which can be measured by electronic devices. A piezoelectric biosensor has been developed for organophosphorus insecticide by incorporating acetylcholine esterase, for formaldehyde by incorporating formaldehyde dehydrogenase and for cocaine in gas phase by attaching cocaine antibodies to the surface of piezoelectric crystal.

3.2.7 Whole Cell Biosensor

In the whole cell biosensor or microbial biosensor, immobilized whole cell of microorganisms or their organelles are used. These biosensors may employ live or dead microbial cells. The microbial cells are easily available with less cost and they are less sensitive to variations in pH and temperature compared to isolated enzymes. The specificity and sensitivity of whole cell biosensors may be less compared to that of enzymes.

3.3 APPLICATIONS OF BIOSENSORS

Biosensors are widely applied in many fields such as pharmaceutical industries, medicine, food industry, pollution control, military etc. They are very popular in many areas due to the small size, easy handling, low cost, and better stability and sensitivity.

Pharmaceutical and biomedical applications:

Biosensors are mainly used for the quantitative estimation of biologically important substances in body fluids e.g. glucose, cholesterol, urea etc. Glucose biosensors are used for diagnosis of diabetes mellitus. Optical biosensors can be used for measurement of patient's blood glucose level by combining bacterial magnitude with a chromophoric system. Blood gas monitoring for pH, pCO_2 and pO_2 is carried out by optical biosensors during critical care and surgical monitoring of patients. Mitomycin, an aflatoxin, causes cancer in inborne infants. Mutagenicity of such chemicals can be detected by using biosensors. Several toxic compounds produced in the body can also be detected by biosensors.

Biosensors are being used in the medical field to diagnose infectious disease mainly urinary tract infections. A novel biosensor (hafnium oxide, HfO_2) has been used for early stage detection of human interleukin-10. Interaction between recombinant human IL-10 with corresponding monoclonal antibody is studied for early detection of cytokine. Fluroescent biosensors can probe ions, metabolites, and protein biomarkers with great sensitivity. They are used in protein localization, probing gene expression and conformation in fields such as signal transduction, transcription and apoptosis. Fluorescent biosensors can be used for detection of cancer, inflammatory diseases, cardiovascular and neuro-degenerative diseases and viral infections.

Fluorescent biosensors are also used in drug discovery for the identification of drugs by high thorough put and high content screening approaches. These are considered potent tools for preclinical evaluation and clinical validation of active drug molecules. These biosensors are effectively used for early detection of biomarkers in molecular and clinical diagnostics, for monitoring disease status and response to treatments.

Potentiometric biosensors are developed with Ion-Selective Field Effect Transistors (ISFETs) for different applications such as chiral amine salt detection, enzyme inhibitors of acetyl choline esterase, detection of pharmaceutical preparations such as procaine, tetracaine and lidocaine, and detection of anionic surfactants like sodium dodecyl sulfate (SDS) and dodecyltrimethyl ammonium bromide. Biosensors can be used in fermentation industry for monitoring fermentation products, biomass, enzymes and estimation of various ions. Biosensors are commonly used to control the fermentation process and produce reproducible results. In fermentation process, glucose biosensors are used to monitor the process to saccharification to produce glucose. Glutamate biosensors are used to conduct experimentation on ion exchange retrieval of an isoelectric liquor supernatant of glutamate.

Non-medical applications:

Biosensors are used in many non-medical fields such as food industry, environmental monitoring, defense, agriculture and related industries.

Food industry:

Biosensors are commonly used in food industry to detect the odour and freshness of food. Freshness of stored fish can be detected by ATPase. ATP is not found in spoiled fish and this can be detected by using ATPase. Biosensors are used for the detection of pathogens in food. *E. coli* contaminated in food or vegetables can be measured by detecting variation in pH caused by ammonia using potentiometric alternating biosensing systems. Enzymatic biosensors are used in the dairy industry. The automated flow-based biosensor is used to quantify the three organophosphate pesticides in milk. Biosensors are also used to defect artificial sweeteners in food additives.

Food safety is one of most important parameters and quality of food refers to the appearance, taste, smell, freshness, flavour, nutitional value and chemicals. Nanotechnology and electromechanical systems are striding in to make sensing technology imminent for use in ensuring food quality and safety. Biosensors are commonly used to detect pesticides such as organophosphtes and carbamic insecticide species. Biosensors also detect pesticides in wine and orange juice.

Environmental Monitoring:

Biosensors are very helpful in environmental monitoring and pollution control. They are useful for monitoring pollutants, chemical residues, pesticides, toxins or microbes in marine water, rivers and reservoirs. The concentration of pesticides and the biological oxygen demand (BOD) can be measured by biosensors. Biosensors coupled with oxygen electrode and immobilized *Trichosporon cutaneum* is used for measuring BOD. The whole cell biosensor in conjugation with oxygen electrode and immobilized *Salmonella typhimurium* and *Bacillus subtilis* can be used to measure mutagenicity or carcinogenecity of several chemical compounds.

Defense:

Biosensors are used by the infantry to detect and identify the toxic gases and other chemical agents used during war.

QUESTIONS

(A) Objective Type Questions:

1. What is biosensor? Explain.
2. Explain general principle and components of biosensor.
3. Write the principle of conductimetric biosensors.

(B) Short Answer Questions:

1. Write the principle and applications of amperometric biosensor.
2. Write notes on:
   (a) Potentiometric biosensor
   (b) Principle of optical biosensor

(C) Long Answer Questions:

1. Explain different types of biosensors used in diagnostics.
2. Write the applications of biosensors in pharmaceutical industry.

(D) Multiple Choice Questions:

1. _______ biosensors are based on the principle of sound vibrations.
   (a) Piezoelectric (b) Optical
   (c) Calorimetric (d) Potentiometric
2. Principle of fibre optic lactate biosensor is based on the measurement of changes in molecular oxygen and this reaction is catalyzed by _______
   (a) Lactate hydrolase (b) Lactate gelatinase
   (c) Lactate monooxygenase (d) Lactate cellulase

■■■

Chapter ... 4

PROTEIN ENGINEERING

♦ LEARNING OBJECTIVES ♦

After completing this chapter, reader should be able to understand:

- *Introduction*
- *Techniques of Protein Engineering*
  - o *Genetic Modifications*
  - o *Chemical Modifications*
- *Applications of Protein Engineering*
  - o *Pharmaceutical or Medical Applications*
  - o *Food and Detergent Industry*
  - o *Environmental Applications*
  - o *Other Applications*

4.1 INTRODUCTION

Protein engineering is the process of developing useful or industrial important proteins. Protein engineering can be defined as the modification of protein structure with rDNA technology or chemical treatment to get a desirable function for better use in pharmaceuticals and other applications. Rational protein design and directed evaluation are general strategies for protein engineering. Protein engineering involves synthesis of new proteins or to make changes in the existing protein sequence or structure to achieve desired functions. The most classified method in protein engineering is the 'rational design' approach which involves 'site-directed mutagenesis' of proteins. Site-directed mutagenesis allows addition of specific amino acids into a target gene. Directed evaluation is a most important method to alter the function of an enzyme without the exhaustive structural and functional data. Direct evaluation introduces desired properties into the proteins by random mutation or gene recombination. Functional variants with desired properties are identified from libraries through screening. Computational protein design uses molecular modeling programs to predict amino acid sequences and to study structure-function relationship of proteins. The main objective of protein engineering is to develop more stable and catalytic efficient enzymes. It introduce new active sites, modify substrate specificity and improve the thermostability. Protein engineering technology is used to produce hybrid enzymes or tailor made enzymes in large quantities by expression of relevant structural genes. This techniques are used to produce more specific, more potent active pharmaceutical proteins and to get humanized antibodies with less immunogenicity. Basic principle of protein engineering is shown in Fig. 4.1.

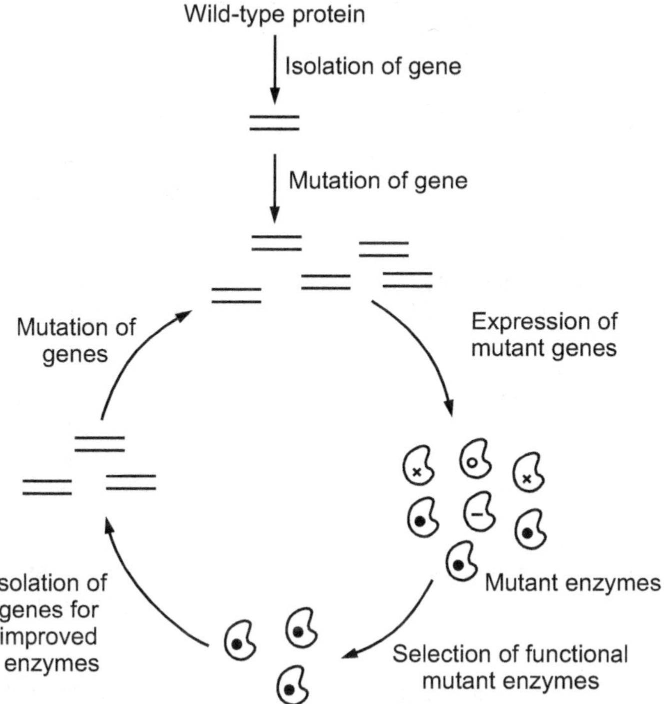

Fig. 4.1: Basic principle of protein engineering

4.2 TECHNIQUES OF PROTEIN ENGINEERING

Different protein engineering methods are used to design the active and stable protein components for wide applications. The most common method in protein engineering is the 'rational design' approach (Fig. 4.2) which involves 'site-directed mutagenesis' of proteins. Random methods includes random mutagenesis and evolutionary methods which involve "DNA shuffling". Protein engineering techniques are also classified into two basic categories such as genetic modifications and chemical modifications.

4.2.1 Genetic Modifications

Modifications of proteins through genes is an easiest and more efficient approach compared to chemical modifications. The basic method of genetic engineering is the modification of responsible gene and generate the proteins with novel properties. Rational design plays a main role in protein engineering and manipulate different processes such as regenerative medicine, protein delivery system, tissue engineering etc. Rational design has been improved by modification in the site directed mutagenesis techniques, protein-protein interaction and protein 2D, 3D structure modeling. The concept of 3D modeling is based on relating a structure to the possible expected functions of amino acid residues and replacing them with other functions.

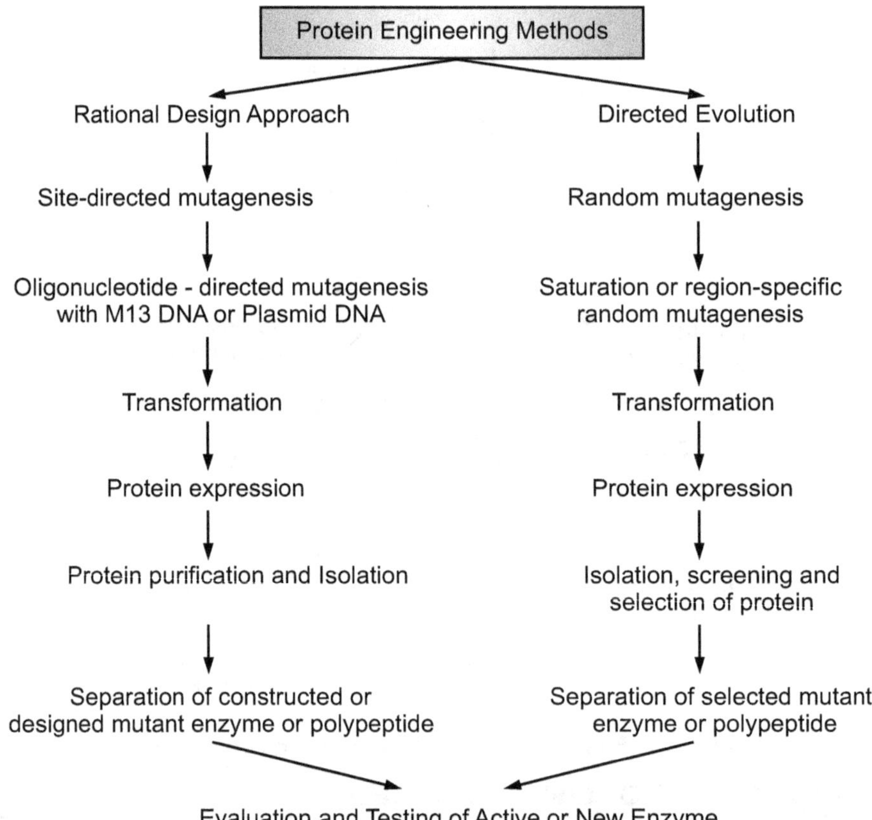

Fig. 4.2: Principle of rational design approach and directed evolution

Site-directed mutagenesis is a *'in-vitro'* technique which allows introduction of specific amino acids into a target gene. It involves the change of cloned target DNA either by deletion, substitution or inseration of the same into the host cell for the production of a functional protein. The simplest method of site directed mutagenesis is the single-prime method. This method involves priming *in-vitro* DNA synthesis with a chemically synthesized oligonucleotide (7 to 20 nucleotide) that carries a base mismatch with the complementary sequence. A single stranded clone of the wild type gene is produced by using an M13 phage based vector. A synthetic oligonucleotide with a desired sequence change at one position is hybridized to a single stranded copy of the gene. The hybridized clone as a primer in the presence of DNA polymerase, synthesizes second DNA strand. The slightly mismatched duplex recombinant plasmid is used to transform bacteria. The duplex DNA replicates in bacterial cell and produce either wild type or mutant plasmids (Fig. 4.3). The clones can be screened by DNA hybridization with ^{32}p-labelled oligonucleotide as probe. Oligonucleotide directed mutagenesis is a method for producing defined point mutations in a cloned gene.

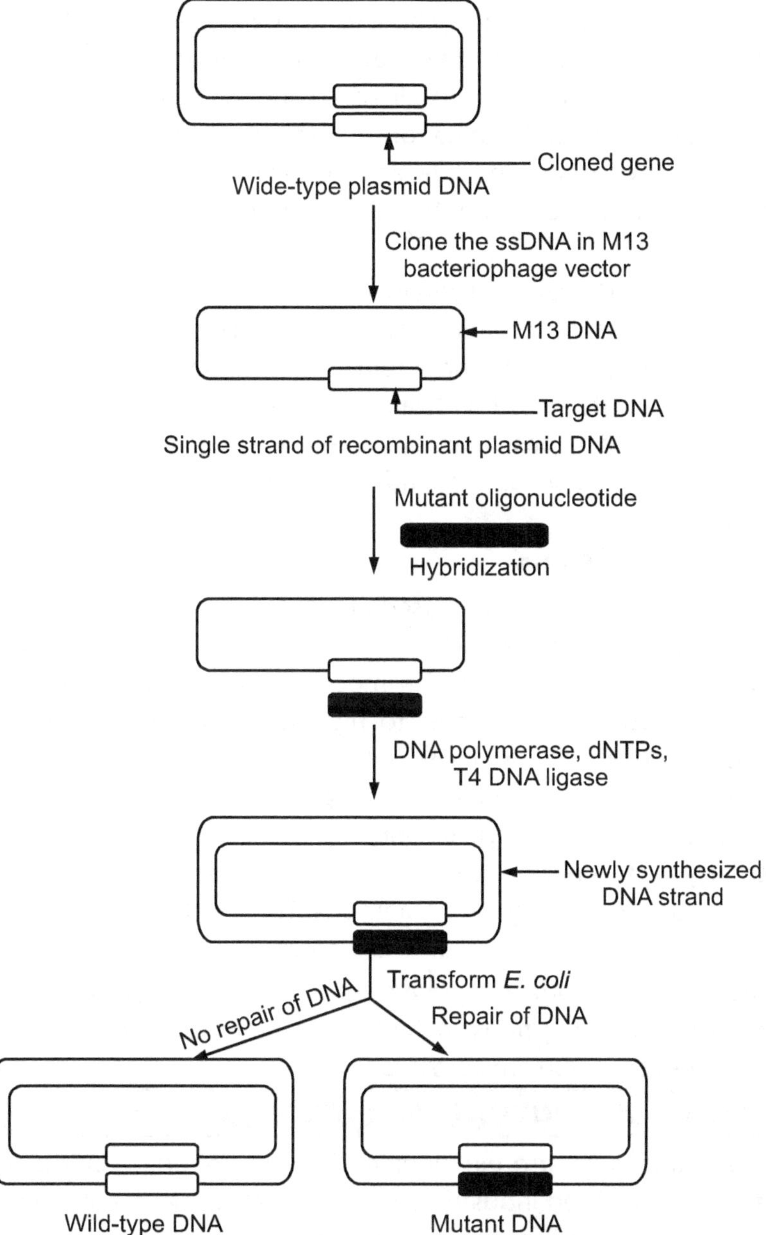

Fig. 4.3: Oligonuclotide site-directed mutagenesis

Random mutagenesis become a best choice when there is a limited information on the structure and mechanisms of the protein. Saturation mutagenesis is a common technique for random mutagenesis. It involves the replacement of a single amino acid within a protein with each of natural amino acids and provides all possible variations at the site. Region-specific or localized random mutagenesis is another technique which is a combination of rational and random approaches of protein engineering. It includes the simultaneous replacement of a few amino acid residues in a specific region to obtain proteins with new specifications.

Directed evolution is an approach of changes in the existing genetic material to modify its structure or functions. It has been developed using controlled or designed selection to introduce new selected functions. It is obtained through the design of successful selection protocol for new mutants. Directed evoluation method is commonly used to improve protein properties and their applications in different industries. The main purpose of directed evoluation is the random mutagenesis of the gene of interest with a selection scheme for the new desired function.

Enhancement of knowledge about protein structures and functions encourage researcher to design proteins *de novo* or protein from scratch. They used information about the molecular recognition, conformational preferences and structure analyses of native proteins together with latest software for data analysis and manipulations. Obtaining *de novo* enzymes from scratch has been possible by *in silico* rational design, utilizing the understanding of a reaction mechanism, and empirical search of large protein libraries by using mRNA display.

4.2.2 Chemical Modifications

Chemical modification is most widely used and had more importance before advances in site directed mutagenesis. In this method, functional group on side chain of natural enzymes may be changed or parts of original protein modified and replaced. Protein modification is used for increase the stability of enzymes to high temperature and organic solvents. The amino acid lysine residues can be cross-linked by use of chemical linkers. The most commonly used protein cross linker or stabilizer is glutaraldyhyde. Chemical modification of surface amino groups of α-chymotrypsin enhances 120 times greater stability of enzyme. Attachment of coenzyme to enzyme is possible by chemical modifications and this method can be applied in conjunction with genetic methods. This method is only applicable to amino acids that have reactive side chains and surface proteins.

Peptide synthesis can be produced chemically using organic synthesis methods. Chemical ligastion is used to produce peptides in high yield. Chemical synthesis is only useful for polypeptides having less than 300 amino acids.

4.3 APPLICATIONS OF PROTEIN ENGINEERING

A different applications of protein engineering are reported in the field of pharmaceutical sciences or medical, food industry, environmental sciences, nanobiotechonolgy, etc.

4.3.1 Pharmaceutical or Medical Applications

Protein engineering has been used to produce therapeutic pharmaceutical proteins with high solubility and stability. This technique is widely used for production of biotechnology drugs and treatment of diseases by vaccines, gene therapy, antisense technology and antibodies derived from 'humanised' transgenic mice. Making protein drugs which are more specific, more potent and coupling them to targeting mechanism.

The use of protein engineering for cancer treatment is a major area of interest in the field of protein biotechnology. Advances in protein engineering and rDNA technology are expected to increase the use of pretargeted radioimmunotherapy. Novel antibodies are used as anticancer agents, where the ability of antibodies to select antigens specifically with high affinity. Protein engineering methods are used to modify antibodies to target cancer cells for clinical applications. Multifunctional and smart drug vehicles can be produced at the nanoscale by protein engineering.

Many protein based drugs, vaccines and scaffolds with more safety, improved efficacy, reduced immunogenicity and improved delivery have been designed as novel biomedical formulations. Fast acting insulin (lispro and aspart) is engineered through mutagenesis to create monomeric forms. Conversely, another form of insulin (glargine) is created by mutagenesis to precipitate upon injection and produce sustain release action. Protein engineering is widely used in development of secreted proteins such as insulin, interferon, erythropoietin as biotherapeutic agents.

Bacteriophage display libraries have been introduced as a alternative to hybridoma technology for antibody production with desired antigen binding characteristics. Phage display has become a important method in protein engineering and immunology. Pharmacokinetic properties of antibodies have been improved, and antibody variants of different size and antigen binding sites have been produced by protein engineering.

4.3.2 Food and Detergent Industry

Industrial important properties of enzymes are improved by protein engineering by modifying thermostability, specificity and catalytic efficiency. Wheat gluten protein is one of best examples of protein engineering in food industry. The heterogeneous expression and protein engineering has been studied using different expression systems (*E. coli*, yeasts). Wild-type and mutant gluten proteins are isolated to compare each other for protein-function studies. The activity or properties of food-processing enzymes (amylases, lipases) are improved by protein engineering and rDNA technology.

Proteases, amylases and lipases are important enzymes for industrial, food and detergent applications. Proteases are commonly used for food industry in milk clotting, flavours and low allergenic infant formulae. The protein engineering is responsible for stability, improvement of catalytic efficiency and changes in washing conditions. New alkaline protease (Durazym, Maxapem) are produced by site directed mutagenesis. Classical mutation and protein engineering techniques are commonly used for production of new enzymes with improved properties.

Thermostability, activity and productivity of amylases are improved by protein engineering and recombinant enzyme technology. Amylases are commonly used for saccharification of starch, and bread softness in food industry. It is also used in detergent industry for removal of starch strains.

Lipases are used for the stability and cheese flavour applications in food industry. It is also used in detergent industry for removal of lipase strains. Protein engineering methods such as lid swapping and DNA shuffling are used for production of C. *rugosa* lipase isoforms.

4.3.3 Environmental Applications

Protein engineering or pathway engineering techniques are used for improvement of microbial strains and their enzymes in bio-remediation applications. Oxygenases, peroxidases and laccases are important enzymes for the treatment of organic pollutants. These enzymes easily catalyze the oxidation of a wide range of toxic organic compounds. Organic pollutants (azo dyes, phenols, polycyclic aromatic hydrocarbons, etc.) are detoxified using enzymatic oxidation. Protein engineering and rational enzyme design are commonly used for modification of enzymes for waste management and pollution control. Fungal enzymes (peroxidases) can used to transform xenobiotics and many pollutants. Wide range of protein engineering strategies are used for improvement of enzyme stability and availability.

4.3.4 Other Applications

Redox proteins and enzymes can be modified by protein engineering to be used as nanodevices for biosensing. Industrial important enzymes such as nitrilases, aldolases, β-D-xylosidases can be modified by different protein engineering techniques. Protein engineering to create and improve protein domains can be used for production of new biomaterials for medical and engineering applications. It is used to produce peptide based biomaterials such as elastin-like polypeptides, silk-like polymers, etc.

Proteins are important components of biological systems for regulation of tissue formation, physical performance and biological functions. They are suitable components for controlled synthesis and assembly of nanotechnological studies. Combinatorial biology methods such as phage display and bacterial cell surface display technologies are used to select polypeptide sequences which selectively bind to inorganic compound surfaces. Virus particles may be modified by protein engineering and used in medicine, as a new vaccines, gene therapy, targeted drug delivery vectors or molecular imaging agents. Protein engineering methods are used to improve physical stability of virus particles.

QUESTIONS

(A) Objective Type Questions:

1. What is protein engineering?
2. Write the principle of protein engineering.

(B) Short Answer Questions:

1. What is rational design approach? Explain.
2. Write a note on:
   (a) Site directed mutagenesis.
   (b) Biomedical applications of protein engineering.

(C) Long Answer Questions:

1. Explain different protein engineering methods used to design stable protein.
2. Write the applications of protein engineering.

(D) Multiple Choice Questions:

1. _____ is a '*in-vitro*' technique which allows introduction of specific amino acids into a target gene.
   (a) Site-directed mutagenesis (b) Chemical modification
   (c) Chemical synthesis (d) None of above
2. Site directed mutagenesis can be achieved by _____.
   (a) RAS (b) LCR
   (c) PCR (d) RT-PCR

■■■

Chapter ... 5

CLONING VECTORS AND ENZYMES

♦ LEARNING OBJECTIVES ♦

After completing this chapter, reader should be able to understand:

- *Introduction*
- *Cloning Vectors*
  - *Plasmid Vectors (pBR 322 Plasmid), Bacteriophase Vectors*
  - *Cosmid Vectors, Shuttle Vector, Yeast Vector, Expression Vector*
- *Enzymes acting on DNA*
  - *Restriction Endonucleases, DNA Ligase*

5.1 INTRODUCTION

The deliberate modification in genetic material of an organism by changing the nucleic acid directly is called gene manipulation or genetic engineering or gene cloning and is accomplished by several methods which are collectively known as rDNA (recombinant DNA) technology. DNA cloning is an important technique that allows specific DNA sequences to be separated from other sequences and copied so that they can be obtained in large amounts permitting detailed analysis. DNA cloning is used to isolate new genes allowing them to be investigated and characterized. In 1997, world's first mammalian clone (Dolly) was developed from a non-reproductive cell of an adult animal through cloning by nuclear transplantation.

The various strategies outlined for gene cloning along with the basic steps are discussed as follows:

- Isolation of target DNA or DNA fragment.
- Insertion of target DNA into suitable vector.
- Cloning vectors.
- Isolation and identification of recombinant genes.

The DNA fragments to be cloned are called foreign DNA or passenger DNA or DNA insert. The desired DNA inserts can be obtained from genomic library, cDNA libraries, chemical synthesis and amplification through PCR (polymerase chain reaction). All these processes are possible only due to enzymes such as restriction endonucleases, S1 nuclease, alkaline phosphatase, DNA polymerase, ligase, reverse transcriptase etc.

5.2 CLONING VECTORS

The vectors are the DNA molecules that carry of foreign DNA segment and replicate inside the host cell. Cloning vectors are also called vehicle DNA because they act as carrier of genes. All vectors used for propagation of DNA inserts in a suitable hosts are called cloning vectors. Any extra-chromosomal small genome is used as a vector e.g. plasmid, bacteriophage, cosmid, bacterial artificial chromosome, phagemid, yeast, shuttle, expression etc. These vectors must possess the following characteristics.

- It must be replicate (ori gene) autonomously in host cell.
- It must be easy to isolate, purify and introduce into the host cells.
- The vector should contain suitable marker genes (tet^R, kan^R, amp^R) that allow easy selection of transformed cells.
- It must have the ability of integrate either itself or the DNA insert.
- The vector must contain specific control systems like promoters, terminators, operators, etc.

5.2.1 Plasmid Vectors

Plasmids are the extra chromosomal, self replicating, double stranded and circular DNA molecules present in the bacterial cell. Naturally, occurring bacterial plasmids size range is 5000 to 400,0000 bp. Plasmids are widely used as cloning vehicles. The number of plasmids in a bacterial cell can be increased to about 1000 per cell. This process of increasing the number of plasmids is called amplification.

Plasmids are introduced into bacterial cells by a process called transformation. The plasmid is digested with a restriction enzyme and converted into a linear molecule with sticky ends. The foreign DNA is also digested with the restriction enzyme to produce the same sticky ends. Plasmid and foreign DNA are mixed to form circular recombinant plasmids. These recombinant plasmids are introduced into host cells (*Escherichia coli*) by the process of transformation. In this process, a naked DNA from donor strain is transported into cell cytoplasm of the host cell. Plasmid DNA and host cells (*E. coli*) are mixed and incubated at 0°C in a $CaCl_2$ solution. These cells are given heat shock treatment by shifting the temperature to 38 to 42°C. Some cells are treated by the process of electroporation. In this method, host cells are incubated with the plasmid DNA and subjected to a high-voltage. The transformed bacteria are spread on surface of agar plates. Individual colonies are cultured in conical flask containing liquid medium and large amounts of plasmids are produced. Some of the important plasmid cloning vectors are given in the Table 5.1. The small size of the plasmids (about 3 kbp) enhances the transformation efficiency and easy to purify from bacterial cultures. The plasmid contains two genes (tet^R, amp^R) that shows the resistance to antibiotics such as tetracycline and ampicillin. Hence, it is easy to isolate the antibiotic resistant colonies on surface of agar plates. The pBR 322 is one of earliest, popular and most widely used plasmid of 4362 bp.

Table 5.1: Plasmid cloning vectors

Vectors	Selective markers	Cloning sites
pBR 322	amp^R, tet^R	*Eco*RI, *Bal*I, *Bam*HI, *Sal*I, *Sph*I, *Pvr*I
pBR 325	amp^R, tet^R, cm^R	*Eco*RI, *Pst*I, *Hind*III, *Bam*HI, *Sal*I
pMB 9	tet^R	*Eco*RI, *Sma*I, *Hind*III, *Bam*HI
pACYC 184	tet^R, cm^R	*Eco*RI, *Bam*HI, *Hind*III
pRK 2501	tet^R, kan^R	*Eco*RI, *Bgl*I, *Hind*III
pBD 6	kan^R, str^R	*Bam*HI
pBC 16-1	tet^R	*Eco*RI, *Hind*III

pBR 322 plasmid: The pBR 322 is the first artificial vector developed by **Bolivar** and **Rodriguez** (1977) from *Escherichia coli* plasmid ColEl. In the name pBR, p stands for plasmid, B is for **Bolivar** and R is for **Rodriguez**, the scientists who developed cloning vector pBR 322. Some plasmid names are derived from the places they were developed.

Plasmid pBR 322 consists of genes for origin of replication for resistance to amplicillin (amp^R) and tetracycline (tet^R) unique recognition for 20 restriction enzymes. Structural features of pBR 322 plasmid are shown in Fig. 5.1. Out of 20 sites, six of these sites (*Bam*HI, *Sph*I, *Sal*I, *Xma*III, *Nru*I and *Eco*RIV) are present within the gene coding for tetracycline resistance, two sites (*Hind*III and *Cla*I) are located within the promoter of the tetracycline resistance gene and three sites (*Pst*I, *Pvu*I and *Sca*I) within the gene that provide resistance to ampicillin. Insertion of the DNA fragment into the plasmid using restriction enzyme *Pst*I or *Pvu*I, places the DNA insert within ampicillin resistance gene (amp^R). Cells containing such as pBR 322 recombinant plasmid may grow in presence of tetracycline but not in presence of ampicillin. In *Bam*HI or *Sal*I restriction enzymes are used then the DNA insert in placed within the tetracycline resistance gene. Bacterial cells containing such type of recombinant plasmid may grow on ampicillin but not on tetracycline. This characteristics allows on easy selection of a single bacterial cell having recombinant pBR 322 from other types of cells. **Messings** and collegues (1983) developed the pUC vector as a derivative of pBR 322.

pUC19: pUC19 is a commonly used plasmid cloning vector in *E. coli*. The pUC name is obtained from University of California. The molecule is a small double-stranded circle, 2686 base pairs in length, and has a high copy number. pUC19 carries a 54 base-pair multiple cloning site polylinker that contains unique sites for 13 different hexanucleotide-specific restriction endonucleases. Vector pUC19 (Fig. 5.2) is smaller and it contains all the essential parts of pBR 322.

It has one ampicillin resistance gene and an N-terminal fragment of β-galactosidase (*lacZ*) gene of *E. coli*. The multiple cloning site (MCS) region is split into the *lacZ* gene (codons 6–7 of *lacZ* are replaced by MCS), where various restriction sites for many restriction endonucleases are present. The *ori* site, or origin of replication, is derived from

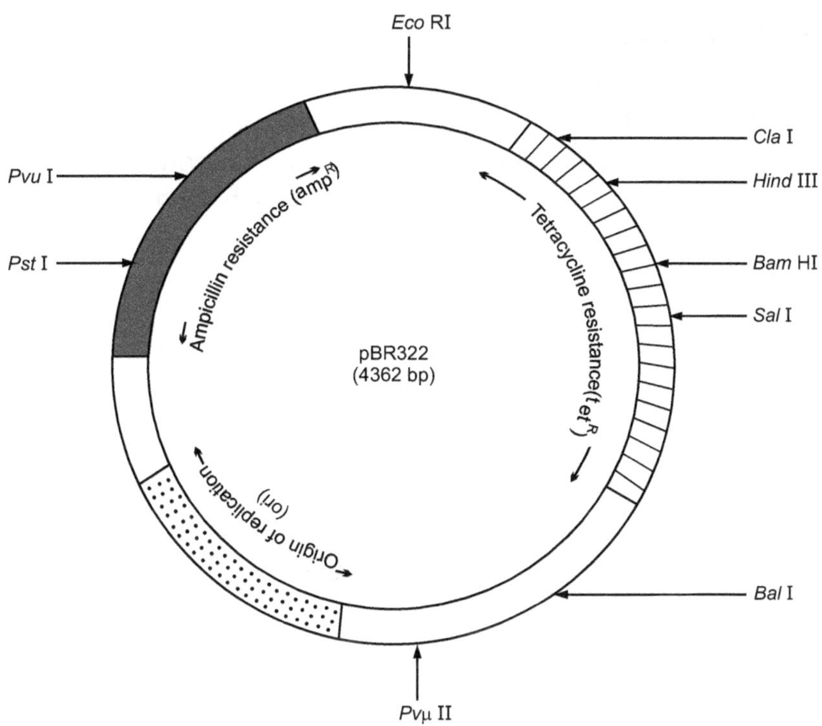

Fig. 5.1: Structural features of pBR 322 vector

the plasmid pMB1. The high copy number is a result of the lack of the *rop* gene and a single point mutation in the ori of pMB1. The *lacZ* gene codes for β-galactosidase. The recognition sites for *Hind*III, *Sph*I, *Pst*I, *Sal*I, *Xba*I, *Bam*HI, *Sma*I, *Kpn*I, *Sac*I and *Eco*RI restriction enzymes have been derived from the vector M13mp19. Due to the presence of MCS and several restriction sites, a foreign piece of DNA of choice can be introduced into it by inserting it into place in MCS region. The cells which have taken up the plasmid can be differentiated from cells which have not taken up the plasmid by growing it on media with ampicillin. The plasmid containing the ampicillin resistance gene will survive and multiply. Transformed cells containing the plasmid with the gene of interest can be distinguished from cells with the plasmid but without the gene of interest (colour of colony), on agar media supplemented with IPTG and X-gal. Recombinants are white, whereas non-recombinants are blue. This is the most notable feature of pUC19. pUC18 contains identical multiple cloning site (MCS) as pUC19 vector except that it is arranged in opposite orientation.

5.2.2 Bacteriophage Vectors

Bacteriophages (phages) are the viruses that infect bacterial cells by injecting their genetic material (DNA or RNA). Most of bacteriophages lyse the bacterial cells by the infection (lytic cycle). Some phage chromosome integreates into the bacterial chromosome and multiplies as lysogenic cycle. The prophage may dissociate from the

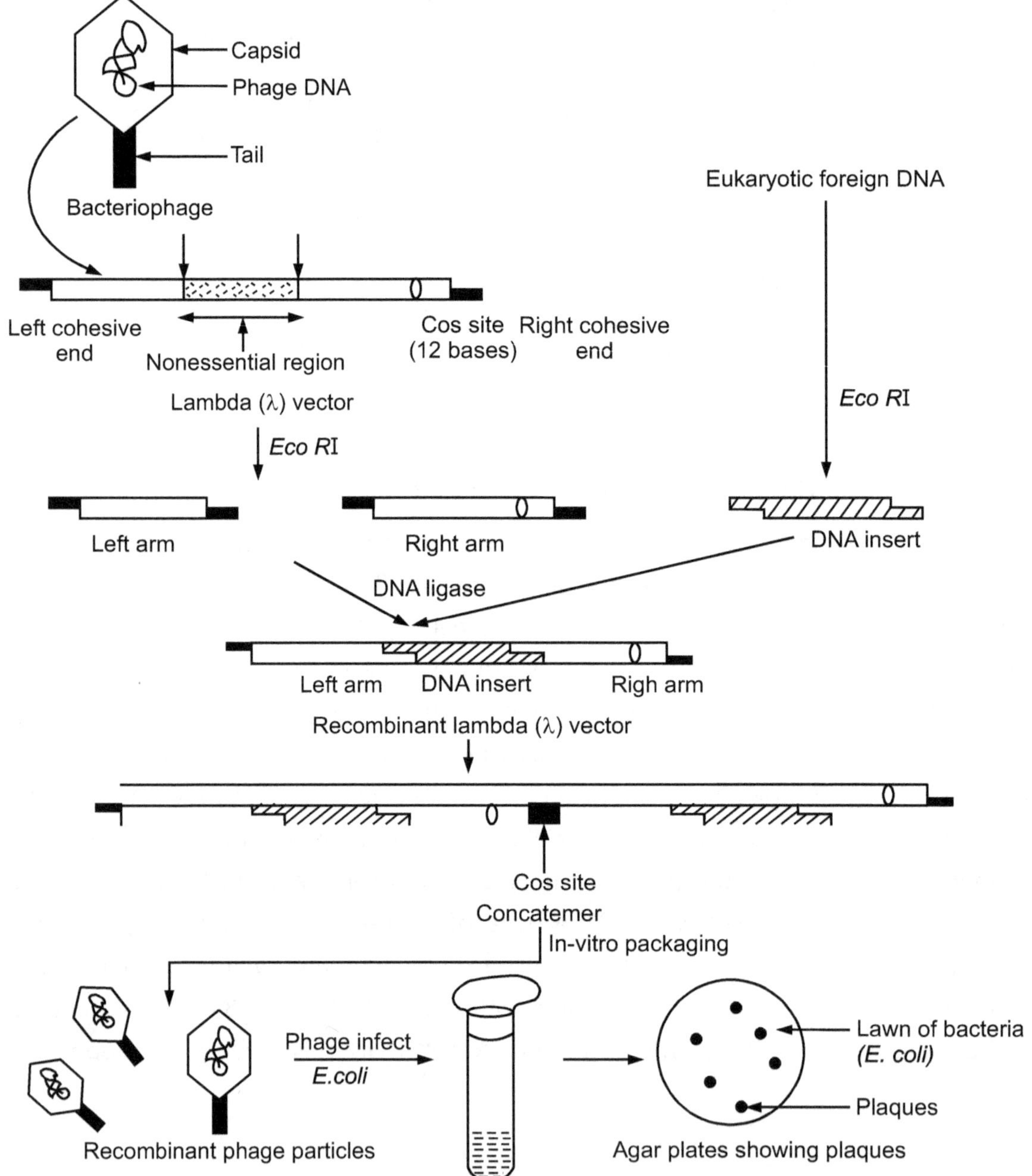

Fig. 5.2: Cloning target DNA with bacteriophage lambda (λ) vector

bacterial chromosome and follow the lytic cycle. Most commonly used *Escherichia coli* phages are λ (lambda), M13 and Fd phages. Phage vectors are most efficient than plasmids (15 kb) for cloning of large fragments of over 25 kb. These vectors are easy to screen in large number of phage plaques than bacterial colonies.

Bacteriophage lamda (λ) DNA has been widely used as cloning vectors. The phage λ is contained within the head attached to a tail. DNA exists as a linear double stranded molecule (48.5 kbp) in the phage head but in host cells, the cohesive ends anneal to form a circular molecule necessary for replication. The sealed cohesive ends are called cos sites (sites of cleavage). It amplifies by rolling mechanism into several genomes joined end to end forming a concatemer (Fig. 5.2) which is the precursor for packaging of λ genome into phage heads. The recombinant phage DNA is inserted (*in-vitro*) into phage capsids by a process called packaging. It involves mixing the recombinant DNA with a packaging extract containing phage capsid proteins and processing enzymes. *E. coli* cells are infected by recombinant phage particles and then these cells are spread on agar plate. It produces a continuous sheet of bacteria called a lawn which contains small clear areas. These correspond to areas of lysis produced by infection with bacteirophage and are called plaques (Fig. 5.2). The plaques are isolated and used to generate large amounts of recombinant DNA by infection of fresh cultures of *Escherichia coli*.

5.2.3 Cosmid Vectors

Cosmids (cos site + plasmid) are the hybrid vectors derived from plasmids which contain *cos* site of phage lambda. Cosmids has unique restriction sites, replication origin and selectable markers from the plasmid (Fig. 5.3). It is prepared using recombinant DNA techniques. The cos sequences occur at one end of lambda DNA molecule and it is

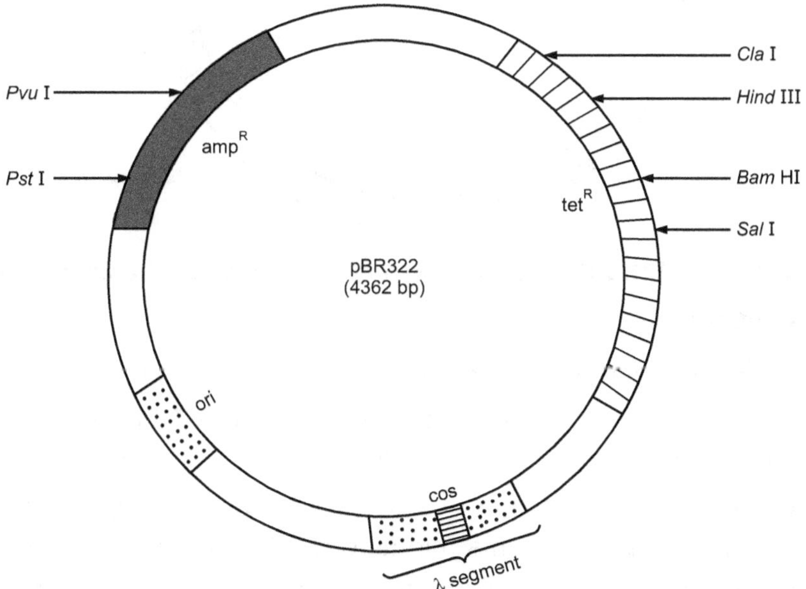

Fig. 5.3: Cosmid vector containing pBR 322 modules and a λ segment

responsible for its insertion into the phage capsid. The presence of cos sites on cosmids allows them to be packaged into phage capsids. The recombinant cosmid is packaged into lambda capsids and used to infect *E. coli*. Cosmids are small 7 kb or less and lambda capsid can accommodate upto 52 kb. Hence, cosmids can accommodate upto 45 kb long DNA inserts.

5.2.4 Shuttle Vector

Specific recombinant plasmids incorporate multiple replication origins and other elements that allow them to be used in more than one species (*E. coli* or yeast). Plasmids which are propagated in cells of two or more different species are called shuttle vectors. Such vectors (Fig. 5.4) possess two origin for replication (ori^{E}, ori^{Euk}). The ori^{E} functions in *Escherichia coli* and ori^{Euk} functions in eukaryotic cells like yeast. The important genes are *ori* (origin for replication in *E. coli*), amp^{R} (ampicillin resistance), ars (autonomously replicating sequence), cen (centromere of yeast) and *leu*-2 (complements of a defective gene encoding for leucin).

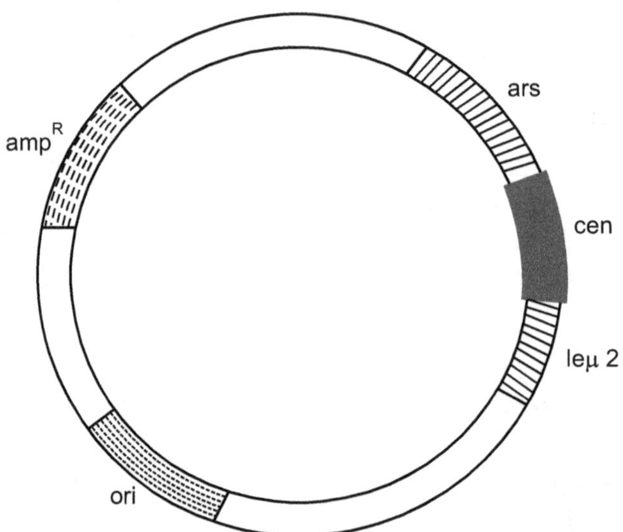

Fig. 5.4: A typical shuttle vector constructed for yeast and *Escherichia coli*

5.2.5 Yeast Vectors

Yeast is a unicellular eukaryotic microorganism. It reproduces sexually as well as asexually by budding. Yeast cells contain their own plasmid (6318 bp long) known as 2 μm plasmid. It is present in many strains in 50 to 100 copies/cell and used as a vector for foreign genes. Yeast plasmid contains an origin of DNA replication (ori), cis-action region (REP 3) and two genes (REP1 and REP2). This plasmid (about 50%) of the 2 μm plasmid is essential for its replication and maintenance in high copy number. The half part of the plasmid is combined with a portion of pBR 322 to form a shuttle vector (Fig. 5.5).

The pBR 322 plasmid segment contains the origin of replication (ori) for *E. coli*, amp^R selectable marker gene and HIS 3 yeast gene. This plasmid vector contains several restriction sites for insertion of DNA segments.

David and colleagues (1987) developed yeast artificial chromosome (YAC) by using new techniques where DNA segment of several thousand base pairs (1 Mb) can be cloned. Yeast artificial chromosome contains all the essential features of a chromosome required for its propagation in a yeast cell. A typical linear YAC contains origin of replication, a centromere, selectable marker gene and telomeres to stabilize the ends of the chromosome (Fig. 5.6). For cloning, yeast artificial chromosome is digested with restriction enzyme such as a *Bam*III and *Eco*RI. Recombinant YAC are produced by inserting a large fragment of genomic DNA. Digestion with restriction enzymes generates two separate DNA arm.

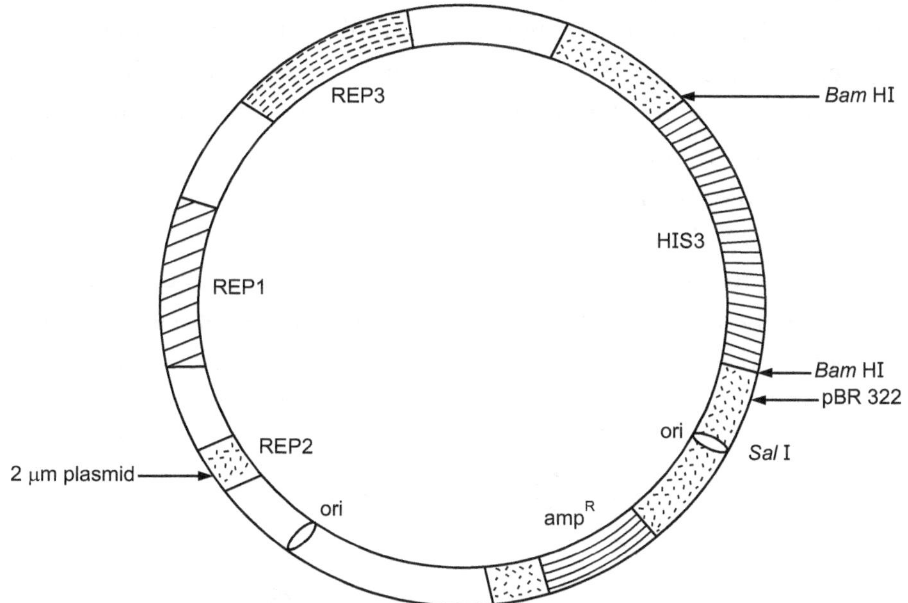

Fig. 5.5: Yeast plasmid (shuttle) vector for *Escherichia coli* and yeast

Each separate arm contains telomeric end and one selectable marker. A large segment of DNA (upto 2×10^6 bp) is ligated to the two arms to create a yeast artificial chromosome (YAC). The YAC is transferred in yeast cells prepared by removal of the cell wall (spheroplasts). The transformants that contain YAC can be identified by change in colour of colonies (red colour – transformed colonies, white colonies – non transformed colonies).

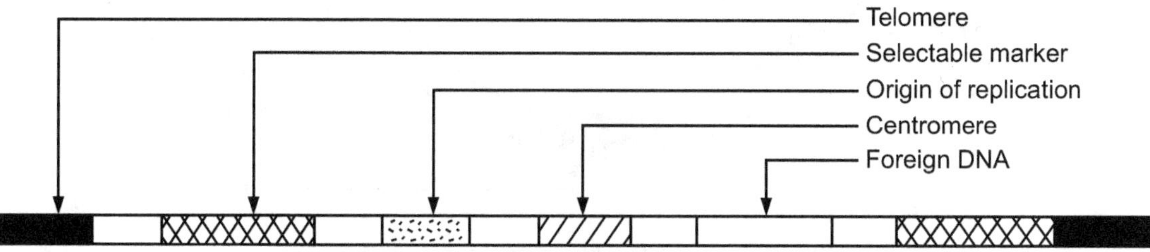

Fig. 5.6: Linear yeast artificial chromosome (YAC)

Yeast artificial chromosomes have been widely used to construct maps of parts of the human genome. It is mainly used for cloning of very large (upto 100 kb) DNA segments for mapping of complex eukaryotic chromosomes. Bacterial artificial chromosomes (BAC) and P1 artificial chromosomes (PAC) vectors are used similar to yeast artificial chromosomes.

5.2.6 Expression Vector

Recombinant DNA technology is used to produce high amount of proteins by addition of desired gene into the blast cell. Expression of cloned genes is carried out by inserting a 'promoter sequence' and a 'terminator sequence'. The cloning vectors which contain the signals for protein synthesis are called expression vectors (Fig. 5.7). Plasmids have been extensively modified to incorporate control elements designed for high level expression of inserted target gene. These control elements contain ribosomes, promoters, polylinkers and terminator sequence. The gene to be expressed is inserted into one of the restriction sites in the polylinker. The promoter allows efficient transcription of the inserted gene. The transcription termination sequence mainly improves the amount of stability of the mRNA produced. The ribosome binding site provides sequence signals needed for efficient translation of the mRNA derived from the gene. In addition, origin of replication and a marker gene (resistant to antibiotic) is incorporated in expression vectors. Lambda PL, lac Z, trip and lac promoters are commonly used to construct expression vectors. The trc and tac promoters are also used which are hybrid promoters derived from lac and trp promoters.

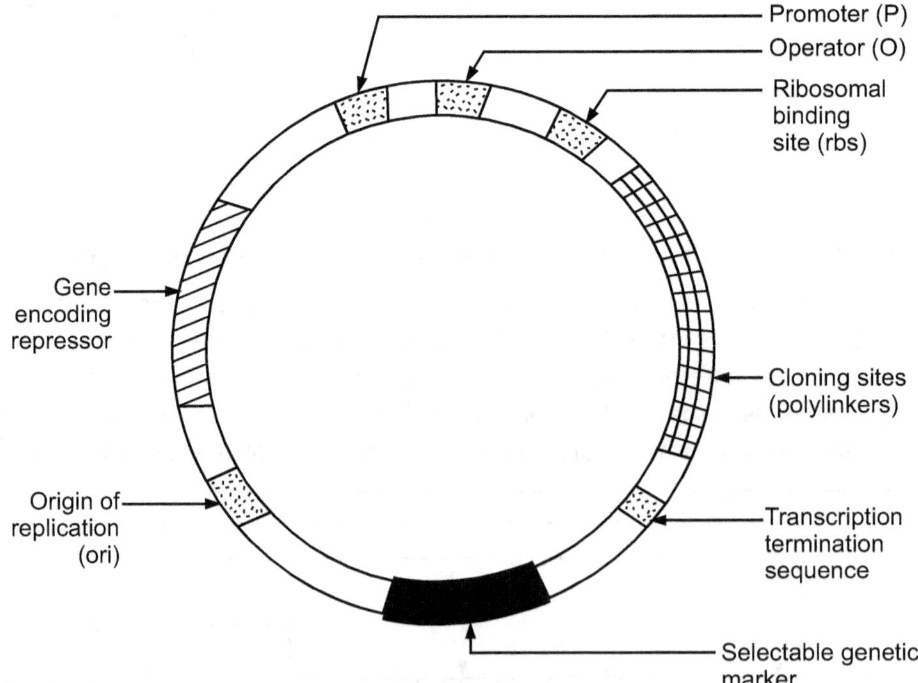

Fig. 5.7: Ideal *E. coli* expression vector

The most commonly used organism for protein expression is the bacterium *Escherichia coli*. The expression host of choice for the expression of many proteins is *Escherichia coli* as the production of heterologous protein in *E. coli* is relatively simple rapid, and convenient. *Bacillus subtilis* is also choice *for* protein expression. Examples of *E. coli* expression vectors are the pGEX series of vectors where glutathione-S-transferase is used as a fusion partner and protein expression is under the control of the tac promoter, and the pET series of vectors which uses a T7 promoter. The promoters used for these vector are usually based on the promoter of the *lac* operon or the T7 promoter, and they are normally regulated by the *lac* operator. These promoters may also be hybrids of different promoters, for example, the tac promoter is a hybrid of *trp* and *lac* promoters.

A yeast commonly used for protein expression is *Pichia pastoris*. Examples of yeast expression vector in *Pichia* are the pPIC series of vectors (pPIC3.5K, pPIC6, pPIC6α, pPIC9K, pPIC3.5K, pPICZ, pPICZα), and these vectors use the AOX1 promoter which is inducible with methanol. The plasmids may contain elements for insertion of foreign DNA into the yeast genome and signal sequence for the secretion of expressed protein. Proteins with disulphide bonds and glycosylation can be efficiently produced in yeast. Another yeast used for protein expression is *Kluyveromyces lactis* and the protein is expressed driven by a variant of the stronglactase LAC4 promoter.

pPICα A, B, and C vectors are 3.6 kb vectors used to express and secrete recombinant proteins in *Pichia pastoris*. Recombinant proteins are expressed as fusions to an N-terminal peptide encoding the *Saccharomyces cerevisiae* á-factor secretion signal. These vectors allow high-level, methanol inducible expression of the gene of interest in Pichia, and can be used in any *Pichia* strain including X-33, SMD1168H, and KM71H.

Saccharomyces cerevisiae is particularly widely used for protein expression studies in yeast. The vectors used in yeast two-hybrid system contain fusion partners for two cloned genes that allow the transcription of a reporter gene when there is interaction between the two proteins expressed from the cloned genes.

Baculovirus, a rod-shaped virus which infect insect cells, is also used as the expression vector. Insect cell lines derived from Lepidopterans (moths and butterflies), such as *Spodoptera frugiperda*, are used as host. Many plant expression vectors are based on the Ti plasmid of *Agrobacterium tumefaciens*. In these expression vectors, DNA to be inserted into plant is cloned into the T-DNA, a stretch of DNA flanked by a 25-bp direct repeat sequence at either end, and which can integrate into the plant genome. The T-DNA also contains the selectable marker.

Mammalian expression vectors offer considerable advantages for the expression of mammalian proteins over bacterial expression systems - proper folding, post-translational modifications, and relevant enzymatic activity. Cultured mammalian cell lines such as the Chinese hamster ovary (CHO), HEK, HeLa, and COS cell lines may be used to produce protein. Vectors are transfected into the cells and the DNA may be integrated into the genome by homologous recombination in the case of stable transfection. Examples of mammalian expression vectors include the adenoviral vectors, the pSV and the pCMV series of plasmid vectors, vaccinia and retroviral vectors, as well as baculovirus. The promoters for cytomegalovirus (CMV) and SV40 are commonly used in mammalian expression vectors to drive protein expression.

Chinese hamster ovary (CHO) cells are a cell line derived from the ovary of the Chinese hamster and it is used in biological and medical research and commercially in the production of therapeutic proteins. CHO cells can be modified to produce proteins with "mammalian" post-translational modifications, and through gene amplification can selectively produce high levels of recombinant proteins. Process development, using CHO cell lines, focuses on achieving the maximum amount of active product. Optimization of the amount of active product can be achieved in at least two basic ways. The first way is to increase the specific productivity (i.e., the product per cell) through cell line development. Cell line development may include both sub-cloning the cell line to select higher producing clones and use of gene amplification. Drug resistance has been the tool of choice in the biopharmaceutical industry to induce gene amplification. By combining the gene of interest with a selectable gene, increased production levels can be accomplished. Using productivity-per-cell approaches, scientists have increased expression levels more than 1,000-fold. Two gene amplification systems used in CHO cells are the dihydrofolate reductase (DHFR) system using methotrexate (MTX) resistance, and the glutamine synthetase (GS) system using methionine sulfoxamine (MSX) resistance. The DHFR enzyme catalyzes the conversion of folate to tetrahydrofolate.

Most peptide and protein pharmaceuticals are now produced through recombinant DNA technology using expression vectors such as hormones, vaccines, antibiotics, antibodies, and enzymes. In recent years, expression vectors have been used to introduce specific genes into plants and animals to produce transgenic organisms. Expression vectors have been used to introduce a vitamin A precursor, beta-carotene, into rice plants to produce golden rice.

5.3 ENZYMES ACTING ON DNA

Genetic engineering is based on different types of enzymes. Some enzymes used in gene cloning are given in Table 5.2.

5.3.1 Restriction Endonucleases

The ability to join DNA molecules together for cloning is dependent on the type of enzymes occur in bacteria. These restriction enzymes are called restriction endonucleases or molecular scissors. Restriction endonucleases recognize specific sequences in the incoming DNA and cleave the DNA into fragments.

The existence of these enzymes was first postulated by **Werner Arber** in the early 1960s while studying bacterial viruses. He found that when virus DNA entered in the bacteria, it was cut into small pieces. **Arber** also proposed that the restriction enzymes act at specific sites on the viral DNA. **Hamilton Smith** and his colleagues (1970) isolated the first restriction enzyme (*Hind* III) from *Haemophilus influenzae*. This enzyme recognizes a particular target sequence in a duplex DNA molecule and breaks the polynucleotide chain.

Table 5.2: Enzymes used in DNA cloning

Enzyme	Function
Restriction enzyme	Cuts both strands of dsDNA within a symmetrical recognition site resulting in blunt or sticky ends.
Alkaline phosphatase	Removes terminal phosphates (PO_4) from either the 5' or 3' end (or both).
Reverse transcriptase	Synthesize of DNA copy of an RNA molecule.
S1 Nuclease	Cleaves a strand opposite to a nick on the complementary strand.
DNA polymerase I	Fills gaps in duplexes by stepwise addition of nucleotides to 3' ends.
Exo nuclease III	It cleaves from the end of linear DNA and digest dsDNA from 3' end.
Terminal transferase	Adds homopolymer tails to the 3'–OH ends of a DNA strand.
Polynucleotide kinase	Adds a phosphate to the 5'–OH end of dsDNA or ssDNA or RNA.
Bacteriophage λ exonuclease	Removes nucleotide from the 5' end of a duplex to expose single-stranded 3' ends.
Taq polymerase	DNA polymerase isolated from *Thermus aquaticus* which operates at 72°C (in PCR) and stable above 90°C.
DNA ligase	It joins two DNA molecules or fragments.

The restricton enzymes name is designated by a three letter abbreviation for the host organism (e.g. *Escherichia coli* – *Eco*). A strain or type identified is written as subscript (e.g. *Eschierichia coli* strain K – *Eco* K). Roman numerals are used to indicate the different restriction – modification systems in a strain, when more than one enzyme is obtained from the same organism (e.g. *Haemophilus influenzae,* serotype d, enzyme III – *Hind* III). Some commonly used restriction enzymes are given in Table 5.3. Arrows indicate in the table are the recognition sites.

There are three distinct types of restriction endonucleases: Type I, Type II and Type III. These enzymes are differentiated by their mode of action. Type I restriction endonucleases cleave DNA at random sites that can be more than 1000 base pairs (bp) from the recognition sequences. This type of enzymes are most complex and not useful in gene cloning as their cleavage sites are non-specific e.g. *Eco* K, *Eco* B, etc. Type (II) restriction endonucleases enzymes cut within the recognition sequence and are used for gene cloning studies giving rise to discrete DNA fragments of defined length and sequence. The first type (II) enzyme to be isolated was *Hind* III by **Hamilton Smith** in 1970. They are most stable enzymes that require Mg^{++} as cofactor. The recognition sequences are usually 4 to 6 bp long and palindromic. Type (II) restriction endonucleases are used for restriction mapping and gene cloning. Type (III) restriction endonucleases are intermediate between the type (I) and type (II) enzymes. They cleave to DNA about 25 bp from the recognition sequence e.g. *Eco* P1, *Eco* P15 etc. Type (I) and type (III) restriction enzymes are not used in gene cloning.

Type (II) enzymes are the most important and they cut DNA molecules at specific sequences usually 4 to 8 bases. The sequences recognized are palindromes. In a palindrome, the base sequence in the second half of a DNA strand is the mirror image of the sequence in its first half (Fig. 5.8 a). In a palindrome with rotational symmetry, the base sequence in the first half of one strand of the DNA double helix is the mirror image of the second half of its complementary strand [Fig. 5.8 (b)]. Some restriction enzymes make staggered cuts on the two DNA strands, leaving two to four nucleotides of one strand unpaired at each resulting end. These unpaired strands are called as cohesive ends or sticky ends [Fig. 5.9 (a)].

Table 5.3: Source and cleavage sites of restriction enzyme

Restriction endonuclease	Source	Cleavage sites
Hind III	*Haemophilus influenzae* – d	↓ 5' – AAGCTT – 3' 3' – TTCGAA – 5' ↑
Eco RI	*Escherichia coli* RY 13	↓ 5' – GAATTC – 3' 3' – CTTAAG – 5' ↑
Hpa I	*Haemophilus parainfluenzae*	↓ 5' – GTTAAC – 3' 3' – CAATTG – 5' ↑
Kpn I	*Klebsiella pneumoniae*	↓ 5' – GGTACC – 3' 3' – CCATGG – 5' ↑
Bam HI	*Bacillus amyloliquefaciens* H	↓ 5' – GGATCC – 3' 3' – CCTAGG – 5' ↑

contd. …

Bgl II	*Bacillus globiggi*	↓ 5' – AGATCT – 3' 3' – TCTAGA – 5' ↑
Sal I	*Streptomyces albus* G	↓ 5' – GTCGAC – 3' 3' – CAGCTG – 5' ↑
Sau 3AI	*Staphylococcus aureus* 3AI	↓ 5' – GATC – 3' 3' – CTAG – 5' ↑
Pst I	*Providencia stuartii*	↓ 5' – CTGCAG – 3' 3' – GACGTC – 5' ↑
Nla III	*Neisseria lactamica*	↓ 5' – CATG – 3' 3' – GTAC – 5' ↑
Taq I	*Thermus aquaticus* YTI	↓ 5' – TCGA – 3' 3' – AGCT – 5' ↑

Certain type (II) restriction enzymes cleave both strands of DNA at the same base pairs but In the centre of recognition sequence. These DNA fragments are called flush ends or blunt ends [Fig. 5.9 (b)].

5' – GAA ↑ AAG – 3'
3' – CTT | TTC – 5'

(a) Sequence in a DNA double helix

5' – GAA | TTC – 3'
3' – CTT ↓ AAG – 5'

(b) Palindrome with rotational symmetry

Fig. 5.8: A palindrome sequence (the arrow represents the axis of symmetry)

↓			
5' – GAATTC – 3'	*Eco* RI	5' – G	AATTC – 3'
3' – CTTAAG – 5'	⇌	3' – CTTAA +	G – 5'
↑	Ligation		Sticky ends

(a) Cohesive or sticky ends

↓			
5' – GGCC – 3'	Cleavage	5' – GG +	CC – 3'
3' – CCGG – 5'	⇌	3' – CC	GG – 5'
↑	Ligation		Blunt ends

(b) Flush or blunt ends

Fig. 5.9: Cohesive and flush ends of DNA fragments

DNA ligase:

DNA ligases seal the cut ends of two DNA molecules. **Mertz** and **Davis** (1972) demonstrated that cohesive termini of cleaved DNA molecules could be covalently sealed with *Escherichia coli* DNA ligase and it produce recombinant DNA molecules (Fig. 5.10). These enzymes were originally isolated from viruses. They also occur in *E. coli* and eukaryotic cells.

There are two types of DNA ligases: *E. coli* DNA ligase and T_4 DNA ligase. DNA ligase catalyses the formation of phosphodiester bonds between 3'–OH and 5'–PO_4 group of a nick and turns into an intact DNA. The T_4 DNA ligase enzyme requires ATP as co-factor while the *E. coli* DNA ligase enzyme requires nicotinamide adenine dinucleotide (NAD^+) as a co-factor for joining reaction of the nick. The cofactor splits and forms an enzyme – adenosine monophosphate (AMP) complex. The complex binds to the nick which must expose a 5'–PO_4 and 3'–OH group and makes a covalent bond in the phosphodiester chain. T_4 DNA ligase enzyme has the ability to join the blunt ends of DNA fragments while *E. coli* DNA ligase joins the cohesive ends produced by restriction enzymes. These enzymes actively participated in cellular DNA repair process.

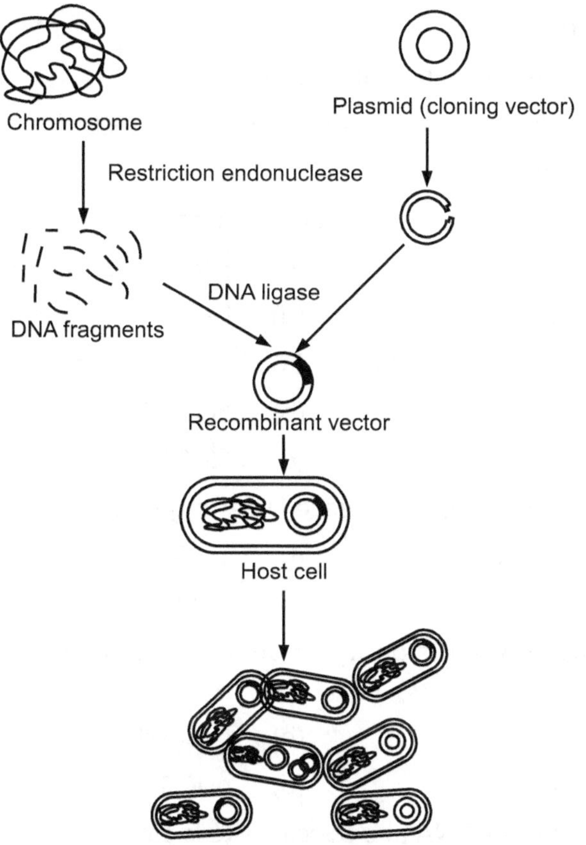

Fig. 5.10: DNA cloning and role of DNA ligase

QUESTIONS

(A) Objective Type Questions:

1. Define vector. Write the features of a good vector.
2. Write the role of following in gene cloning
   (a) Cosmid vector
   (b) DNA ligase
3. List different enzymes used for gene cloning.

(B) Short Answer Questions:

1. Explain the role of restriction enzymes in gene cloning.
2. Write notes on:
   (a) Plasmid vectors
   (b) Yeast vectors

(C) Long Answer Questions:

1. Explain various types of vectors for *E. coli.*
2. Explain the importance of expression vectors in rDNA technology.

(D) Multiple Choice Questions:

1. The pBR 322 is the first artificial vector developed from ______.
   (a) *B. subtilis* (b) *Saccharomyces cerevisiae*
   (c) *Escherichia coli* (d) Hepatitis B virus
2. Which one of the following is a restriction endonuclease?
   (a) *Taq* pol (b) *Bam* HI
   (c) *Eac* HII (d) *Sta* PII
3. Sequence specific enzymes that cleave DNA to give sticky ends are ______.
   (a) Restriction endonucleases (b) DNA ligases
   (c) Beta-lactamases (d) DNA methylases
4. _____ are the hybrid vectors derived from plasmids which contain *cos* site of phage lambda.
   (a) Plasmids (b) Cosmids
   (c) Bacteriophage λ DNA (d) pUC 19
5. An enzyme that cleaves DNA at a specific site is called _____
   (a) Trypsin (b) Restrictive ribonuclease
   (c) Restriction endonuclease (d) All of the above

■■■

Chapter ... 6

RECOMBINANT DNA TECHNOLOGY

♦ LEARNING OBJECTIVES ♦

After completing this chapter, reader should be able to understand:

- *Introduction*
- *Principles of Genetic Engineering*
- *Applications of Genetic Engineering in Medicine*
- *Application of rDNA Technology*
    - *Interferon*
    - *Vaccines: Hepatitis-B*
    - *Hormones- Insulin*

6.1 INTRODUCTION

The most important application of molecular genetics in biotechnology is genetic engineering or recombinant (rDNA) technology. Genetic engineering is the process of producing an organism that contains a gene or genes not naturally present in that organism. This technique has tremendous potential of developing microorganisms that are able to produce many useful products which are difficult or impossible to produce by other methods. This is a useful tool for the production of vaccines and antigens. Recombinant DNA technology has also been used for the production of proteins of therapeutic interest such as human insulin, interferons, human growth hormone, tissue plasminogen activator, tumour necrosis factor, interleukin-2, fibroblast growth factor, erythropoietin and other biologicals.

6.2 PRINCIPLES OF GENETIC ENGINEERING

The basic technique of recombinant DNA technology is simple. Plasmid DNA from *Escherichia coli* and chromosomal DNA from another organism are cleaved (Fig. 6.1) with a restriction enzyme, mixed and ligated with DNA ligase. The recombinant DNA molecule is then introduced into *Escherichia coli* where foreign chromosomal DNA can replicate. It is linked to a plasmid which has an origin of replication and the genes in the donor segment are said to be cloned and the DNA molecule that carries it is known as vector.

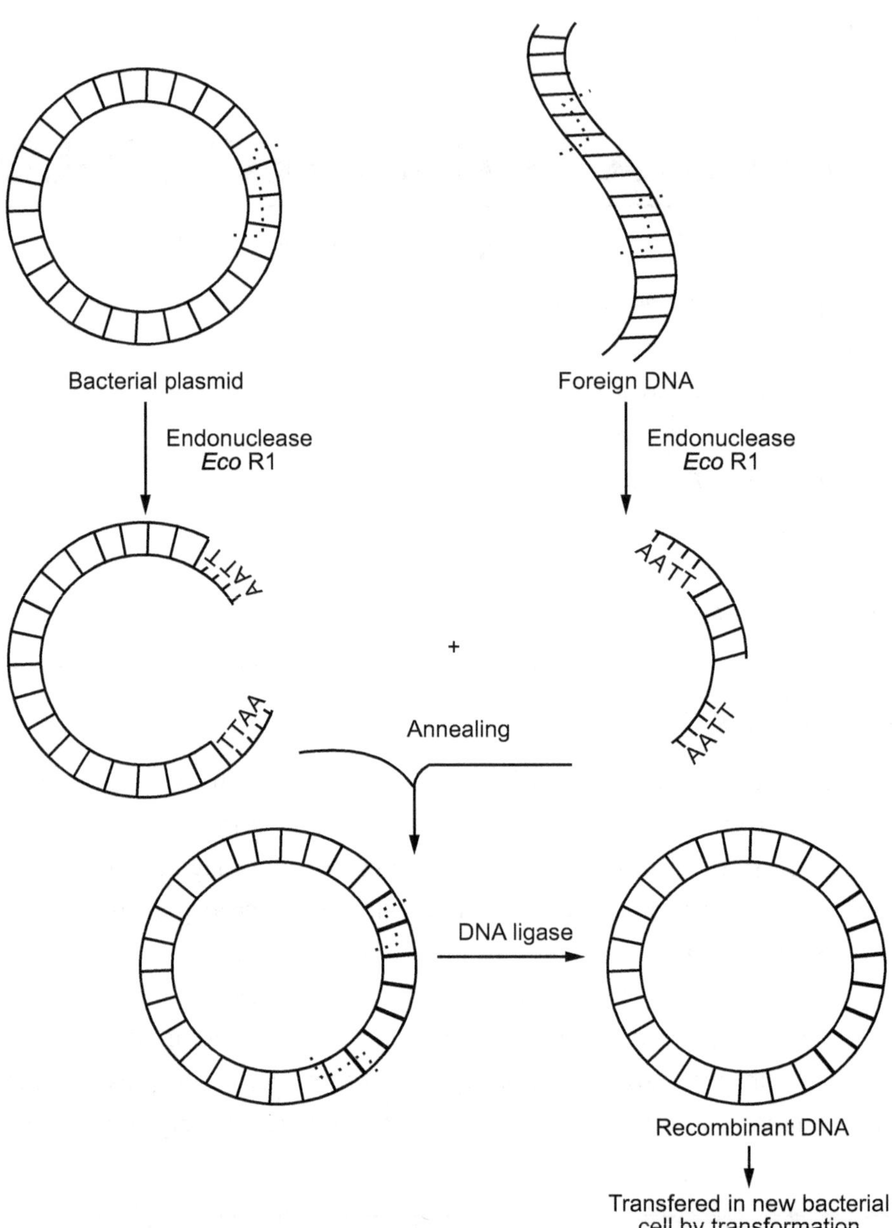

Fig. 6.1: Preparation of recombinant DNA by genetic engineering

Insertion of the gene into the DNA carrier molecule is done with restriction endonucleases. These enzymes are present in bacteria and naturally function to protect against invading DNA molecules. Restriction endonucleases *Eco* RI, *Hind* III, *Bgl* H, *Pst* I and *Sma* I are obtained from *Escherichia coli, Haemophilus influenzae, Bacillus globigii, Providencia stuarti* and *Serratia marcescens* respectively. These enzymes cut DNA molecules at specific base sequences that occur in palindromic order. Type I restriction endonucleases recognises a specific sequence but makes cuts only within the recognition sites. Type II restriction endonucleases are used in genetic engineering. These enzymes make two single strand breaks, one break in each strand. These breaks may be at the centre of symmetry (flush or blunt ends) or at same relative location in each strand generating complementary or cohesive or sticky ends that can overlap for two to four bases. Fragments of DNA cut can be rejoined by a sealing or ligating enzyme known as DNA ligase. The most commonly used ligase commercially available is that encoded by phase T_4.

6.3 APPLICATIONS OF GENETIC ENGINEERING IN MEDICINE

Cloned genes are utilized in production of pharmaceuticals, medical sciences, agriculture and different industries for synthesis of active chemicals.

Production of Pharmaceutical Products:

The pharmaceutical products of recombinant DNA technology are broadly divided as human protein replacements, therapeutic agents for human diseases and vaccines. The synthesis of the cellular proteins is ultimately under the control of genes. The recombinant DNA technology can be employed to produce human proteins that can be used for the treatment of genetically liked diseases. Human insulin (humulin) is the first therapeutic product produced by rDNA technology by Eli Lilly and company in 1980. Shreya Life Sciences, Pune has started producing the second generation rDNA-based insulin without using DNBr with the name 'Recosulin'. Second generation recombinant proteins (muteins) are produced by site-directed mutagenesis and protein engineering. Human growth hormone (hGH) can synthesize by genetic engineering. Recombinant hGH was approved for human use (1985) and marketed as protropin by Genetech company and Humatrope by Eli Lilly company. Tissue plasminogen activator (tPA) is a naturally occurring protease enzyme that helps to dissolve blood clots. It was the first pharmaceutical product to be produced by mammalian cell culture. Recombinant tPA has been used for treatment of patients with acute myocardial infarction or stroke. Interferons are used for the treatments of a large number of viral diseases and cancers. Alpha interferon (IFN-α) and Beta interferon (IFN-β) were successfully produced from genetically engineered *E. coli* cells. The yeast *Saccharomyces cerevisiae* is more suitable for production of recombinant interferons. Hybrid interferons can be produced by using appropriate hybrid genes. Amgen Inc. first marketed enythropoietin (Epogen) for treating patients with severe anaemia that accompanies kidney diseases.

Recombinant Vaccines:

Vaccines are another important group of pharmaceutical products of rDNA technology. Recombinant vaccines may be classified as subunit recombinant vaccines, attenuated recombinant vaccines and vector recombinant vaccines. Recombinant hepatitis B vaccine (subunit vaccine) is produced by cloning hepatitis B surface antigen (HBsAg) gen in yeast cells. It was marketed by trade names Recombivax and Engerix-B. Transgenic plants (tomato, potato) have been developed for expressing antigens derived from animal viruses. The first clinical trials (1997) in humans were conducted using plant-derived vaccines. This involved the ingestion of transgenic potatoes with a toxin of *E. coli* causing diarrhoea. Vaccinia virus is basically the vaccine that was used for the eradication of smallpox. The genome of this virus can accommodate stretches of foreign DNA which can be expressed along with the viral genes. Recombinant vaccinia viruses carries genes encoding different antigens which are used for vaccinating individuals against different diseases.

Diagnosis and Cure of Disease:

Genetic engineering have solved the problem of diagnosis of diseases by using DNA probe, monoclonal antibodies and antenatal diagnosis. DNA probes used for diagnosis of pathogens contain the most specific DNA sequences of genetic material of parasite. Specific DNA probes have been designed for diagnosing the infection caused by bacteria, protozoa or viruses. Tuberculosis caused by *Mycobacterium tuberculosis* is diagnosed by DNA probe method.

Monoclonal antibodies are produced against a variety of proteins, glycoproteins, glycolipids, nucleic acids, etc. These antibodies are useful in diagnosis of cancer, viral diseases, pregnancy, ABO blood groups and certain hormones. Monoclonal antibodies (MAb) are also used to detect the location and the degree of damage of the heart by using radiolabeled antimyosin MAb. MAbs are used in the treatment of cancer, autoimmune diseases, cardiovascular diseases and transplantation of bone marrow. It is also used for the appropriate delivery of drugs and isotopes to the targeted tissues. Antenatal diagnosis is performed by taking amniotic fluid sample from the foetus of about 16-18 week pregnant women. Genetic counseling is possible on the basis of antenatal diagnosis and treatment or remedies for progeny.

Gene Therapy:

Gene therapy is the process of inserting genes into cells to treat diseases. The newly introduced genes will encode proteins and correct the deficiencies that occur in genetic diseases. Somatic or non-reproductive cell gene therapy involves the insertion of a fully functional gene into a target somatic cell to correct a genetic disease permanently. Germ or reproductive gene therapy involves the introduction of DNA into germ cells and it is passed on to the successive generations.

Transgenic Plants and Animals:

Plants and animals are the best sources of foods and pharmaceuticals. Crop improvement by genetic engineering helps for improvement of yield or disease resistance. *Agrobacterium tumifaciens* can be used as a vector for transferring the desired genes into plant cells. The most important application of transgenic plant is to develop plant bioreactors for inexpensive manufacture of proteins, drugs or pharmaceutical compounds.

Transgentic animals serve as good models for understanding the human diseases. Several proteins produced by transgenic animals are important for medical and pharmaceutical applications. Transgenesis is important for improving the quality and quantity of milk, meat, eggs and wool production.

6.4 APPLICATIONS OF rDNA TECHNOLOGY

The development of recombinant technology has created an enormous potential for the pharmaceutical industries. Cloned genes are utilized commercially in medicals, agriculture, and pharmaceuticals for the production of valuable products. Genes are responsible for the expression of the proteins and these proteins and peptides are easily prepared by using recombinant technology. The recombinant proteins provide a high level of sensitivity and specificity as compared to natural proteins which are isolated from plants, animals and microorganisms. The biological activity of expressed protein is dependent on the choice of host, type of host cell, characters of host cell substrate, recombinant culture etc. Preparation of recombinant proteins by transgenic animals is most important system for production of pharmaceutical useful proteins. Erythropoietin (EPO), human insulin, somatotropin, somatostatin, interferons, tissue plasminogen activator, interleukins, hepatitis B vaccine, granulocyte colony stimulating factor (G – CSF) etc. are the important biologicals (Table 6.1) prepared by recombinant DNA technology.

Table 6.1: Important recombinant proteins and their applications

Proteins/Peptides	Applications
Human insulin	Diabetes mellitus
Interferons	Hepatitis, cancers, hairy cell leukemia, genital warts
Tissue plasminogen activator	Coronary thrombolysis (anticoagulant)
Erythropoietin	Anemia associated with renal failure
Hepatitis B vaccine	Vaccination
Granulocyte colony stimulating factor (G – CSF)	Bone marrow transplantation
Human growth hormone	Pituitary dwarfism
DNase	Cystic fibrosis
Tumour necrosis factor	Cancer treatment
Interleukins – 1, 2, 3	Immune disorder and tumours

6.4.1 Interferon

Interferon is an antiviral substance and is the first line of defense against viral attacks. **Alec Issacs** and **Jean Lindermann** (1957), two British scientists discovered a glycoprotein naturally produced by cells called interferon. Interferons are the set of small proteins which are secreted by cell in response to viral infections. Human interferons are about 145 amino acid long and its molecular weight is between 20,000 to 30,000 daltons. They are classified into three types based on their physicochemical and antigenic properties.

(i) Alpha interferon (IFN-α) or leukocyte interferon

(ii) Beta interferon (IFN-β) or fibroblast interferon.

(iii) Gamma interferon (IFN-γ) or immune interferon.

Interferons mainly inhibit viral replication (antiviral agent) and also protect the cell from other intracellular parasites. It activates natural killer cells and macrophages, stimulates B cells and increases cell resistance to many microbial infections. They have a significant role in treatment of hepatitis B, cancer and other viral diseases.

Human interferon genes are inserted in *Escherichia coli* for production of interferon by recombinant DNA technology. The complementary DNA was synthesized from the mRNA of a specific interferon. This is inserted to a plasmid vector and then transferred to the cells. The interferon can be isolated from culture medium. Interferons are glycoprotein in nature and hence, production of interferons are relatively less in bacterial cell. Bacterial cell do not possess the machinery for glycosylation of proteins.

The yeast is most suitable for production of recombinant interferons. Yeast cells possess the mechanism to carry out glycosylation of proteins. The DNA sequence coding for human leukocyte interferon is attached to the yeast alcohol dehydrogenase gene in a plasmid. The recombinant plasmid is introduced into yeast cells of *Saccharomyces cerevisiae*. In yeast cell, plasmid grows easily to replicate into glycoproteins. Plasmids are also successfully replicate in *Escherichia coli* but production is slow as compared to yeast cells.

Hybrid interferons are more reactive in performing their functions and that is produced by creation of hybrid genes from the genes of different interferons. These genes are digested by restriction endonucleases and resulting fragments are ligated to generate hybrid genes. The appropriate hybrid genes can be selected and transferred to bacterial cell to produce hybrid interferons.

6.4.2 Vaccines: Hepatitis-B

A subunit vaccine that is produced using recombinant techniques is called a recombinant vaccine. This method is used to prepare highly pure component vaccine (subunit vaccine) e.g. Hepatitis B surface antigen (Hbs Ag). Hepatitis B surface antigen gene from hepatitis B virus is isolated, sequenced and cloned by using yeast cells. The yeast system has its complex membrane and ability of secreting glycosylate protein. It is possible to build an autonomously replicating plasmid containing hepatitis B surface antigen gene near the yeast alcohol dehydrogenase (ADH) I promoter. The gene contains 6 bp vector long sequence preceding the AUG that synthesises N-terminal methionine. This is joined to ADH promoter cloned in the yeast vector pMA-56 (Fig. 6.2).

Genetic material is extracted from hepatitis B virus and individual genes are analysed and identified. Genes that directs production of surface protein is located and removed from viral DNA. This gene is inserted into plasmid and then plasmids are inserted into yeast cells. The recombinant yeast cells are grown in fermenters to reproduce and generate more surface protein. These cells are harvested and disrupted to release the recombinant surface antigen which is then purified by biochemical methods. Surface proteins are combined with preserving agent and other ingredients to make vaccine. First recombinant vaccine was developed in India by Shantha Biotechnics Pvt. Ltd. Hyderabad in 1997.

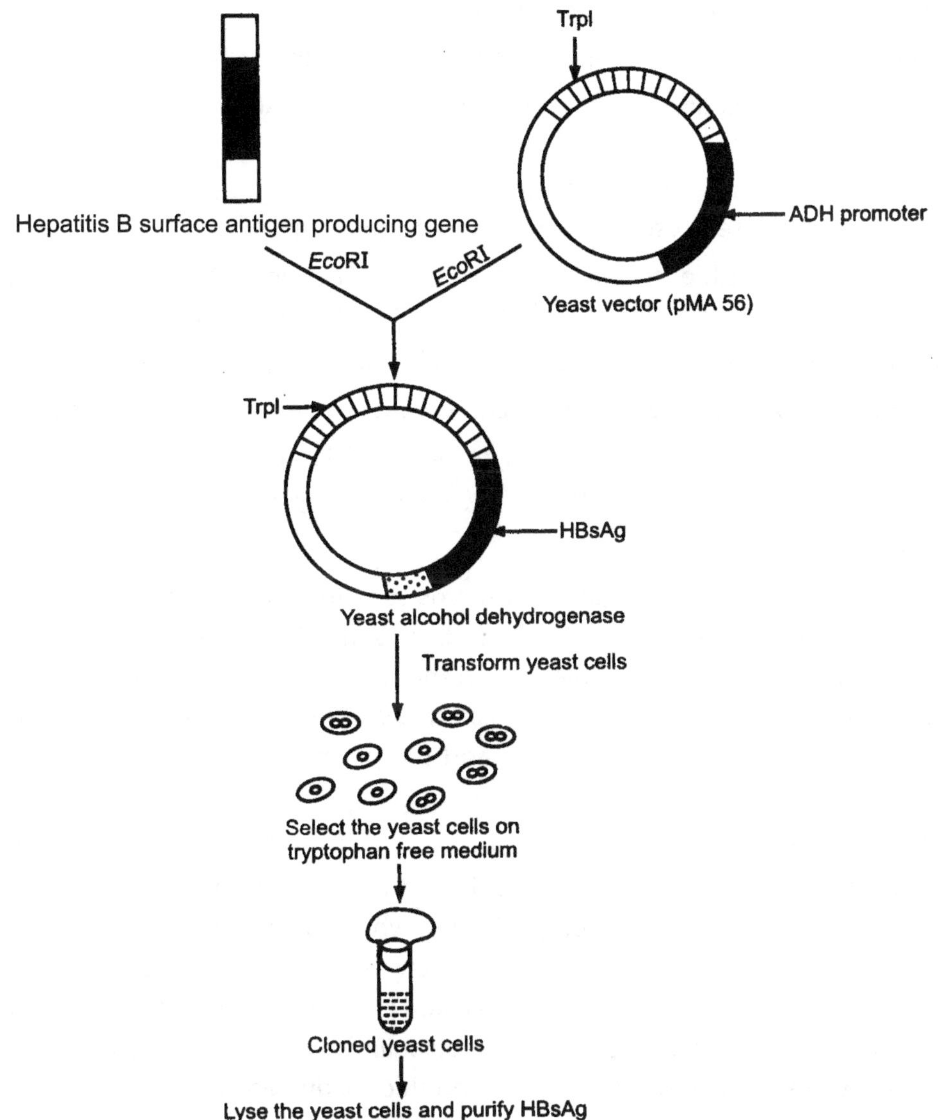

Fig. 6.2: Preparation of recombinant antigen vaccine using yeast cells

Foreign genes are incorporated into viral and bacterial vectors in recombinant vector vaccines. This class of vaccines utilizes attenuated versions of certain micro-organisms as recombinant vectors to express target antigen from other pathogens. Vaccinia virus, adenoviruses, attenuated poliovirus, *Mycobacterium bovis* and *Salmonella* (attenuated strains) are used for vector vaccines. A vaccinia virus with several genes from the human immuno deficiency virus (HIV) is currently being tested as a vaccine for acquired immuno deficiency syndrome (AIDS). A close relative of vaccinia, canary pox virus, engineered with harmless fragments of HIV is being tested in human volunteers as a vaccine for AIDS.

Advantages of recombinant vaccines are as follows:

1. Large amount of antigen can be produced in less cost.
2. Genetic manipulation of the antigen itself is possible after availability of gene sequence.
3. Viral recombinant vector vaccines produce strong humoral and cell-mediated immune responses, resulting in immunological memory.
4. It may be possible to encode for several antigens from different pathogens, introducing the possibility of a single vaccine for several diseases.

Limitations of recombinant vaccines are as follows:

1. Immune response generated by recombinant antigen vaccines is primarily humoral.
2. In viral vector vaccines, live virus being used is an attenuated form of a human pathogen. There is always a risk of reversion to virulence.

6.4.3 Hormones - Insulin

Human insulin is one of the smallest proteins secreted by Islet of Langerhans (β-cells) of pancreas which catabolizes glucose in blood. It is used for the patients suffering from diabetes mellietus who is not capable to metabolize sugars. Insulin was first derived using recombinant technology from *Escherichia coli* in 1982 for human use. The basic technique consisted of inserting human insulin gene and the promoter gene of lac operon on to the plasmids of *Escherichia coli.*

Insulin is composed of two polypeptide chains (A and B) linked via disulfide bonds. Polypeptide chain A contains 21 amino acids and chain B contains 30 amino acids. Insulin chains (A and B) are derived from preproinsulin which is synthesized in β-cells of Islets of Langerhans containing 109 amino acids. When preproinsulin passes through the cell membrane of the synthesizing cells, then delinked first 23 amino acids and forms proinsulin containing 86 amino acids (Fig. 6.3). Finally, proinsulin is converted to insulin by the action of proteolytic enzymes such as endopeptidase and thiol-activated carboxypeptidase.

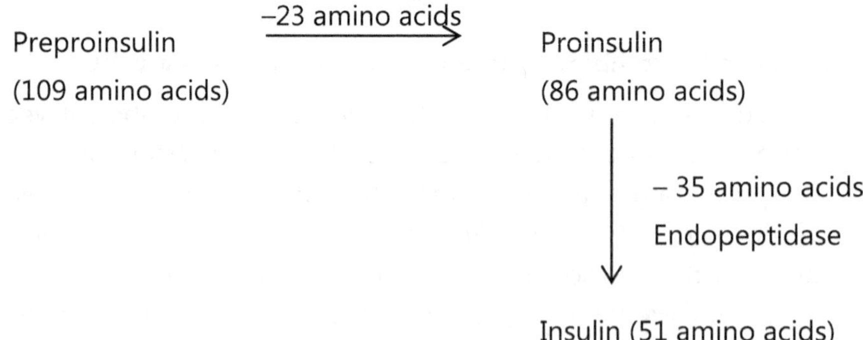

Fig. 6.3: Conversion of preproinsulin to insulin

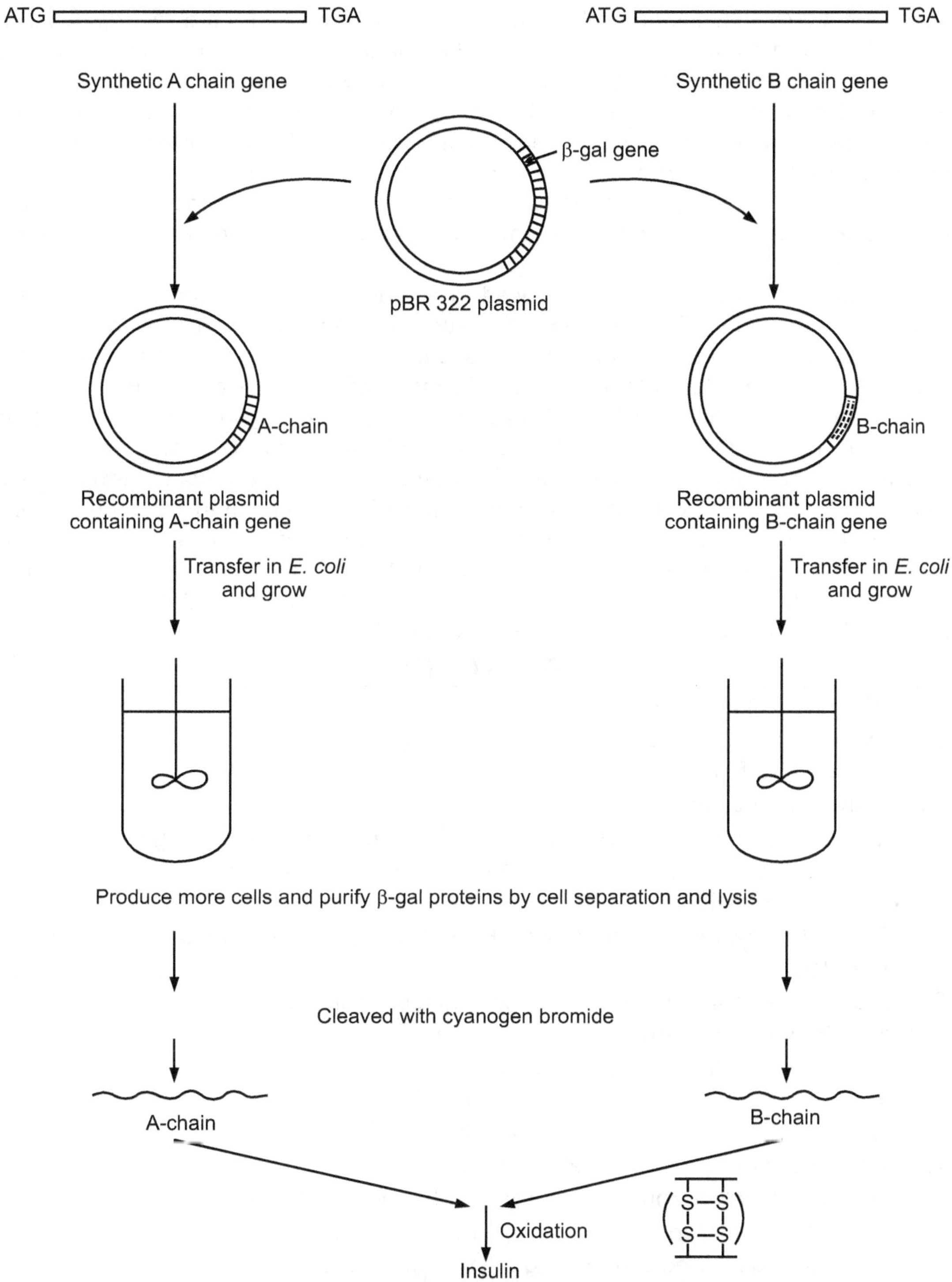

ATG TGA

Synthetic A chain gene

ATG TGA

Synthetic B chain gene

β-gal gene

pBR 322 plasmid

A-chain

Recombinant plasmid containing A-chain gene

B-chain

Recombinant plasmid containing B-chain gene

Transfer in *E. coli* and grow

Transfer in *E. coli* and grow

Produce more cells and purify β-gal proteins by cell separation and lysis

Cleaved with cyanogen bromide

A-chain

B-chain

Oxidation

S—S

S—S

Insulin

Fig. 6.4: Production of insulin by recombinant DNA technology

Insulin is easily prepared by recombinant DNA technology from synthetic gene or from mRNA separated from rat pancreas. **Itakura et al** (1977) chemically synthesized DNA sequence for A and B chains of insulin. The synthetic A and B genes are separately inserted into two pBR 322 plasmids by the side of β-galactosidase gene. The recombinant plasmids are separately transferred into *Escherichia coli* cells (Fig. 6.4). The bacterial cells are grown in large fermenter by using proper nutrients and optimized physical conditions. The product contains large chimeric protein consisting of the A chain or B chain attached to naturally occurring *Escherichia coli* protein. These two chains (A and B) are obtained by detaching from β-galactosidase through cyanogen bromide (CNBr). The chain A and chain B are joined (*in-vitro*) to form insulin by sulphonating the two peptides with sodium disulphonate and sodium sulphite.

Second generation insulins are produced in recent years by site directed mutagenesis and protein engineering. The second generation recombinant proteins are termed as muteins. A large number of insulin muteins have been prepared with an objective of faster dissociation of hexamers to biologically active forms. Insulin lispro is prepared with modified amino acid residues at position 29 and 30 of the B-chain of insulin. Porcin (Pig) insulin is different from human insulin just by one amino acid-alanine in place of threonine at the C-terminal and of B-chain of human insulin The Researcher have developed methods to alter the chemical structure of porcin insulin to make it similar to human insulin. The chemically modified porcin insulin can also be used for the treatment of diabetes mellitus. It is estimated that clones of *Escherichia coli* are capable of producing about one million molecules of insulin per bacterial cell. Human insulin (humulin) is the first therapeutic product produced by recombinant technology by Eli Lilly and Company.

QUESTIONS

(A) Objective Type Questions:

1. What is recombinant technology?
2. What are interferons?

(B) Short Answer Questions:

1. How will you prepare Hepatitis-B vaccine by recombinant technology?
2. Write the role of yeast cells in preparation of interferons by recombinant technology.

(C) Long Answer Questions:

1. What is healthcare biotechnology? How will you prepare human insulin by rDNA technology?
2. Write in detail applications of genetic engineering in medicine.

(D) Multiple Choice Questions:

1. Insulin is made up of .... amino acids.
   (a) 119 (b) 51
   (c) 86 (d) 35
2. Fibroblast interferon is also called ....
   (a) Immune interferon (b) Leukocyte interferon
   (c) Alpha interferon (d) Beta interferon
3. The most widely used carrier for gene therapy is ....
   (a) Adenovirus (b) *Escherichia coli*
   (c) *Saccharomyces cerevisiae* (d) *Bacillus subtilis*

■■■

Chapter ... 7

POLYMERASE CHAIN REACTION

♦ LEARNING OBJECTIVES ♦

After completing this chapter, reader should be able to understand:

- *Introduction*
- *Polymerase Chain Reaction Technique*
- *Types of PCR*
- *Applications of PCR*

7.1 INTRODUCTION

The development of polymerase chain reaction (PCR) or gene amplification method in 1983 was a major breakthrough in molecular biology. This technique was developed by **Kary Mullis** at Cetus Corporation (biotech company) in Emery Ville, California. The details of PCR techniques are described by **Erlich** (1989) in his edited book 'PCR Technology'. It is an *in-vitro* method for producing large amounts of specific DNA fragment of defined length and sequence from a small amount of complex template. PCR is now considered as a basic tool for the molecular biologist.

7.2 POLYMERASE CHAIN REACTION TECHNIQUE

PCR is an *in-vitro* method for producing large amounts of specific DNA fragment. In this technique, microgram quantities of DNA from picogram produce amounts of starting material. Target DNA, primers, polymerase and nucleotides are combined in a test tube for multiplication of genetic material.

DNA is amplified by polymerase chain reaction (Fig. 7.1) in an enzymatic reaction which undergoes multiple incubations at three different temperatures. Each PCR contains four important components.

DNA Template: Any source that contains one or more target DNA molecules to be amplified can be taken as template. RNA can also be used for PCR by first making a DNA copy using the enzyme reverse transcriptase.

Primers: Each PCR requires a pair of oligonucleotide primers. These are short single-stranded DNA molecules obtained by chemical synthesis. These primers are designed to anneal on opposite strands of target sequence so that they will be extended towards each other by addition of nucleotides.

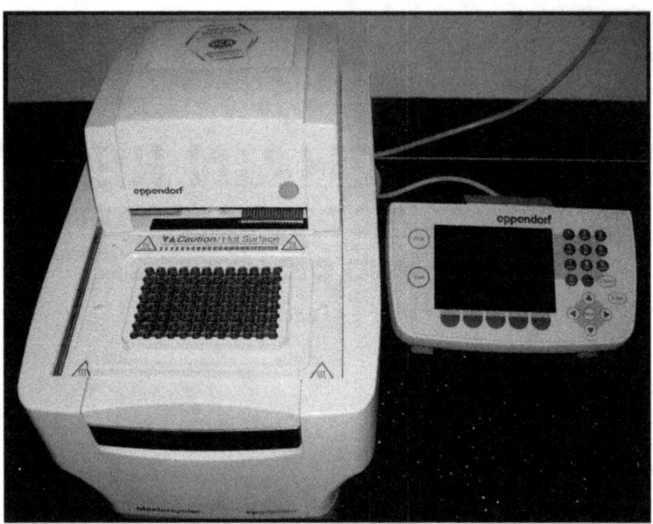

Fig. 7.1: Polymerase chain reaction (PCR) machine (thermal cycler)

DNA polymerase: The most commonly used enzyme in PCR is *Taq* DNA polymerase isolated from a thermostable bacterium called *Thermus aquaticus*. It survives at 95°C for 1 to 2 minutes and has a half life for more than 2 hours at same temperature. The DNA polymerase binds to a single-stranded DNA and synthesizes a new strand complementary to the origin strand. The role of this enzyme in PCR is to copy DNA molecules.

Deoxynucleotide triphosphates: PCR requires four deoxynucleotide triphosphates, dNTPs (dATP, dGTP, dTTP, dCTP) which are used by the DNA polymerase as building blocks to synthesize new DNA.

Polymerase chain reaction (PCR) involves three stages which are as follows (Fig. 7.2):

1. Melting of DNA (95°C) to convert double stranded DNA to a single stranded DNA (denaturation).
2. Promoting the primers (at 50 - 65°C) to attach themselves to either end of the target strip (annealing of primers).
3. Extension of the primers by DNA polymerase to form new double-stranded DNA across the segment by sequential addition of deoxynucleotides (primer extension). When the temperature is again raised the new strands separate and the process begins again. Temperature profile of typical PCR cycle is shown in Fig. 7.3.

The oligonucleotide primers are designed to hybridise the region of DNA flanking a desired target gene sequence. The primers are then extended across the target sequence using DNA polymerase derived from *Thermus aquaticus* (Taq) in the presence of free deoxynucleotide triphosphate. These three steps constitute one cycle of the reaction. These steps are repeated by manipulating the temperature, by using the PCR machine. A cycle takes about 3 to 5 minutes and after 30 cycles (about 3 hours), a single copy of DNA can be multiplied into 1,000,000 copies.

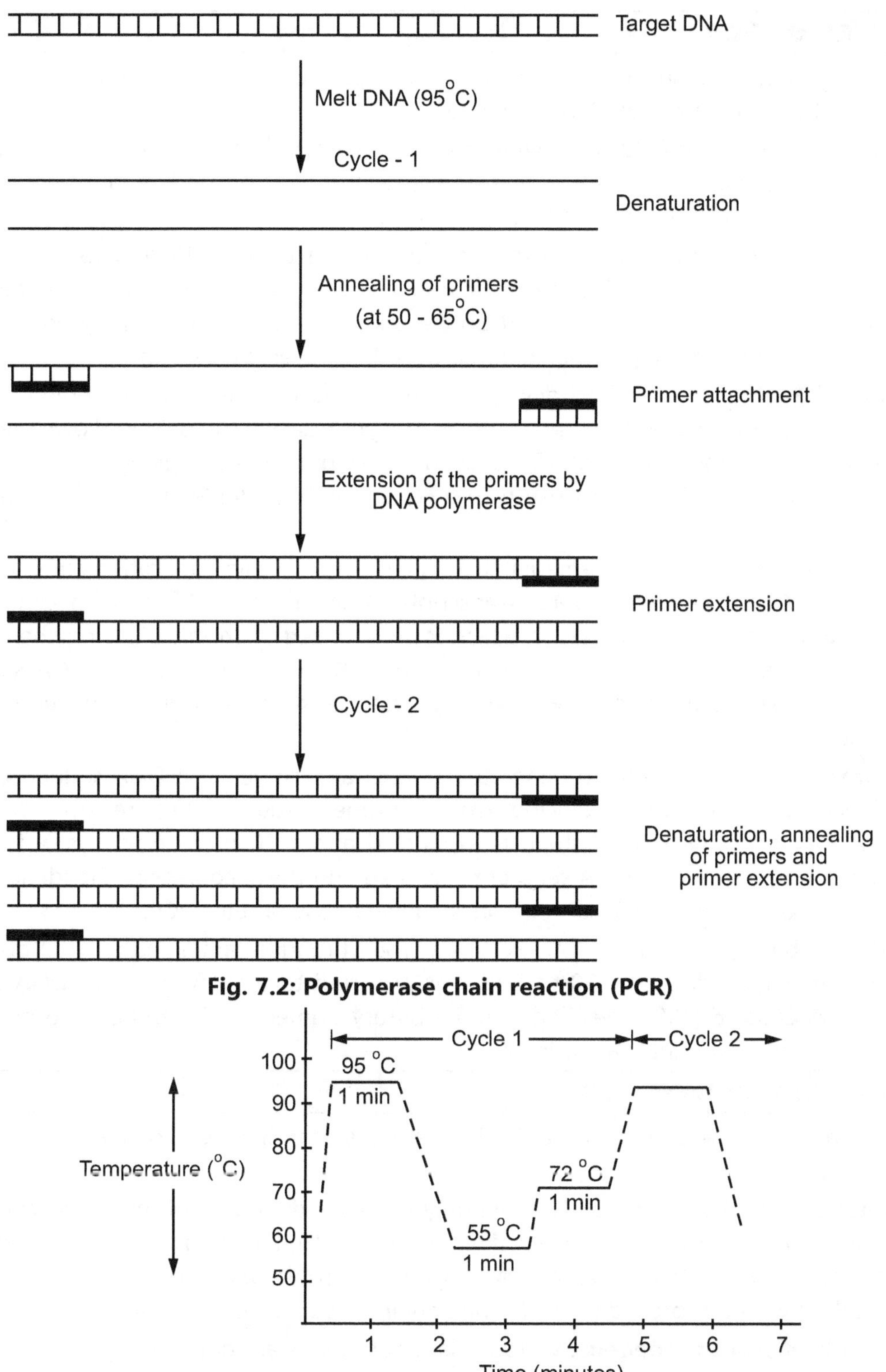

Fig. 7.2: Polymerase chain reaction (PCR)

Fig. 7.3: Temperature profile of a typical PCR cycle

7.3 TYPES OF PCR

RNA polymerase chain reaction is a modification of PCR technique which allows amplification beginning from an RNA template.

Recent research in the field of polymerase chain reaction has led to the development of the techniques contributing to the effectiveness of the method. PCR is a highly versatile technique. Important variations of PCR are as follows:

Inverse PCR: PCR can be used to the amplification of those DNA sequences which are away from the primer and not of those which are flanked by the primer. The sequences to be amplified may be cloned in a vector and border sequence of the vector may be used as a primer in such a way that the polymerization proceeds in reverse direction.

Anchored PCR: In this method only one primer is used. One strand is copied first and then poly G tail is attached at the end of the newly synthesized strand. This allows the use of complementary homopolymer, poly-C, to be used as primer for copying the DNA single strands generated by PCR. It gives rise to the complete DNA duplex that can be amplified normally.

RT-PCR: Reverse transcription-mediated PCR includes a single application combining the process of cDNA synthesis (by reverse transcription) and PCR amplification. It can also be applied to double stranded cDNA also which is synthesized from mRNA using the enzyme reverse transcriptase. Thermostable enzyme rT_{th} uses RNA templates from cDNA synthesis and thus allows single enzyme RT-PCR viral reverse transcriptase from avian murine virus (AMV RTase).

Asymmetric PCR: It is used to generate single-strand copies of a DNA sequence which can be directly used for DNA sequencing. The two primers (100 : 1 ratio) are such adjusted in the reaction mixture that one of them is exhausted about 10 or more cycles. After these cycles, only a single strand of DNA segment is copied and these copies are the ideal starting materials for DNA sequencing. This variation is known as asymmetric PCR.

AP-PCR: Arbitrary primed PCR (AP-PCR) is a type of random amplified polymorphic DNA (RAPD) where single primers of 10 to 50 bases are used to amplify genomic DNA in PCR. **Welsh** and **McCleland** (1990) developed the arbitrary primed – PCR and carried out finger printing of genomes with arbitrary primers.

7.4 APPLICATIONS OF PCR

Polymerase chain reaction is useful in diverse areas of molecular biology, medicines and biotechnology.

Diagnosis of pathogens: PCR is commonly used for diagnosis of infections caused by viruses (e.g. HIV–1, HIV–2, Herpes simplex virus, Hepatitis B virus etc.), bacteria (*Mycobacterium tuberculosis, Helicobacter pylori, Mycoplasma pneumoniae* etc), fungi (*Candida albicans*) and protozoa (*Toxoplasma gondii, Trypanosoma cruzi* etc).

Diagnosis of plant pathogens: Various plant pathogens are detected by using PCR such as viruses (plum pox virus, cauliflower mosaic virus), fungi (*Verticillium* spp., *Laccaria* spp.,

Phytophthora spp. etc), mycoplasms bacteria (*Agrobacterium tumifaciens, Rhizobium leguminosarum, Xanthomonas* compestris etc.) and nematodes (*Meloidogyne incoginta*) etc.

Inherited diseases: Inherited disorders are caused by gene mutations passed on from parents to their children e.g. hemophilia, cystic fibrosis etc. PCR is used to amplify gene sequences which can then be screened for disease causing mutations.

Research: PCR is used extensively as a research tool for identification of new species. Many bioactive microbial species are isolated from various extreme environment such as soil, water, air, sediments etc. DNA fingerprinting of new microorganisms is carried out to confirm their identity by comparing with the DNA sequences of known microorganisms.

Cancer research: Polymerase chain reaction has been widely used in studies for the role of genes in cancer. Tumour-supressor genes and mutations in oncogenes have been identified in DNA from tumors using PCR-based strategies.

Biotechnology: PCR has played major role in the production of recombinant proteins. Insulin and growth hormones are recombinant proteins, widely used as drugs and recombinant vaccines are developed for hepatitis B virus. It is an important tool in the biotechnology industries of research institutes.

Forensic science: PCR is most applicable in forensic science where it is being used in search of criminals through DNA fingerprinting technology. PCR allows amplification of DNA from individual hairs, stains of blood or seminal fluid having partially degraded DNA. Analysis of variable sequences is also used in tissue typing to match organ donors with recipients.

DNA polymorphism: PCR is used to study DNA polymorphism in the genome using known sequences as primers. PCR can be used to study RFLPs (restriction fragment length polymorphisms) as well as RAPDs (random amplified polymorphic DNA).

Gene therapy: PCR proves to be immense help in monitoring a gene in gene therapy experiments. This PCR technology provides shortcuts for many cloning and sequencing applications.

QUESTIONS

(A) Objective Type Questions:

1. Explain the role of primer in PCR.
2. Write the role of DNA Polymerase in PCR.

(B) Short Answer Questions:

1. Write in short different types of PCR.
2. Explain the importance of temperature profile in PCR.

(C) Long Answer Questions:

1. Explain in detail method of PCR.
2. Explain the applications of polymerase-chain reaction.

(D) Multiple Choice Questions:

1. Polymerase chain reaction is useful in the diagnosis of ______ .

   (a) HIV (b) Fever

   (b) Diabetes (d) None of the above

2. The polymerase chain reaction is ______ .
   (a) A method of gene amplification
   (b) A type of DNA repair
   (c) Require for ligation of DNA ends
   (d) Essential for chromosome replication
3. RT-PCR stands for ______.
   (a) Random temperature PCR (b) Random template PCR
   (c) Reverse transcriptase PCR (d) Real time PCR
4. Polymerase chain reaction (PCR) technique was discovered by ______.
   (a) Louis Pasteur (b) Robert Koch
   (c) George Kohler (d) Kary Mullis
5. A technique used for amplifying RNA *in-vitro* is known as ______.
   (a) Western blotting (b) Transcription
   (c) ELISA (d) RT-PCR

■■■

Chapter ... 8

IMMUNITY

♦ LEARNING OBJECTIVES ♦

After completing this chapter, reader should be able to understand:

- *Introduction*
- *Types of Immunity*
- *Cellular and Humoral Immunity*
- *Structure of Immunoglobulins*
- *Structure and Function of MHC*

8.1 INTRODUCTION

The resistance offered by the host to the harmful effects of pathogenic microbial infection is called 'immunity'. Lack of power of the body to resist infection is called 'susceptibility'. The study of immunity is called 'immunology' and the preparations used to produce immunity are called 'immunological preparations'. Immunological mechanisms are involved in the protection of the body against infectious agents but they can also cause damage periodically.

The immune system protects an individual against invasion by foreign bodies specially microbial agents and their toxic products. The activities of this system are not always useful to the body. The immune defence may have pathological consequences because of the phenomenon of allergies, inflammatory tissue damage, autoimmune diseases and reactions to grafts.

An antigen is any substance which, when introduced into the vertebrate host, stimulates the production of antibodies and reacts with preformed antibodies, if they are already present. The antigen had earlier been associated with production of immunoglobulins and immunity and hence accordingly named as immunogen (generator of immunoglobulins and immunity). Most antigens are proteins but some are carbohydrates, lipids or nucleic acids. Two important characteristics of antigens are immunogenicity or ability to stimulate the specific immune response and reactivity or ability to react specifically with antibodies. An antigen with both these characteristics is called a 'complete antigen'. An antigen which has reactivity but no immunogenicity is called a 'incomplete antigen or hapten'. A hapten can be converted to a complete antigen by combining it with a larger carrier molecule such as a protein.

Antibodies or immunoglobulins are γ-globulins which are produced in response to antigenic stimulation. Antibodies are found in serum, lymph and other body fluids and they serve as protective agents against microorganisms. Antibodies are synthesised by plasma cells and also by lymphocytes. Antibodies constitute 20 to 25 per cent of the total serum proteins. An antibody is a biological and functional concept while the term immunoglobulins provide a structural and chemical concept. All antibodies are immunoglobulins but all immunoglobulins may not be antibodies. On the basis of physicochemical and antigenic structures immunoglobulins (Ig) can be divided into five distinct classes (IgG, IgM, IgA, IgD and IgE).

8.2 TYPES OF IMMUNITY

Immunity against infectious diseases is mainly classified into two types:

(i) Innate or natural immunity.

(ii) Acquired immunity.

These immunities may be subdivided into different groups (Fig. 8.1).

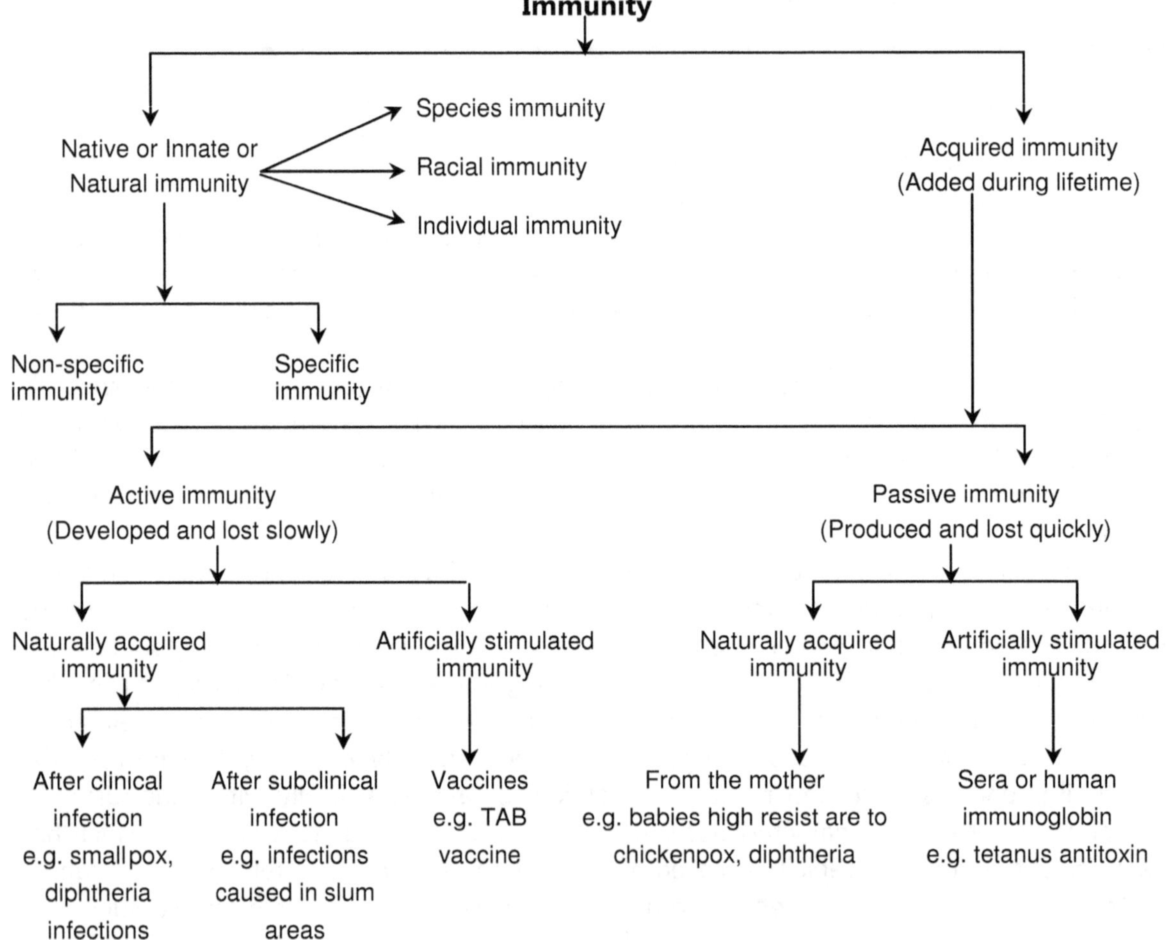

Fig. 8.1: Types of immunity

(i) Innate or natural immunity:

Innate or native or natural immunity is the resistance to infections which an individual possesses by virtue of his genetic and constitutional make up. It may be non-specific, when it indicates a degree of resistance to infections in general or specific when resistance to a particular pathogen is concerned. It results in differences between species, races and individuals (Note: For details, please refer 'Defence mechanism of host').

(ii) Acquired immunity:

Natural immunity is inadequate for protection against many microbial diseases and during the lifetime additional immunity is acquired either actively or passively. Acquired or adaptive immuity is classified into two types 'active immunity' and 'passive immunity'.

8.3 CELLULAR AND HUMORAL IMMUNITY

The lymphocyte is the basic cell responsible for both cellular and humoral immunity. Lymphocytes are found in high concentrations in the lymph nodes, spleen and at the sites where they are manufactured and processed (bone marrow and thymus). Lymphoid organs contain lymphocytes at various stages of development and are classified as primary or central lymphoid organs (thymus, bone marrow) and secondary or peripheral lymphoid organs (lump nodes, spleen, adenoids, tonsils, appendix etc.). The bone marrow hemopoietic stem cells are the ultimate origin of erythrocytes and all leukocytes including the lymphocytes (Fig. 8.2). Many lymphocytes pass through the thymus where they become processed by the hormonal microenvironment prior to release. The lymphocytes are now called thymus-derived lymphocytes or T-lymphocytes. The majority of the bone-marrow derived lymphocytes which do not enter or become processed by the thymus are called 'B cells'. Cellular and humoral immunity is mediated by two distinct types of lymphocytes. B-lymphocytes respond to antigens by differentiating into antibody producing plasma cells while T-lymphocytes are responsible for cell mediated immunity. Difference between T-cells and B-cells is given in Table 8.1.

Table 8.1: Differences between T and B lymphocytes

Characteristics	T-cell	B-cell
Site of production	Thymus	Bursal equivalent tissue
Type of immunity	Cell mediated	Humoral (Antibody-mediated)
Secretory product	Lymphokines	Antibodies
Sub-population	Helper, suppressed, delayed hypersensitivity, killer cells.	Plasma cells, memory cells.
Effect	Against intracellular viruses, fungi, protozoa and cancer cells.	Against bacteria, viruses present in body fluids.
Type of response	Engulfment, cytotoxic	Agglutination, precipitation, neutralization, complement fixation.
CD3 receptor	+	–
Thymus specific antigens	+	–
Receptor for F_C piece of IgG	–	+
Surface immunoglobulins	–	+

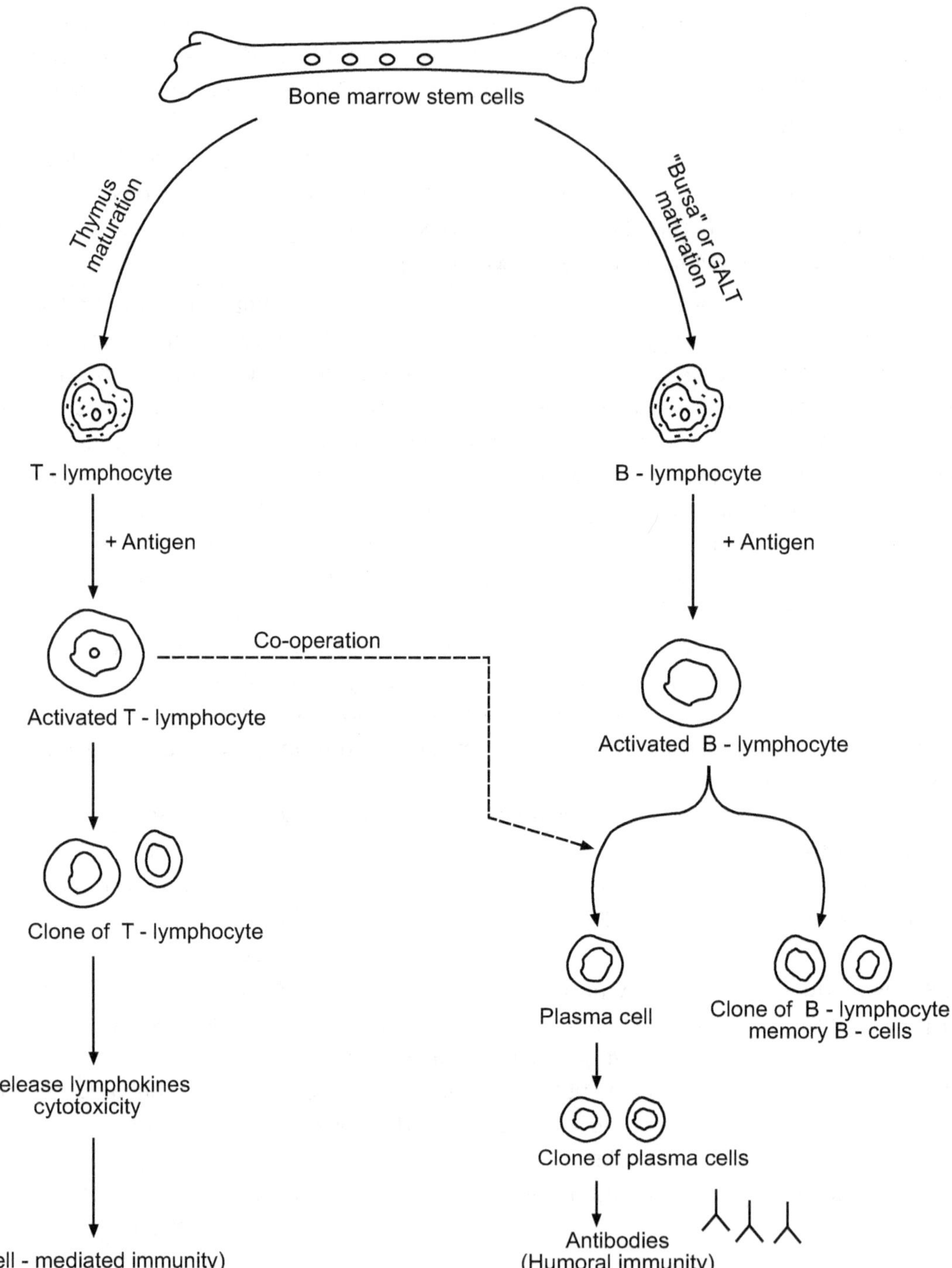

Fig. 8.2: The generation of humoral and cell-mediated immune responses

Immunity mediated by antibodies contained in body fluids is called 'Humoral immunity'. Humoral immunity or response is carried by a special group of cells called B cells. These B cells are responsible for the production of antibodies. B cells which are produced in the bone marrow, mature and migrate into the lymphoidal organ, where they encounter antigens (Fig. 8.2). When an appropriate antigen contacts the antigen receptor antibodies on a B-cell, the B-cell proliferates into a large clone of cells. This phenomenon is known as 'clonal selection'. Sometimes, the production of antibodies by a B cell depends on other cells. Production of antibodies against T-dependent antigens requires the help of certain macrophages and T-cells. Humoral immunity is effective against extracellular pathogens and their products because antibodies can bind to these structures and cause their destruction.

The cellular or cell-mediated immune response depends on lymphocytes called T-cells, which are located both in the blood and in the lymphoid tissues. T-cells do not secrete antibodies into body fluids but they do make antibody like molecules that remain attached to cell surfaces. The principal cells involved in cell-mediated immunity and their functions are given in Table 8.2. Lymphocytes which do not express either B or T-cell markers or functions are called null lymphocytes or large granular lymphocytes.

Table 8.2: Cells involved in cell-mediated immunity and their functions

Cell	Functions
Helper T cell (T_H)	Necessary for B cells activation by T-dependent antigens.
Suppressor T cell (T_S)	Regulates immune response and helps in maintaining immune tolerance.
Cytotoxic T-cell (T_C)	Destroys target cells.
Delayed hypersensitivity T cell (T_D)	Provides protection against infectious agents.
Killer cell (K)	Attacks antibody-coated target cells.
Natural killer cell (NK)	Attacks and destroys target cells.

8.4 STRUCTURE OF IMMUNOGLOBULINS

Antibodies were shown by **E.A. Kabat** and **A. Tiselius** (1939) to belong to a class of serum protein called gamma globulins. It is now possible to isolate specific antibody molecules and to investigate their structures by biochemical techniques. The basic immunoglobulin molecule is composed of two light (L) polypeptides and two heavy polypeptides joined by disulfide bonds. It is a Y-shaped four polypeptide chain molecule (Fig. 8.3). These chains are designated as light or heavy based upon their molecular weight which is 50,000 to 70,000 daltons for heavy (H) chains and 20,000 to 25,000 daltons for light (L) chains. Heavy chains are composed of 446 amino acid residues or more whereas light chains have 213 or 214 residues. Some antibody molecules exist as monomers, whereas others are composed of more than one of these basic structural units.

The structure can be studied in detail by employing reduction and acidification, pepsin and papain. The antibody molecule can thus be split by papain to yield two identical fragments, each with a single combining site for antigen. This is called 'antigen binding fragment (F_{ab})'. The third fragment which lacks the ability to bind the antigen is called 'crystallizable fragment (F_c)'. The F_{ab} fragment binds to an antigen because it contains the antibody's binding site. The antigen combining site of the molecule is at its aminoterminus. The portion of the H chain present in the F_{ab} fragment is called F_d piece. The antibody (IgG) treated with reducing agent such as mercaptoethanol in the presence of urea, the disulfide bonds are reduced releasing four peptide chains (two heavy and two light).

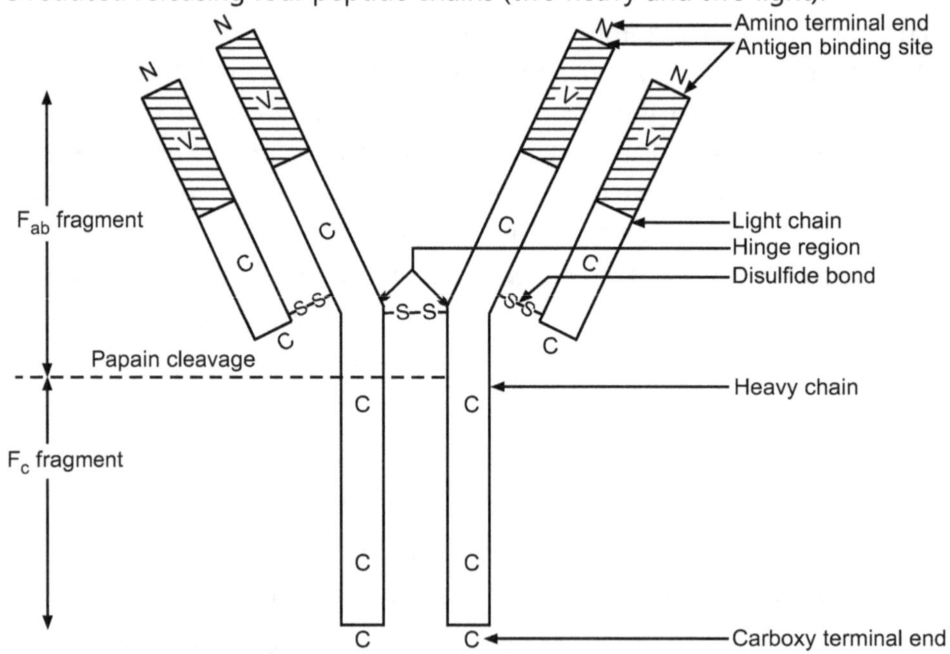

Fig. 8.3: Basic structure of immunoglobulin

The F_c fragment is composed of the carboxyterminal portion of the H chains. It does not possess antigen combining activity but determines the biological properties of the immunoglobulin molecule such as complement fixation, placental transfer, skin fixation and secretion into body fluids. Each heavy or light chain has a variable (V) region at the aminoterminal end and a constant (C) region at the carboxyl terminal end. The amino acid sequences in the variable regions differ from the amino acid sequences in the constant region. Antibody molecule is flexible because of a hinge region and it may convert to T-shape structure, when it is not in combination with an antigen. The area of heavy chain between CH_1 and CH_2 is the hinge region. The polypeptide chains are folded and held by interchain disulfide bonds. The folding produces compact globular regions known as 'domains' (Fig. 8.4). The light chains have only two domains, one variable (VL) and one constant (CL). There are four domains in each heavy chain of IgG, IgA and IgD, one in the variable region (VH) and three in the constant region (CH_1, CH_2, CH_3). IgM and IgE have four in the constant region (CH_4).

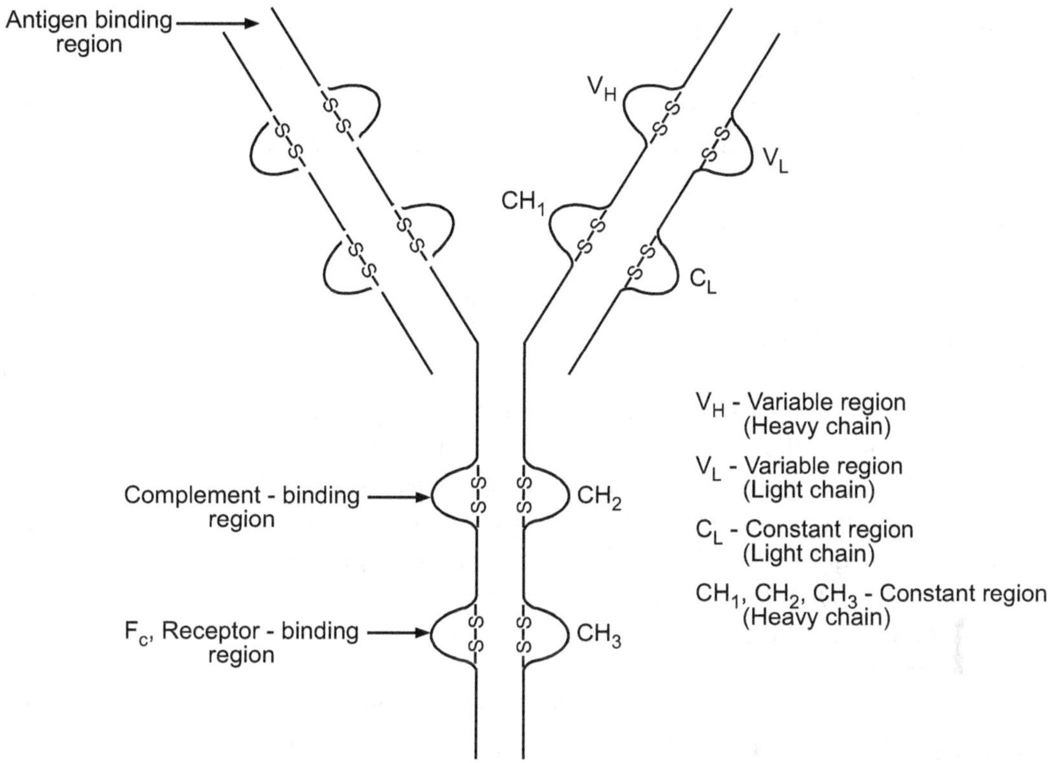

Fig. 8.4: Variable and Constant region of immunoglobulin molecule

8.5 STRUCTURE AND FUNCTIONS OF MHC

The major histocompatibility complex (MHC) is a set of molecules displayed on cell surfaces that are responsible for lymphocyte recognition and antigen presentation. MHC is set of genes that code for cell surface proteins essential for the acquired immune system to recognize foreign molecules in vertebrates. The main function of MHC molecules is to bind to antigens derived from pathogen's and display them on the cell surface for recognition by the T-cells. The MHC determines compatibility of donors for organ transplant and susceptibility to an autoimmune disease. The MHC is very large genetic complex containing over 100 genes. The few genes which are directly involved with graft rejection are referred as the histocompatibility genes. It also determines overall response to antigenic challenge in terms of antigenic presentation, processing and the overall immunological response. It determines the characteristics of the immune response to a given antigen.

The name of the MHC varies with the species. The human MHC is also called the human leukocyte antigen (HLA) complex or HLA and the MHC in mice is called the H-2 complex or H-2. In humans, the MHC genes encode the HLAs on the cell surface. Proteins inside the cell are broken into short fragments that can be displayed as peptide antigens by MHC molecules on the surface of the cell. MHC molecules display both peptides such as self peptides and foreign peptides. The immune system is constantly monitoring the surface of cells and the MHC-presented peptides help immune cells to differentiate normal antigens and foreign antigens. The immune system also monitors the amount of MHC-presented antigens which helps them to target and kills cancerous cells. Defects in certain MHC genes lead to cause autoimmune disorders in which body fail to recognize self-antigens. It may cause diseases like arthritis, multiple sclerosis, inflammatory bowel disease etc.

Classification of MHC:

Three classes of MHC molecules (glycoproteins) are known in human beings. MHC class I molecules are found on almost all the nucleated cells of the body. MHC class II molecules are associated only with leukocytes involved in cell-mediated immune response. Class III molecules are the secreted proteins possessing immune functions.

MHC Class I:

The MHC class I molecules are made up of two polypeptide chains. It consist of one membrane - spanning a chain (heavy chain) produced by MHC genes and one b chains (light chain) produced by the b_2-microglobulin gene. The MHC encoded alpha or heavy chain is about 43 kDa in molecular weight while the non-MHC encoded beta chain is lighter (12 kDa). The alpha chain is glycosylated and folds into three separate domains called α-1, α-2 and α-3. The β_2-microglobulin is non-covalently associated with α-3 domain (Fig. 8.5). MHC class I molecules have β_2-microglobulin subunit which can only be recognized by CD8 co-receptors. The region between α-1 and α-2 domains is in the form of groove and it is helpful for interaction of the two alpha domains. The floor of the groove is formed of 8 stranded β-pleated sheet and this groove plays a major role in presenting the antigen. The α-3 domain is highly conserved and structurally resembles the immunoglobulin constant domains. The β_2-microglobulin is a highly conserved protein and it resembles the constant domains of immunoglobulins. The α-3 domain is transmembrane, anchoring the MHC class I molecule to the cell membrane.

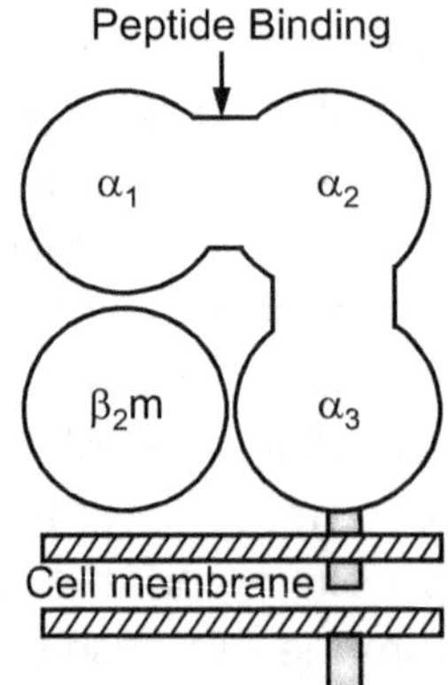

Fig. 8.5: Structure of MHC Class-I molecule

MHC class I glycoproteins are present on almost every cell in the body, acting to present endogenous antigens that originate from the cytoplasm. These antigens contains self proteins as well as foreign proteins produced within the cell. MHC class I proteins work to present the types of proteins being synthesized within a cell, which can be monitored by killer T-cells. MHC class I helps to mediate cellular immunity for intracellular pathogens such as viruses and some bacteria.

MHC Class II:

MHC class II molecules are composed of two polypeptide (α and β) chains. The α-polypeptide has a molecular weight of 34 kDa while β is 28 kDa. The α polypeptide folds into two domains, α-1 and α-2 while the β also folds into two domains, β-1 and β-2. The α-1 and β-1 domains create almost a similar groove as like MHC class I molecules (Fig. 8.6). Class II molecules have β-1 and β-2 subunits and can be recognized by CD4 co-receptors. The α-2 and β-2 domains give rise to the immunoglobulin like region similar to MHC Class I molecules. The α-2 and β-2 chain having a transmembrane domain, anchoring the MHC class II molecule to the cell membrane.

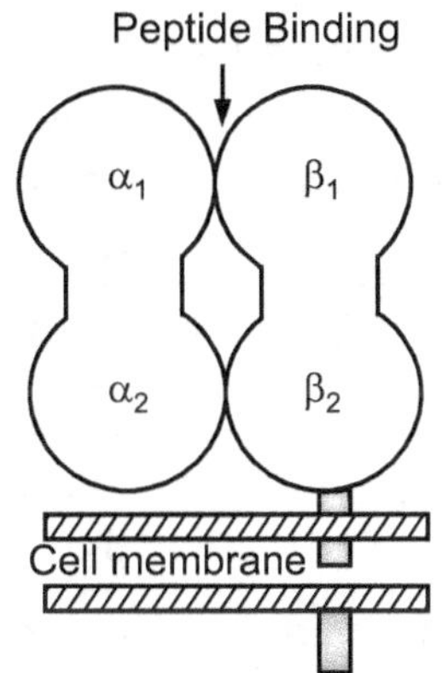

Fig. 8.6: Structure of MHC Class II molecule

MHC class II glycoproteins are only present on specialized antigen-presenting immune cells. MHC class II proteins present exogenous antigens that originate extracellularly from foreign bodies such as bacteria. MHC class II can be expressed by professional antigen-presenting cells (APCs), macrophages, B cells and dendritic cells (DCs). Exogenous antigens are usually fragments of viruses or bacteria engulfed and processed by macrophages or other phagocytic cells. These exogenously derived antigens are presented to helper T-cells. The helper T-cells activate B cells to produce antibodies that lead to the destruction of the pathogen.

MHC class I and MHC class II molecules appear structurally somewhat similar and both present antigens to T-cells. The functions of both class antigen are really quite distinct. The main differences of class I and Class II molecules are given in Table 8.3.

MHC Class III:

MHC Class III molecules have physiologic roles unlike classes I and II, but are encoded between them in the short arm of human chromosome. Class III molecules include several secreted proteins with immune functions such as components of complement system (C_2, C_4 and B factor), cytokines (TNF-α, LTA and LTB) and heat shock proteins.

Table 8.3: Differences of MHC Class I and MHC Class II molecules

MHC Class I	MHC Class II
• They are found on virtually every cell in the human body.	• They are found only on B cells, macro-phages and other antigen presenting cells.
• Class I molecules present antigens to cytolyltic T-lympocytes ($CD8^+$).	• Class II molecules present antigens to the helper T-lympocytes ($CD4^+$).
• These molecules present endogenously synthesized antigens.	• These molecules present exogenous derived antigens.
• Comprises essentially of single polymorphic trans-membrane poly-peptide chain (α, 3 domains α_1, α_2, α_3) and β_2 microglobulin	• Comprises of two trans-membrane polymorphic polypeptides α and β each made up of two extracellular domain pairs α_1 and α_2 and β_1 and β_2.
• β_2-microglobulin not coded in MHC.	• α, β chains are usually encoded in MHC.
• Immunoglobulin (Ig) resembles α_3 and β_2.	• Immunoglobulin (Ig) resembles α_2 and β_2.
• α_1 and α_2 the two outermost domains help in binding.	• α_1 and β_1 the two outermost domains form the groove for binding.
• Bonded peptide has a chain of 8 to 10 amino acids.	• Bound peptide has a chain of 15 to 24 amino acids.
• Genetic loci in humans (HLA-A, B and C) and in mice (H-2K, 2D and 2L).	• Genetic loci in humans (HLA-DP, DQ, DR) and in mice (H-2A, 2E clusters).

QUESTIONS

(A) Objective Type Questions:

1. Define:
   (a) Immunity
   (b) Antibody
   (c) MHC
2. Differentiate the following:
   (a) Cellular immunity and humoral immunity.
   (b) T-lymphocytes and B-lymphocytes.

(B) Short Answer Questions:

1. Explain the structure of MHC.
2. Write the functions of MHC.
3. How will you differentiate MHC Class I and MHC Class II molecules.

(C) Long Answer Questions:

1. Explain the structure of immunoglobulin.
2. Explain different types of immunity.

(D) Multiple Choice Questions:

1. The first line of general defence is ______.
   (a) Specific (b) Non-specific
   (c) Antigen-specific (d) None of the above
2. B-lymphocytes are processed in ______.
   (a) Bone marrow (b) Liver
   (c) Lung (d) Brain
3. ______ molecules have β2 microglobulin subunit which can only be recognized by CD8 co-receptors.
   (a) MHC Class I (b) MHC Class II
   (c) MHC Class III (d) MHC Class IV
4. Heavy chains in immunoglobulin are composed of ______ amino acid residues.
   (a) 50,000 (b) 20,000
   (c) 446 (d) 214

■■■

Chapter ... 9

HYPERSENSITIVITY REACTIONS

♦ LEARNING OBJECTIVES ♦

After completing this chapter, reader should be able to understand:

- *Introduction*
- *Hypersensitivity Reactions*
  - *Type I Hypersensitivity*
  - *Type II Hypersensitivity*
  - *Type III Immune-Complex Mediated Hypersensitivity*
  - *Type IV or Cell Mediated Hypersensitivity*
  - *Type V or Stimulatory Hypersensitivity*
- *Immune Stimulation*
- *Immune Suppressions*

9.1 INTRODUCTION

Hypersensitivity is an abnormal immune response which produces physiological or histopathological damage in the host. Hypersensitivity reactions have been classified into 'immediate' and 'delayed' types, based on the time required for a sensitised host to develop clinical reactions on re-exposure to the antigen. The differences between immediate and delayed reaction are listed in Table 9.1. **Coombs and Gell** (1963) classified hypersensitivity reactions into five types based on the different mechanisms of pathogenesis:

(i) Type I: Anaphylactic, immediate, IgE or reagin dependent: e.g. anaphylaxis, atopy etc.

(ii) Type II: Cytotoxic or cell stimulating: e.g. thrombocytopenia, hemolytic anemia etc.

(iii) Type III: Immuno complex or toxic complex: e.g. Arthus reaction, serum sickness etc.

(iv) Type IV: Delayed or T-cell mediated: e.g. tuberculin type, contact dermatitis etc.

(v) Type V: Stimulatory or antireceptor: e.g. autoimmune orchitis in guinea pigs.

Type I, II, and III hypersensitivity depend on the interaction of antigen with humoral antibodies and are known as immediate type reactions. Type IV hypersensitivity or delayed hypersensitivity is mediated by T-lymphocytes.

Table 9.1: Differences between Immediate and Delayed Hypersensitivity

Immediate hypersensitivity	Delayed hypersensitivity
• Appears rapidly and lasts for a shorter time.	• Appears slowly, lasts longer
• Induced by antigens or haptens	• Induced by infection, injection of antigens or haptens.
• Passive transfer possible with serum	• Passive transfer possible with T-lymphocytes.
• Circulating antibodies present (antibody mediated reaction)	• Circulating antibodies may be absent (cell mediated reaction)
• Desensitization easy but short lived.	• It is difficult but long lasting.
• Lesions are acute, exudation and fat necrosis.	• Mononuclear cell collection around blood vessels.
• Immediate hypersensitivity reactions develop in less than 12 hours.	• Delayed hypersensitivity reactions develop in 24 to 48 hours.

9.2 TYPE I – HYPERSENSITIVITY

Type I hypersensitivity is also known as immediate hypersensitivity or anaphylactic hypersensitivity because of the speed with which the immunologic reactions take place which may culminate into anaphylaxis within minutes following antigen challenge. Antibodies are fixed on the surface of tissue cells (mast cells and basophils) in sensitized individuals. The antigens combine with the cell-fixed antibodies, leading to release of pharmacologically active substances (vasoactive amines) which produce the following clinical reactions.

Anaphylaxis:

This is a classical immediate hypersensitivity reaction. It is mediated by IgE antibody and is due to the powerful effects of histamine and other vasoactive amines. Hypersensitivity may be local or generalised, depending upon the amount of histamine released, the site of its release and route of stimulating antigens. Antigens administered to mucous membrane or skin will induce local anaphylaxis (hay fever, asthma), whereas larger amounts may induce a generalised reaction. Insect venoms, horse serum and injected drugs are associated with systemic reactions involving the cardiovascular system (anaphylactic shock).

In order for immediate hypersensitivity reactions to occur, an individual must first come in contact with an antigen and produce IgE antibodies in response to that antigen. These antibodies bind to mast cells and basophils. Basophils are found in the circulation while mast cells are located in lymphoid regions of the respiratory tract, gastrointestinal tract, reproductive tract, skin and blood capillaries. After a second exposure the allergen travels to the mast cells and basophilis, where it binds to antigen-binding site of IgE molecule (Fig. 9.1). Antigen-antibody binding triggers the process of degranulation through which the mast cell explosively discharges its pharmacologically active agents. This include histamine, serotonin, slow-reacting substances of anaphylaxis, platelet-activating factors, eosinophil chemotactic factor of anaphylaxis and prostaglandins. Histamine is the most abundant and fastest acting agent. It induces smooth muscle contraction, release of mucus, vasodilation and increased capillary permeability. Serotonin is a base derived by decarboxylation of tryptophan. It causes smooth muscle contraction, increased capillary permeability and vasoconstriction. The eosinophil chemotactic factors of anaphylaxis are acidic tetrapeptides released from mast cell granules which are strongly chemotactic for eosinophils. Heparin is an acidic mucopolysaccharide and it mainly contributes to anaphylaxis in dogs.

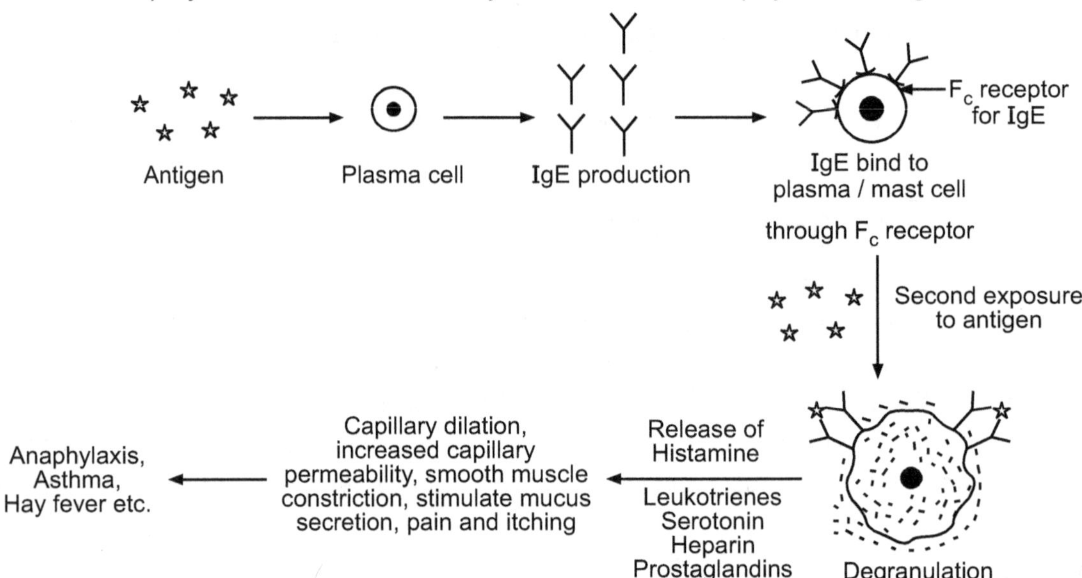

Fig. 9.1: Mechanisms of type I hypersensitivity

Prostaglandins and leukotrienes (secondary mediators of anaphylaxis) are derived by two different pathways from arachidonic acid, which is formed from disrupted cell membranes of mast cells and other leukocytes. Cyclooxygenase pathway leads to the formation of prostaglandins and thromboxane, while the lipoxygenase pathway leads to leukotrienes. A substance originally demonstrated in lungs, produces slow, sustained contraction of smooth muscles and is therefore termed as slow reacting substance of anaphylaxis. Prostaglandin E_2 is a bronchodilator. Prostaglandin F_{2a} and thromboxane A_2 are powerful but transient bronchoconstrictors. Platelet activating factor (PAF) is a low moleculer weight lipid released from basophils during immediate hypersensitivity. It causes aggregation of platelets and release of their vasoactive amines.

Cutaneous Anaphylaxis:

When a small shocking dose of an antigen is administered intradermally to a sensitised host, there will be a local wheal and flare response (local anaphylaxis). Wheal is a pale central area of puffiness due to edema (caused by increased capillary permeability) which is surrounded by flare caused by hyperemia due to vasodilation. The reaction becomes maximum in 10 to 30 minutes and fades away in a few hours. Cutaneous anaphylaxis (skin test) is useful for testing hypersensitivity and in identifying the allergen responsible for atopic diseases.

9.3 TYPE II - HYPERSENSITIVITY

Type II hypersensitivity is often referred to as cytotoxic hypersensitivity because in these reactions IgG or IgM antibodies directed against cell surface components cause damage or lysis of the affected cell. Complement can participate in these reactions by affecting cell lysis or through opsonisation of the antibody coated cell.

In cytotoxic type II reaction, antibodies (IgG or IgM) can bind to the surface of cell antigens. If the antibody is IgM, IgG1, IgG2 or IgG3, then C1q component is bound and activated. This initiates complement activation by classical pathway and terminates in lysis of the affected cell. The complement split product facilitates uptake of entire cell-antibody C3b complex by phagocytic cells (Fig. 9.2). Antibody coated cells can also lead to destruction of target cells by the killer cells through antibody dependent cell mediated cytotoxicity.

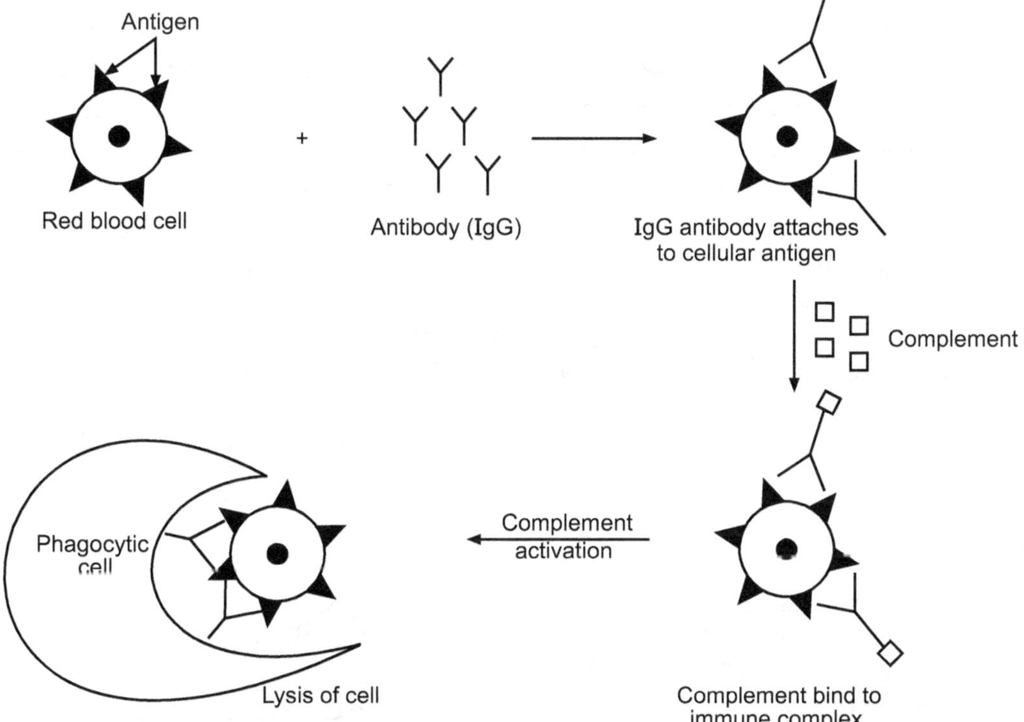

Fig. 9.2: Mechanism of type II hypersensitivity

Examples of type II hypersensitivity reactions are described as follows:

(i) Drug induced immune haemolytic anaemia: Autoimmune haemolytic anaemia is an important example of type II hypersensitivity. Haemolytic anaemia may be induced by administration of certain drugs such as penicillin, alpha-methyldopa etc. These drugs can bind to the surface of red blood cells and form an antigenic complex with the cells. This can bring about the production of complement fixing antibodies. Reaction of these antibodies with the RBC - bound drug, activates the complement system, resulting in RBC lysis and anaemia.

(ii) Rh - incompatibility: Rh antibodies are the main cause of haemolytic disease of newborns (erythroblastosis foetalis). Antibodies responsible for erythroblastosis fetalis arise when an Rh - ve mother carries an Rh + ve foetus (Rh D). During the birth of the baby, foetal erythrocytes are released into maternal circulation which stimulate the mothers immune system to produce IgG antibodies against the RhD antigens. During subsequent pregnancies involving any Rh + ve foetus, anti Rh D antibodies cross the placenta and cause red cell destruction. The first Rh + ve child born to an Rh - ve mother is usually unaffected but subsequent children are at considerable risk from erythroblastosis foetalis.

9.4 TYPE III – IMMUNE–COMPLEX MEDIATED HYPERSENSITIVITY

Type III hypersensitivity reactions are due to the combination of antigens with circulating antibodies, with the formation of immune complexes. This combination leads to the formation of micro-precipitates in and around small blood vessels which leads to inflammation and mechanical blockage of vessels. Type III hypersensitive reactions develop when immune complexes activate the complement systems array of immune effector molecules. Tissue damage in this type of reaction is due to the release of lytic enzymes by neutrophils as they attempt to phagocytose immune complexes (Fig. 9.3).

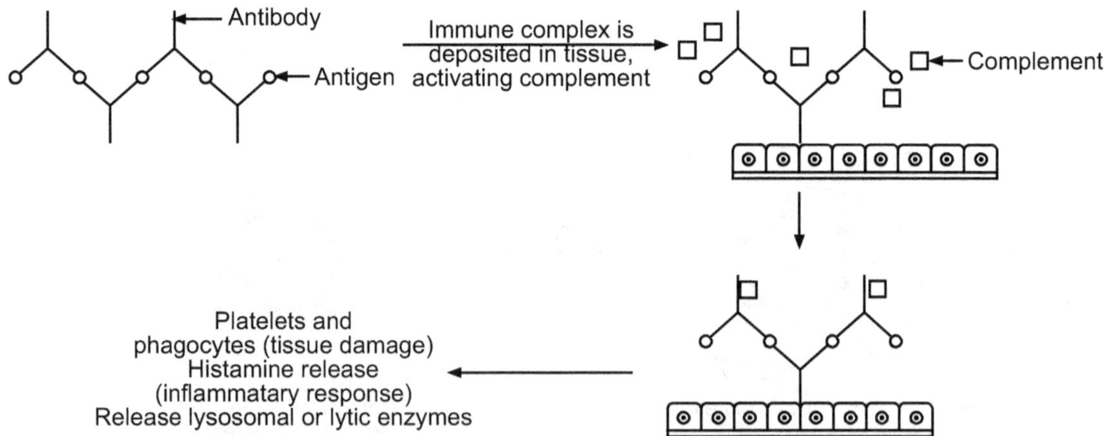

Fig. 9.3: Mechanism of type III (immune complex) hypersensitivity

Arthus or Localised Reaction:

Arthus (1903) observed that when rabbits were repeatedly injected subcutaneously with normal horse serum, the initial injections were without any local effect, but with later injections, there occurred intense local reaction consisting of edema and haemorrhagic necrosis. This is known as 'Arthus reaction'. Antigen-antibody precipitates are deposited on the walls of blood vessels and damage the tissues. There is activation of the vasoactive amines such as histamine, with resulting increase in vascular permeability and consequent edema. Leucocyte - platelet thrombi are formed which leads to tissue necrosis. The Arthus reaction can be passively transferred with sera containing precipitating antibodies (IgG, IgM) in high titres.

Serum Sickness or Systemic Reaction:

Serum sickness develops in normal human beings who receive a single injection of bovine or horse antitoxin against tetanus, gas gangrene, rabies, diphtheria or other toxins for prophylactic or therapeutic purposes. The clinical syndrome consists of fever, lymphadenopathy, arthritis, endocarditis, abdominal pain, nausea and vomiting. The pathogenesis is the formation of immune complexes which get deposited on the endothelial lining of blood vessels in various parts of the body.

Immune complexes occur in many diseases, including bacterial, viral and parasitic infections. The nephritis and arthritis seen in these conditions may be caused by deposition of immune complexes.

9.5 TYPE IV OR CELL MEDIATED HYPERSENSITIVITY

Type IV hypersensitivity is also known as delayed hypersensitivity since the signs of reactions are observed after 24 hours or more after contact with antigens. Unlike types I to III, this hypersensitivity reaction is mediated by T-lymphocytes and macrophages. T-lymphocytes, sensitised by prior contact with antigens, become activated upon reexposure to allergens and release soluble mediators known as lymphokines (Fig. 9.4). Most lymphokines exhibit multiple biological effects and the same effect may be caused by different lymphokines. These lymphokines can cause biological effects on leucocytes, macrophages and tissue cells. Delayed hypersensitivity cannot be passively transferred by serum but can be by lymphocytes or by the transfer factor.

Tuberculin or Infection Type:

The immune response to the tubercle bacillus was observed by **Robert Koch** in 1880. When a small dose of tuberculin or purified protein derivative (PPD) is injected intradermally in an individual sensitized to tuberculoprotein by prior infection or immunization, an indurated inflammatory reaction develops at the site of the injection within 48-72 hours. It is characterised by erythema due to increased blood flow to the damaged area and in duration due to infiltration with a large number of mononuclear cells, mainly T-lymphocytes and macrophages. Tuberculin type of hypersensitivity is developed in many infections with bacteria, fungi, viruses and parasites.

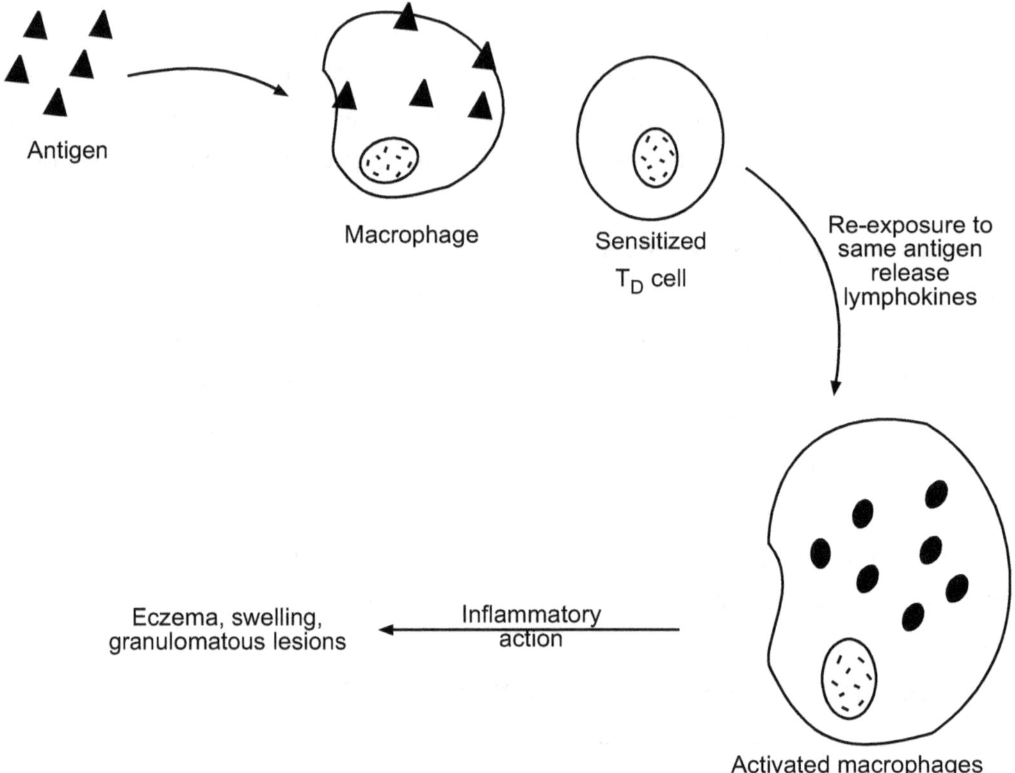

Fig. 9.4: Mechanism of type IV hypersensitivity

Contact Dermatitis Type:

Contact dermatitis is a cell-mediated allergic reaction that occurs when certain chemicals like metals (nickel), dyes (dinitrochlorobenzene) and drugs (penicillin) come in contact with skin. Sensitization is particularly liable to occur when contact is with an inflammed area. Antibiotic ointments applied on patches of dermatitis frequently provoke sensitization.

The substances involved are not antigenic by themselves but may acquire antigenicity on combination with skin proteins. Subsequent contact with allergens in a sensitized individual leads to contact dermatitis. This hypersensitivity can be detected by patch test. The allergen is applied to the skin and sensitivity (itching) is detected in 5 to 6 hours or local reaction (erythema) may be observed in 24 to 30 hours.

The essential differences between type IV reactions with other reactions are summarised in Table 9.2.

Table 9.2: Comparison of hypersensitivity reactions

Characteristics	Type I	Type II	Type III	Type IV
Type of reaction	Immediate	Cytotoxic	Immune complex	Delayed
Antibody involved	IgE	IgE, IgM	IgG, IgM	T-cells
Reaction mediators	Anaphylactic factors, mast cells, eosinophils	Complement	Eosinophils, neutrophils, complement	Macrophages and lymphokines
Antigen	Soluble or particulate	On cell surface	Soluble or particulate	On cell surface
Reaction time	Variable (in seconds or minutes)	Variable (in hours)	4 to 8 hours	24 to 48 hours
Nature of reaction	Local wheal and flare	Clumping of R.B.C.'s	Acute inflammation	Cell mediated cell destruction
Examples	Anaphylaxis, asthma, hay fever, food and insect allergies	Agranulocytosis, thrombocy-topenia, hemolytic anemia, blood reaction	Arthus reaction, serum sickness, glomeruler nephritis	Tuberculosis, contact dermatitis, graft rejection.
Therapy	Desensitization	Steroids	Steroids	Steroids

9.6 TYPE V OR STIMULATORY HYPERSENSITIVITY

It is an antibody mediated hypersensitivity. In this case, an antibody reacts with a key surface component such as a hormone receptor and switches on or stimulates the cell. An example of this type of hypersensitivity is thyroid hyperactivity in Grave's disease due to thyroid stimulating autoantibody. Thyroid stimulating hormones from pituitary gland get attached to thyroid cell receptors thus, activating adenyl cyclase in the membrane. It converts ATP to AMP. The latter stimulates activity of thyroid cells thus secreting thyroxine. The thyroid stimulating antibodies present in the sera of thyrotoxic patients are autoantibodies directed against receptors for thyroid stimulating hormones.

9.7 IMMUNE STIMULATION

Immunomodulators are natural or synthetic components that regulate the immune system and induce innate and adaptive defense mechanisms. Immunomodulators are drugs or components which suppress the immune system (immunosuppressants) or stimulate the immune system (immunostimulants). Immunostimulants or immunostimulators are substance that stimulate the immune response or enhance body's resistance against various infections through increasing the basal levels of immune response. These substances are responsible for increase the oxidative activity of neutrophils, stimulate cytotoxic cells and augment engulfment activity of phagocytic cells. Immunostimulants are used for treatment of autoimmune diseases, chronic infections, viral infections, and cancer like diseases. Immunostimulants induce synthesis of specific antibodies and cytokines for treatment of infectious diseases. Immunostimulants are responsible to develop the non-specific immunotherapy by stimulating the major factors of the immune system. These includes complement systems, phagocytosis, interferon release, T and B lymphocytes, synthesis of specific antibodies, etc. Many immunostimulants activate innate immunity and promote release of endogenous immune mediators (cytokines) in the treatment of immunodeficiency conditions and chronic infections.

There are two main types of immunostimulants:

1. **Specific immunostimulants:** It provides antigenic specificity in immune response. e.g. antigen, vaccines.
2. **Non-specific immunostimulants:** It act irrespective of antigenic specificity to augment immune response of other antigen or stimulate components of the immune system without antigenic specificity. e.g. adjuvants.

There are several types of immunostimulants (Fig. 9.5) such as immunoenhancing drugs, complex carbohydratyes, bacterial products, vaccines, plant extracts, animal extracts, nutritional factors etc. Immunostimulatory drugs are used to induce humoral or cellular immune responses against immunodeficiency diseases and chronic infections. Levamisole, thalidomine, isoprinosine, immunocynin, bestatin and polyribonucleotides are commonly used as immunostimulants. Complex carbohydrates such as glucans, schizophyllan, lentinan, trehalose, prebiotics are important class of immunostimulants. β-glucans is used to stimulate antitumor activity and to enhance host resistance to microbial pathogens. Trehalose dimycolate (TDM), and lipopolysaccharides (bacterial products) promote the production of antibodies and stimulate activation of lymphocytes. Indigestible fibres (prebiotics) such as oligosaccharide, inulin, or β-glucan directly enhance innate immune responses by phagocytosis and activation of complement system.

The immunostimulatory effects of bacterial products are due to the release of cytokines. Several interferons and interleukins are stimulate effective immune responses. Adjuvants are used in vaccine products to enhance and modulate immune responses to antigens. Medicinal plants are well known for immunostimulants, growth promoters and antimicrobial agents to the host immune system. e.g. *Ocimum sanctum* (Tulsi), *Azadirachta indica* (Neem), *Zingiber officinale* (Ginger), *Camellia sinensis* (Green tea), Aloe vera, Saffron, fermented vegetable products, etc. Chitin and chitosan are the non-specific animal originated immune stimulants. These components shows strong antimicrobial activity as well as more effective in enhancing the migratory activity of microphages.

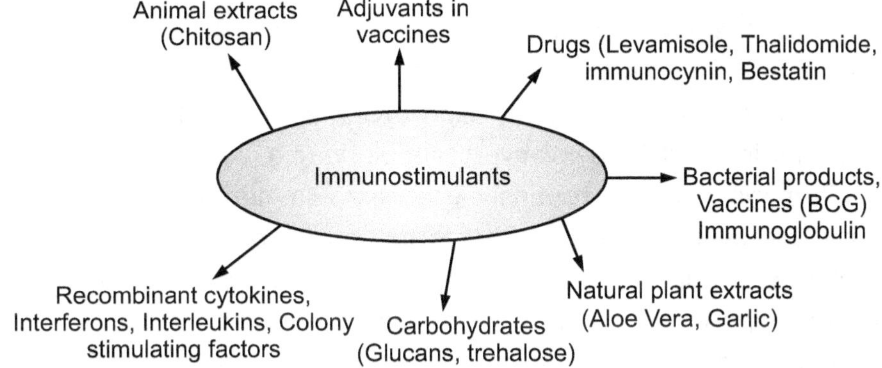

Fig. 9.5: Types of immunostimulants

9.8 IMMUNO SUPPRESSION

Immunosuppression is a reduction of the activation or efficacy of the immune system. It is a phenomenon wherein an organism's ability to form antibodies in response to an antigenic stimulus is reduced or suppressed. This suppression may be the result of a disease that targets the immune system, such as HIV infection or consequence of pharmaceutical agents used to fight cancer. In some cases, immunosuppression may be deliberately induced. The induction may be required for therapeutic interventions of tissue or organ transplantation to reduce the risk of organ rejection. It is also used for treating graft-versus-host disease after a bone marrow transplant or for the treatment of auto-immune diseases such as systemic lupus erythematosus, rheumatoid arthritis, Sjogren's syndrome or Crohn's disease.

Immunosuppression are classified into two types such as non-specific immuno-suppression and specific immunosuppression.

Non-specific immunosuppression:

This immunosuppression invariably takes places particularly in the natural instances related to immune-deficiency disorders or may even be induced by gradual depletion of lymphoid tissue or by the administration of immunosuppressive drugs. It has been observed adequately that the undue exposure to radiation gives rise to significant depletion of lymphocytes. It may cause impairment of the antigens present on the macrophages thereby producing immunosuppression. Non-specific immunosuppression can also be induced by antilymphocyte globulin (ALG) that specifically affects the T-cells by causing inhibition of their normal functionalities or by depleting T-cells dependent areas.

Specific immunosuppression:

Specific immunosuppression is usually induced either by antigen or antibody. Azathiopurine and corticosteroid combination therapy is commonly used in tissue transplantation to inhibit cell-mediated immunity (CMI). Cyclosporine is commonly used in immunosuppressive therapy. Specific class of endogenous corticosteriods such as hydrocortisone, testosterone, corticosterone, prednisone, prednisolone are extensively used to inhibit CMI. Antiproliferative agent (e.g. cyclophophamide), DNA-base analogous (e.g. 6-merceaptopurine and its derivatives), antibiotic (e.g. actinomycin – D) and mitotic poison (e.g. mitomycin – c) are routinely used as a immunosuppressive agents. These substances may act by repression of the formation of precursor cells, destruction of immunocompetent cells, suppression of proliferation and differentiation of lymphocytes and monocytes by inhibition of the biosynthesis of nucleic acids and proteins. Antilymphocyte serum (ATS) is also commonly used to combat specific immunosuppression.

The monoclonal antibody (OKT_3) is also used as immunosuppressive agent after organ transplantation in humans. OKT_3 specifically directed against CD_3 antigen of T-lymphocytes is used in renal and bone marrow transplantations. CD_3 antigen activates T-lymphocytes and plays a key role in organ transplant rejection. This is prevented by use of MAb against CD_3 antigen. AIDS infection is one of major causes of immunosuppression by reduction in CD_4 (Cluster determinant antigen 4) cells of T-lymphocytes.

QUESTIONS

(A) Objective Type Questions:

1. What is hypersensitivity reaction?
2. Write the classification of hypersensitivity reactions.

(B) Short Answer Questions:

1. What is the basis of type II hypersensitivity reactions? Explain with suitable examples.
2. Differentiate the following:
   (a) Immediate hypersensitivity and delayed hypersensitivity.
   (b) Type II hypersensitivity and type III hypersensitivity.
3. Write the importance of immune stimulation and immune suppressions.

(C) Long Answer Questions:

1. Describe the mechanism of type I hypersensitivity reaction with suitable diagrams.
2. Explain different hypersensitivity reactions with suitable examples.

(D) Multiple Choice Questions:

1. Antibody isotypes which can cause erythroblastosis foetalis are ______ .
   (a) IgG (b) IgD
   (c) IgM (d) IgE
2. The immunoglobulin most often associated with immediate type (type 1) allergic reactions ______ .
   (a) IgA (b) IgE
   (c) IgM (d) IgD
3. Delayed hypersensitivity reaction is mediated by ______ .
   (a) T-lymphocytes (b) B-lymphocytes
   (c) Killer cells (d) Natural killer cells
4. Receptor for IgE is present on ______ .
   (a) Plasma cell (b) Basophil
   (c) Eosinophil (d) Polymorphs
5. AIDS infection is one of major causes of immuno-suppression by reduction in ______ cells of T-lympocytes.
   (a) CD_3 (b) CD_4
   (c) CD_6 (d) CD_8

■■■

Chapter ... 10

VACCINES AND SERA

♦ LEARNING OBJECTIVES ♦

After completing this chapter, reader should be able to understand:

- *Introduction*
- *Preparation of Vaccines (General Method)*
- *Quality Control of Vaccines*
  - *In-process Quality Control*
  - *Final Product Quality Control*
- *Storage of Immunological Products*
- *Bacterial Vaccines and Toxoids*
  - *BCG Vaccine, TAB Vaccine, Diphtheria Vaccine, Tetanus Vaccine, Pertusis Vaccine, DPT Vaccine*
- *Viral Vaccines*
  - *Poliomyelitis Vaccine*
- *Antitoxic Sera*
  - *Diphtheria Antitoxin, Tetanus Antitoxin*
- *Antiviral Sera*
  - *Rabies Antiserum*

10.1 INTRODUCTION

Vaccines or sera are biological products which act by reinforcing the immunological defence of the body against foreign agencies (infecting organisms or their toxins). The agents or products through which immunization is achieved are called 'immunizing agents'.

Active immunization is the process of increasing resistance to infections whereby microorganisms or products of their activity act as antigens and stimulate certain body cells to produce antibodies with a specific protective capacity. Biological products comprising vaccines and toxoids confer active immunity. Passive immunization which results in immediate protection of a short duration, may be achieved by the administration of antibodies themselves. Biological products comprising human immune sera and animal immune sera confer passive immunity. These immunological preparations are classified in Fig. 10.1. Vaccines and sera are potentially dangerous products and mostly used in public health programmes. These biologicals are standardised by bioassays and stored in a cold place to maintain potency.

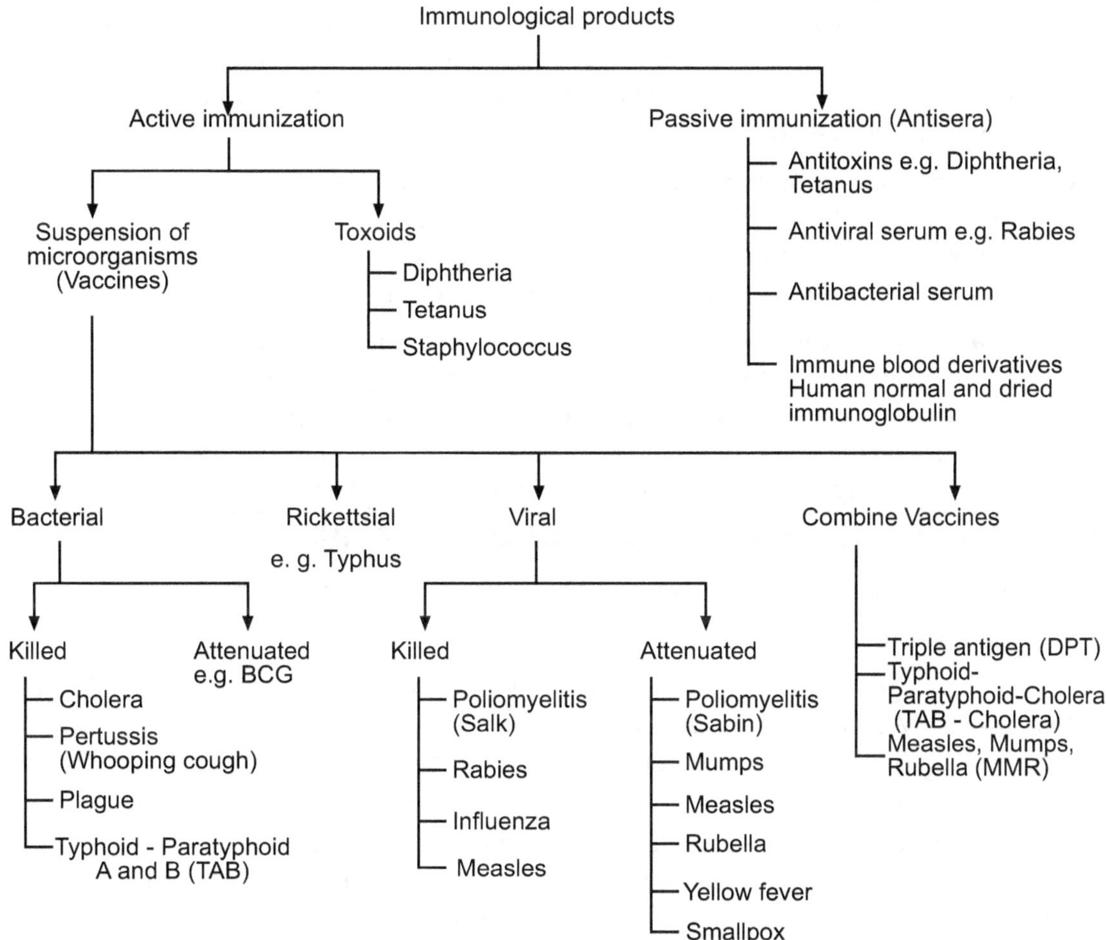

Fig. 10.1: Immunological products

Vaccines are preparations of antigenic materials, which are administered with the objective of inducing in the recipient a specific and active immunity against the infectious microorganisms or toxins produced by them. They may contain living or killed microorganisms, bacterial toxoids or antigenic material from particular parts of the bacterium, rickettsia or virus.

Vaccines may be single-component or mixed component vaccines. Single vaccines are prepared from a single species of microorganisms. Mixed or compound vaccines are prepared from two or more species. Simple vaccines containing only one strain of a species are univalent and those containing two or more strains of the same species are called polyvalent. Vaccines may be classified into five types:

(i) Live attenuated vaccines: Live attenuated vaccines consist of live bacteria or viruses which have been rendered avirulent e.g. B. C. G. vaccine, smallpox vaccine.

(ii) Killed vaccines: Killed vaccines are suspensions of bacteria or of viruses that have been killed by heat or by disinfectants such as phenol or formaldehyde. The best known killed vaccines are pertussis, cholera, plague, influenza and rabbies vaccine.

(iii) Toxoid vaccines: Toxoids may be defined as modified toxins, detoxified by the use of moderate heat and chemical treatment so that their antigenic properties are retained. Toxoids are toxins whose toxicity has been removed e.g. tetanus toxoid, staphylococcus toxoid.

(iv) Bacterial cell component vaccine: Some bacterial vaccines do not contain whole bacterial cells but contain components of bacterial cells. Such vaccines induce a response that is more specific and effective e.g. *Haemophilus influenzae* Type B vaccine, *Neisseria meningitidis* Type A and C vaccine.

(v) Viral subunit vaccines: The influenza vaccines are prepared by treating intact influenza virus particles from embryonated hens eggs, infected with influenza virus with a surface acting agent. The virus particles are disrupted and release the two viral subunits, haemagglutinin and neuraminidase that are required in the vaccine. Another example of viral subunit vaccine is hepatitis B vaccine.

10.2 PREPARATION OF VACCINES (GENERAL METHOD)

Many bacterial and viral vaccines are prepared by the following methods:

The seed lot system:

The starting stage for the preparation of all microbial vaccines is the isolation of suitable microbial strains. Microbial strains are mainly isolated from human infections and in some cases have required elaborate laboratory manipulation and selection. Once a suitable strain is available, a sizeable culture is prepared. It is distributed in a large number of ampoules and then stored at $-70^{\circ}C$ or freeze dried. This culture is called 'seed lot'. The biological properties of seed materials are carefully examined in the laboratory. The seed is then used to make one or more batches of vaccine production. If it is found satisfactory, then it is tested for efficacy and safety in clinical trials. Satisfactory results in the clinical trials validate the seed lot and it is used for production of vaccines.

Production of bacteria and bacterial components for bacterial vaccines:

Bacteria and bacterial components needed for the manufacture of bacterial vaccines are readily prepared by fermentation by using different laboratory media.

Fermentation: The production of a bacterial vaccine batch begins with the resuscitation of the bacterial seed lot stored at $-70^{\circ}C$ or freeze dried. The resuscitated bacteria are first cultivated through one or more passages in preproduction media. Then, sufficient bacterial inoculum are used to inoculate a production medium. Fermentation process is carefully regulated and monitored for temperature, pH and oxidation - reduction potential.

Process of bacterial harvests: The harvest is a complex mixture of bacterial cells and metabolic products. The bacterial harvesting depends on the nature of the component that is required and may involve one or more of the following procedures:

1. **Killing:** Killing is the process in which live bacteria in the culture are killed. Heat or formalin is required to kill the cells of *Bordetella pertussis* (whooping – cough

vaccine). Phenol is very commonly used to kill *Vibrio cholerae* (cholera vaccine) and *Salmonella typhi* (typhoid vaccine).

2. **Separation:** Separation is the process by which bacterial cells are separated from the fermentation medium. Centrifugation or precipitation (by pH reduction) is commonly used for the separation of cells from the culture fluid. In the case of vaccines prepared from cells, the fluid is discarded and the cells are resuspended in a saline solution. If vaccines are prepared from a constituent of the fluid, then the cells are discarded.
3. **Fractionation:** The process by which components are extracted from bacterial cells or from the medium is called fractionation. The antigens of *Pseudomonas aeruginosa* are extracted with water. The polysaccharide antigens of *Neisseria meningitidis* are separated from the cells by treatment with hexadecyltrimethyl ammonium bromide and those of *Streptococcus pneumonia* with ethanol. The purity of an extracted material may be improved by resolubilization in a suitable solvent and precipitation.
4. **Detoxification:** Detoxification is the process by which toxins are converted to harmless toxoids. Formalin is used to detoxify the toxins of *Corynebacterium diphtheriae* and *Clostridium tetani*. Detoxification is generally performed in the fermenter.
5. **Adsorption:** The mineral adjuvants or carriers are used to increase immunogenicity and decrease toxicity e.g. aluminium hydroxide, aluminium phosphate, calcium phosphate etc. Diphtheria vaccine, tetanus vaccine and DPT vaccine are prepared as adsorbed vaccines.
6. **Conjugation:** Conjugation is the linking of a vaccine component (poor immune response), with a vaccine component that induces a good immune response. The immunogenicity for infants of *Hemophilus influenzae* type b is greatly enhanced by the conjugation with diphtheria and tetanus toxoids.

Production of viruses and viral components for viral vaccines:

Viruses replicate only in living cells, hence the first viral vaccines against smallpox and rabies were made in intact mammalian hosts (calves, sheep, rabbits). Today, the only intact host used in advanced production techniques is the developing chick embryo. Almost all virus growth is preferably achieved in cell cultures.

Growth of viruses: The chick embryo is the most convenient host for the growth of viruses that are needed for influenza and yellow fever vaccines. Influenza viruses accumulate in high titre in the allantoic fluid of the eggs and yellow fever virus accumulates in the nervous systems of the embryos.

Processing of viral harvests: Different techniques are used for processing of viral materials. Allantoic fluid is centrifuged to provide a concentrated and partially purified suspension of influenza virus. This concentrated suspension is treated with ether or other age[illegible] to split the virus into its components. Cell cultures provide infected fluids that [illegible]tle debris and that can be separated by filtration. Most viral vaccines are not [illegible]ecause they are made from cultures consisting of live attenuated virus.

But inactivated poliomyelitis virus vaccine is inactivated with dilute formalin or β-propiolactone and rabbies vaccine is inactivated with β-propiolactone. When processing is complete, the bulk materials may be stored (– 70°C) until needed for blending into a final vaccine.

Blending:

Blending is the process in which the various components of a vaccine are mixed to form a final bulk. A single component final bulk is prepared by adding bacterial suspensions or bacterial components e.g. BCG vaccine, cholera vaccine, diphtheria vaccine etc. A multiple component final bulk of a combined vaccine is made by adding each required component e.g. DPT vaccine. Vaccines blended without an adjuvant are called 'plain vaccines' or 'fluid vaccines' (in bacterial toxoids). Those vaccines blended with an adjuvant (e.g. aluminium hydroxide) are called 'adsorbed vaccines'. Preservatives (thiomersal) are added in killed bacterial vaccines in multidose containers.

When viral vaccines are blended, it is necessary to maintain adequate antigenicity or infectivity. After proper mixing a final bulk may be separated into a number of small size containers to facilitate handling e.g. measles vaccine, poliomyelitis vaccine, rabbies vaccine, smallpox vaccine etc. Live attenuated viral vaccines lose potency in the suspension hence, these vaccines are stored at low temperature or a stabilizer may be added. Live attenuated poliomyelitis vaccine is stabilized by using magnesium chloride or sucrose.

Filling and drying:

Bulk vaccines are dispensed into single dose ampoules or into multidose vials. Vaccines that are filled as liquids are sealed and capped in the containers. Vaccines that are dispensed as dry preparations are freeze-dried before sealing.

10.3 QUALITY CONTROL OF VACCINES

The quality control of vaccines is intended to provide assurances of efficacy and safety. Quality of vaccines are checked in two ways: in-process control and final product control.

10.3.1 In-Process Control

In-process quality control is the control exercised over starting materials and intermediates. The quality control of diphtheria and tetanus vaccines requires that the products are tested for the presence of free toxins. Adequate infectivity of the virus from the tissue cultures is an indicator of the adequate virus content of the starting materials and since infectivity is destroyed in the inactivation process. In case of tissue culture substrates, to exclude contamination with infectious agents from the source animal or in the case of human diploid cells, to exclude abnormal cellular characters. Monkey kidney cell cultures are tested for simian herpes B virus, simen virus 40 and mycoplasmas.

10.3.2 Final Product Quality Control

Final product quality control is the quality control exercised by the monographs of a Pharmacopoeia over products in their final containers. All vaccines are tested for identity, potency and safety. Combined vaccines are required to pass tests prescribed for each of the separate components.

Identity tests: The identities of bacterial vaccines can be checked by precipitation and agglutination reactions. Inactivated viral vaccines are tested by observation of the specific antibody responses in vaccinated animals and live viral vaccines by neutralisation of their cytopathic effects by specific antisera.

Potency assay: Vaccines containing killed microbes or their products are tested for potency in which the amount of the vaccine that is required to protect animals form a defined challenge dose of the pathogen. The potency of whooping cough vaccine is estimated by 3 + 3 dose quantal assay method as per Pharmacopoeia. Three logarithmic serial doses of the test vaccine and three logarithmic serial doses of the standard vaccine are inoculated (each) in a group of 16 mice. On the basis of experience, a middle dose of test and standard vaccine that induce a protective response in about 50% of the animals are selected. Fourteen days later all of the mice are infected with *Bordetella pertussis* and after a further 14 days, the number of mice surviving in each of the six group are counted. The number of survivors in each group are then used to calculate the potency of the test vaccine relative to the standard vaccine. Same tests may be used for the estimation of the potencies of diphtheria and tetanus vaccines. Vaccines containing live microorganisms are generally tested for potency by counts of their viable cells e.g. BCG vaccine. The potency of live viral vaccines is estimated by using substrates of living cells. Dilutions of vaccines are inoculated on the tissue culture monolayers in Petri dishes and the live count of the vaccines is calculated from the infectivity of the dilutions and dilution factor involved. Potency of many vaccines are also checked by physicochemical or serological techniques.

Safety tests: Viral vaccines have some problems for safety testing as compared to bacterial vaccines. Killed bacterial vaccines must be completely free from living microbes used in the production process. The final product must provide an assurance that all microorganisms have been killed. Incomplete virus inactivation is detected by inoculation of susceptible tissue cultures and of susceptible animals. The cultures are examined for cytopathic effects and the animals for symptoms of disease.

Some other tests are used for estimation of potency and safety of bacterial and viral vaccines. These tests are as follows:

1. **Sterility test:** All vaccines must be bacteriologically and mycologically sterile. In each batch of a product the number of containers to be tested depends on the batch size and is the subject of pharmacopoeial regulation. Membrane filtration method is commonly used for sterility testing of vaccines.
2. **Free formalin testing:** Inactivation of bacterial toxins (by formalin) may lead to the presence of free formalin in the final product. The concentration of free formalin may not exceed 0.02% which is estimated by colour development with acetylacetone.
3. **Abnormal toxicity testing:** This test is used for detection of toxic contaminant in vaccines. Five mice (approx. 20 gm) and two guinea pigs (approx. 300 gm) are inoculated with one human dose or 1.0 ml (whichever is less) of the test preparation. All must survive for 7 days without sign of illness.
4. **Phenol concentration:** Phenol is used as a preservative in different types of vaccines. Its concentration must not exceed 0.5% w/v.

5. **Presence of aluminium and calcium:** Aluminium hydroxide, aluminium phosphate and calcium phosphate are commonly used in vaccines as an adjuvant. The quantity of aluminium must not exceed 1.25 mg/dose and is estimated compleximetrically. The quality of calcium must not exceed 1.3 mg/dose and is usually estimated by flame photometry.

10.4 STORAGE OF IMMUNOLOGICAL PRODUCTS

Preservation of the potency of immunological products involves maintaining the viability of living cells or preventing the denaturation of proteins. Most vaccines and immunological preparations are stored at 2 to 10°C. Viral vaccines (e.g. smallpox and oral poliomyelitis) are more stable at or below their freezing points but bacterial vaccines or antitoxins are easily deteriorated if they are allowed to freeze. This may be due to mechanical damage by ice crystals or the adverse effects of inorganic salts. Freeze dried vaccines are stable as compared with corresponding liquid forms. Freeze-dried smallpox and yellow fever vaccines must be kept at not more than 10°C and 0°C respectively.

Immunological products must be protected from light because these products usually accelerate decomposition in presence of light. Dilution and the choice of diluent may also influence stability. The diagnostic preparations, undiluted old tuberculin, is stable for 8 years but when diluted, its stability depends on the degree of dilution and the nature of diluent. Good stock control is particularly important for biological preparations.

10.5 BACTERIAL VACCINES AND TOXOIDS

Bacterial vaccines and toxoids may be considered as representing live or killed bacterial cells or purified bacterial components. These vaccines are prepared by using different methods. Preparation techniques of some bacterial vaccines and toxoids are described as follows:

Bacillus Calmette – Guerin vaccine (BCG vaccine):

It is a live bacterial vaccine bearing an attenuated bovine strain of *Mycobacterium tuberculosis*, developed by **Calmette** and **Guerin** (1921) in France. The vaccine is prepared immediately before use by reconstitution from the dried vaccine with a suitable liquid.

Preparation: The strain grown on a suitable culture media, shows not less than 20 million colonies (seed lot system). After suitable growth, they are separated by filtration in the form of a cake. The cake is homogenised in a grinding flask and suspended in a sterile liquid medium designed to preserve the antigenicity and the viability of the vaccine (determined by plate count). The suspension is transferred into the final sterile container and freeze - dried under conditions designed to prevent microbial contamination and finally sealed. It is available as white pellets or powder, which when reconstituted, yields an opalescent and homogeneous suspension.

Storage: BCG vaccine should be stored in sealed light resistant glass containers at a temperature between 2 to 8°C. The reconstituted vaccine should be used immediately after preparation.

Dose: Prophylactic, by intracutaneous injection, as a single dose, 0.1 ml.

Use: BCG vaccine is used as an immunising agent which provides protection against tuberculosis.

TAB vaccine (Typhoid – paratyphoid A, B):

It is a sterile suspension of *Salmonella typhi* and *Salmonella paratyphi* A and B. TABC contains *Salmonella paratyphi* 'C' in addition to TAB.

Preparation: TAB vaccine is a mixed polyvalent vaccine and is prepared by mixing of simple vaccines of *Salmonella typhi, Salmonella paratyphi* A and *Salmonella paratyphi* B. These strains are grown in acid digested agar medium and cultivated for 48 hrs at 37°C. These bacterial strains are harvested with a sterile normal saline solution. Strains are diluted to form 3,000 million organisms/ml of *Salmonella typhi* and 2,250 million organisms/ml of each of *Salmonella paratyphi* A and B. All these strains are killed by addition of 0.1% formalin or by heat treatment. Bacterial strains are incubated at 37°C for 4 days for detoxification and then tested for sterility. Bacterial strains are mixed together to contain 1,000 million organisms of *Salmonella typhi* and 750 million organisms of each of *Salmonella paratyphi* A and B. The suspension is transferred to final sterile containers and freeze dried. Check the sterility and abnormal toxicity of the vaccine.

Storage: Store in well closed containers at a temperature between 2 to 8°C.

Dose: Prophylactic, 0.5 ml (subcutaneous), 2 to 3 injections at 2 to 4 weeks intervals. Booster doses may be given every 1 to 2 years.

Use: TAB or TABC mixed polyvalent vaccine is used in the prophylaxis of enteric infections. TAB is also mixed with tetanus vaccine and cholera vaccine.

Diphtheria vaccine or toxoids:

Diphtheria vaccine or toxoid is a Formol Toxoid prepared from toxins produced by *Corynebacterium diphtheriae.*

Preparation: A suitable strain of *Corynebacterium diphtheriae* is grown on a liquid medium (dextrose veal infusion medium) at 35°C for 7 days. After maximum toxin production, the bulk of the organisms are separated on paper pulp and the filtrate is sterilized using fibrous pads or ceramic candles.

Preparation of diphtheria toxoid:

(i) Formol Toxoid (FT): In the diphtheria toxin, 0.5% formalin is added and the mixture is incubated at 37°C for 3 to 4 weeks to remove toxicity. The toxoid is confirmed for sterility and presence of toxins. The final preparation is known as Formol Toxoid (FT). For many years this product was used in its unpurified form. It was an excellent antigen but it often caused severe reactions. Different purification techniques are used for the purification of toxoids but it reduces its activity and stability.

(ii) Toxin – Antitoxin Floccules (TAF): If suitable quantity of toxoids (100 units) and antitoxins (80 units) are mixed they forms floccules. These floccules contains good antigenic activity. These floccules are separated and washed to remove all contaminations. Floccules are again resuspended in a saline solution containing a bactericide. This product is known as Toxoid - Antitoxin Floccules.

(iii) Alum Precipitated Toxoid (APT): This preparation resulted from the discovery that slow absorption of precipitated toxoids from the site of injection and slow excretion from the body led to increased antigenic activity. High quality Formol Toxoid is treated with charcoal to remove colouring matter and other impurities. The charcoal is separated by filtration and suitable concentration of alum is added. This reacts with bicarbonate, phosphate and protein impurities in the toxoid to produce a precipitate containing aluminium hydroxide and phosphate. Then the precipitate is washed and suspended in saline containing a bactericide. Alum is used to potentiate the effect of antigens (adjuvants). Alum Precipitated Toxoid (APT) produces more antibodies than Formol Toxoid (FT) and Toxoid – Antitoxin Floccules (TAF).

(iv) Purified Toxoid Aluminium Phosphate (PTAP): Purified Toxoid Aluminium Phosphate (PTAP) is a pure toxoid prepared by using a semi-synthetic medium in the preparation of the toxin. It is prepared by using different purification techniques involving the use of magnesium hydroxide, to precipitate colour, phosphate, ammonium sulphate, cadmium chloride and some proteins.

Tetanus vaccine or toxoid:

Tetanus vaccine or toxoid is prepared from the exotoxin of the anaerobe *Clostridium tetani*. This toxoid is prepared by using veal (calves) infusion peptone medium and maintaining anaerobic conditions (anaerobic jar). It is available in the forms of Alum Precipitated Toxoid (APT), Purified Toxoid Aluminium Phosphate (PTAP) and other forms except Toxoid - Antitoxin Floccules (TAF).

Pertusis vaccine or whooping cough vaccine:

Pertusis vaccine is a sterile suspension of killed *Bordetella pertussis*.

Preparation: The *Bordetella pertussis* culture is maintained on a charcoal agar medium. Preinoculum of culture is inoculated in Cohen Wheeler liquid medium and incubated for 48 hours at 37°C on a rotary shaker. The bacteria are harvested and suspended in a saline or other appropriate solution isotonic with blood. The bacteria are inactivated using a suitable chemical agent (0.1% formalin) or by heating at 56°C. The suspension is stored at a temperature of 2 to 8°C for a period of 2 to 3 months to diminish its toxicity. The final suspension is made using a saline or other suitable solution isotonic with blood containing a suitable antimicrobial preservative. The opacity is again adjusted to 40,000 million organisms per CC. The adsorbed vaccine is prepared by addition of aluminium phosphate, aluminium hydroxide or calcium phosphate.

DPT vaccine or Triple vaccine or Diphtheria – Tetanus – Pertussis vaccine:

DPT vaccine is prepared from Diphtheria Formol Toxoid, Tetanus Formol Toxoid and suspension of killed *Bordetella pertussis*. These three components are mixed in the following proportions to form DPT vaccine.

Pertussis vaccine	–	0.5 CC
Diphtheria Toxoid	–	0.2 CC
Tetanus Toxoid	–	0.3 CC

Merthiolate (0.01%) is commonly added as a preservative immediately before mixing and then the preparations to form DPT vaccine are mixed. The antigenic properties of DPT vaccine are adversely affected by exposure to the action of certain antimicrobial preservatives like phenol and some of the quaternary ammonium compounds.

10.6 VIRAL VACCINES

Viral vaccines are prepared by using free living animals, fertile eggs and tissue cultures. Viruses require a living medium for growth unlike bacteria which can grow on non-living media. Viruses are responsible for infectious diseases in man, animals and plants. Important viral diseases are influenza, common cold, measles, mumps, poliomyelitis, smallpox, yellow fever, rabies etc. For preparation of viral vaccines, viruses are usually grown in the chorioallantoic membrane of incubated fertile hen eggs or in whole animals. Preparation techniques of some viral vaccines are described as follows:

Poliomyelitis vaccine (inactivated or salk-formalin vaccine):

Inactivated poliomyelitis vaccine is an aqueous suspension of suitable strains of poliomyelitis virus, type I, II and III, grown in suitable cell cultures and inactivated by a suitable method.

Preparation: The three types of poliomyelitis virus are grown separately in either suspended or fixed cell cultures of monkey kidney tissue (Rhesus monkey kidney). Nerve cells are avoided because these cells have a short life in tissue culture and sometimes cause an allergic reaction in the brain. After the virus suspension has been harvested it is tested to confirm the presence of poliomyelitis virus, good virus titre and absence of viral, bacterial and fungal contaminants. It is passed through filters to remove remaining tissue cells and bacterial cells. The vaccine is inactivated by using formaldehyde (0.01%), under controlled conditions of pH and temperature with constant stirring. Inactivation is usually completed in six days but the absence of active virus should be confirmed. The suspension is refiltered and after 9 to 12 days, the suspension is retested for absence of infective virus.

The univalent vaccines are then blended to give the trivalent product and again tested for sterility and freedom from infective virus.

Finally, formaldehyde is neutralized with sodium metabisulphite and thiomersal is added as a bactericide.

Poliomyelitis vaccine (live oral or sabin vaccine): Sabin poliomyelitis vaccine is an aqueous suspension of suitable live, attenuated strains of poliomyelitis virus, types I, II or III, grown in suitable cell cultures. It may contain any one of the three virus types or a mixture of two or three of them.

It is manufactured essentially in the same way as Salk-Type vaccine except:

(i) Attenuated strains, prepared by rapid passages through tissue cultures of monkey kidney cells are used.

(ii) The virus in the final vaccine must not represent more than three subcultures from a strain that laboratory and clinical tests have shown to be satisfactory.

(iii) There is no inactivation stage.

(iv) Final vaccine is free from bacteria, moulds, viruses as well as virulent poliomyelitis virus.

For primary immunization, oral poliovirus vaccine is generally given at birth and then at 6, 10 and 14 weeks. Booster doses are given between 15 to 18 months. Oral poliovirus vaccine is the vaccine of choice for active immunization of children because it is simple to administer, is well accepted, induces systemic as well as intestinal immunity and is highly efficacious. Simultaneous vaccination of all infants and children upto 5 years age (pulse polio programme) has eradicated the wild virus in many countries.

10.7 ANTITOXIC SERA

Antisera or immunosera are preparations which contain antibodies. If the blood of an immune person or animal is withdrawn and allowed to clot, a large number of antibodies are found in the serum that separates. A serum may contain antitoxic, antibacterial or antiviral antibodies and these are known as antitoxic, antibacterial or antiviral serum respectively. Antitoxic sera are commonly known as 'antitoxins'. Antitoxic sera are more effective than antibacterial or antiviral sera.

Diphtheria antitoxin:

Diphtheria antitoxin is a sterile, non-pyrogenic solution containing the specific antitoxic antibodies obtained from the serum of healthy horses and have the power of neutralizing the toxin formed by *Corynebacterium diphtheriae*.

Preparation: The method of preparation of the Diphtheria antitoxin is divided into the following steps:

(i) Preparation of toxin: A pure culture of *Corynebacterium diphtheriae* is grown in a suitable culture media at 37°C for 4 to 5 days. After incubation, 0.5% phenol is added and the culture media is filtered through bacteria proof filters. The filtrate (crude toxin) is converted into a toxoid.

(ii) Selection of horse: Horses are selected for production of Diphtheria antitoxin because they are easy to handle and readily produce antitoxins. Considerable quantity of blood can be withdrawn at a time without any ill effects.

The horses selected must be free from disease. Horses are kept in an isolated place for 7 days and then carefully examined for infectious diseases.

(iii) Active immunization of the horse: Diphtheria toxoid is given to the selected healthy horses for active immunization. The toxoid is injected into the muscles of the neck by intramuscular injection. The first dose of the toxoid is usually not more than 5 ml which is gradually increased daily or after 1 to 2 days for about 2 months and as much as 600 ml is injected for the final dose.

(iv) Separation of serum from the horse: After about 10 days of the injection of the final dose, about eight litres of blood is withdrawn aseptically into bottles containing an anticoagulant solution. Similarly two more collections each about eight litres of blood are made within the next eight days, after which the horse is given about 15 days rest. Then another course of the toxoid is repeated in similar doses to stimulate further antibody production. Blood is collected in three batches each about eight litres. Further courses of administration of the toxoid and bleeding are continued for 4 to 5 times or till the animal stops producing satisfactory antitoxins.

After the collection of the blood, it is allowed to clot to separate the serum. The serum contains antitoxin alongwith other proteins, such as beta-globulins, gamma globulins and albumins. Antitoxins are largely associated with beta-globulin.

(v) **Concentration and refinement:** Horse serum contains a high concentration of several other proteins which may cause undesirable reactions, such as anaphylactic shock or serum sickness. So these undesirable proteins are separated by fractional precipitation or by fractional proteolytic digestion method.

Diphtheria antitoxin has a potency of not less than 1000 IU/ml, in the case of antitoxins obtained from horse serum and not less than 500 IU/ml for antitoxins obtained from other animals.

Storage: Diphtheria antitoxin is stored in containers protected from light at a temperature between 2 to 8°C. It should not be allowed to freeze.

Dose: Diphtheria antitoxin is administered by subcutaneous or intramuscular injection. For prophylactic use, the dose is not less than 1500 IU and for therapeutic use, the dose is not less than 50,000 IU.

Use: Passive immunising agent for diphtheria.

Tetanus antitoxin:

Tetanus antitoxin is a preparation containing antibodies that have the power of specifically neutralizing the toxins formed by *Clostridium tetani.* It is obtained by fractionation from the serum of horses or other mammals, that have been immunised against Tetanus toxins.

Method of preparation, storage and dose are similar to diphtheria antitoxin.

10.8 ANTIVIRAL SERA

These are used in passive immunization against certain viruses. It acts differently as viruses are intracellular parasites while antibodies can not penetrate the cells. Inactivation of viruses takes place in body fluids or on surfaces at which invasion occurs. The main source of antiviral antibodies is human serum. This is because the horse is not susceptible to many viruses against which protection may be required e.g. measles, rubella, poliomyelitis etc. However, official antiviral sera (e.g. rabies antiserum) is prepared in horses.

Rabies Antiserum or Antirabies Serum (ARS): Antirabies Serum (equine rabies immunoglobulin, ERIG) is a refined, concentrated and lyophilized serum from horses hyperimmunized by repeated injections of fixed rabies virus. Horses are injected with dead virus and when a good level of immunity has developed, are injected with live virus. The methods of protein purification used to refine the serum are designated to separate the gamma-globulin fraction that contains the antiviral antibodies. Antirabies serum is indicated promptly after suspected exposure and is given simultaneously with Rabies vaccine to non-immunized individuals.

QUESTIONS

(A) Objective Type Questions:

1. Define 'vaccines'. Classify the different immunological products.
2. What is a viral vaccine? Give names of two killed or attenuated viral vaccines.
3. Differentiate the following:
   (a) Vaccine and toxoid (b) Killed vaccine and attenuated vaccine

(B) Short Answer Questions:

1. What is a mixed vaccine? Explain in short any one mixed vaccine.
2. Write notes on:
   (a) Quality control of vaccines (b) Formol toxoid
   (c) Storage and stability of official vaccines

(C) Long Answer Questions:

1. Explain the general method for preparation of bacterial vaccines.
2. Explain in short, the method of preparation, storage and dose of Diphtheria Antitoxin.

(D) Multiple Choice Questions:

1. Select polyvalent vaccine ______ .
   (a) DPT (b) MMR
   (c) Polio (d) Diphtheria
2. BCG vaccine is a type of ______ .
   (a) Killed vaccine (b) Live attenuated vaccine
   (c) Recombinant vaccine (d) None of the above
3. Which of the following are live viral vaccines?
   (a) Rabies (b) Cholera
   (c) Influenza (d) Small pox
4. Which of the following vaccines is mainly administered at the birth of a child?
   (a) MMR (b) BCG
   (c) DPT (d) DPTC
5. Killed bacterial vaccine is ______ .
   (a) MMR (b) Small pox
   (c) Rabies (d) Pertussis
6. The main limitation of an attenuated vaccine is ______.
   (a) Stability (b) Storage
   (c) Recombination (d) Reveral of virulence
7. Typhoid vaccine IP is a sterile suspension or a freeze dried solid prepared from______.
   (a) *Staphylococcus aureus* (b) *Pseudomonas aeruginosa*
   (c) *Mycobacterium tuberculosis* (d) *Salmonella typhi*

■■■

Chapter ... 11

HYBRIDOMA TECHNOLOGY

♦ LEARNING OBJECTIVES ♦

After completing this chapter, reader should be able to understand:

- *Introduction*
- *Production of Monoclonal Antibody*
  - *Large Scale Production of Monoclonal Antibodies*
  - *Characterization and Quality Control of Monoclonal Antibodies*
- *Applications of Monoclonal Antibody*

11.1 INTRODUCTION

Antibodies are produced in response to antigens, which are either protein or polysaccharide molecules which may be foreign to the body. Monoclonal antibody means antibody produced by a cell clone derived from a fusion of one antibody producing cell with one myeloma cell. Such a fused cell, which was originally described as hybrid-myeloma, was named as hybridoma. Hybridoma technology for the production of antibodies was introduced by **Cesar Milstein** and **Georges Kolher** (1975). Hybridomas are somatic cells hybrids produced by fusing antibody forming spleen cells with myeloma cells. The antibody produced by lymphocytes is homogeneous because it is all drived from the single homogeneous clone of cells. Hence, it is called a monoclonal antibody or M-protein. These antibodies are conventionally obtained by hybridoma technique and recently by recombinant DNA technology.

The advantages of monoclonal antibodies are as follows:

1. Pure antibodies are produced from crude antigen preparations.
2. Antibodies produced are of single immunoglobulin class and specific for single epitope.
3. *In-vitro* or *in-viro* production is possible with a high production rate.
4. Antiserum titer values obtained are very high.
5. High reproducibility with respect to specificity and avidity.
6. Antibodies with high avidity can be produced.
7. Radiolabelling and fluorescent conjugation or enzyme marking of monoclonal antibodies are easy.
8. Dynamics of mutation in antibody forming cells can be studied.

The limitations of monoclonal antibodies are as follows:

1. Monoclonal antibody production is costly and a time consuming method.
2. Monoclonal antibodies do not form a precipitate in a standard double-immuno-diffusion method.
3. Poor compliment fixation capabilities.
4. The energy of binding to an antigen is strong in case of monoclonal antibodies. It is undesirable for the purification process (chromatography).

11.2 PRODUCTION OF MONOCLONAL ANTIBODY

Monoclonal antibodies are mainly produced by hybridoma technology. Details of conventional hybridoma technology used for the production of monoclonal antibody is described in the following steps:

- Immunization of mice with immunogen.
- Fusion of plasma cells with myeloma cells.
- Selection of hybrid cells.
- Growth and cloning of hybrid cells.
- Purification and storage of hybridoma cells.
- Human monoclonal antibody.

Immunization of mice is achieved by injecting immunogen mixed with an adjuvant (Freund's adjuvant or aluminium salts). The antigen is given by intradermally or subcutaneously at multiple sites repeatedly. Generally, 50 μg of antigen is administered per mouse per injection. The choice of immunization schedule depends on the antigen and the type of antibodies required. Serum of mice is assayed for antibody titre and desired specificity. When concentration of antibodies is found optimum then the animal is sacrificed. The spleen, which contains a large number of plasma cells is dissociated into single spleenocytes by mechanical or enzymatic method.

The spleenocytes are fused *in-vitro* with murine lymphocytic tumour cells (myeloma cells). The fusing agent can be a defective virus (sendai virus), chemicals (e.g. polyethylene glycol, PEG) or electrofusion. Polyethylene glycol binds to glycoproteins on surface of the cells and through complex events, dissolves the plasma membrane resulting in mixing of the contents of both cells to get hybrid cells. Cell fusion is performed by adding 50% polyethylene glycol solution to the cell pellet containing both spleen cells and myeloma cells in equal proportion. All cells are incubated at 37°C for 1 hr. and then plated. The resulting fusion mixture contains hybrid cells as well as unfused lymphocytes and myeloma cells. This separation of the correctly fused cells is done by a chemical way. The fusion cocktail is distributed on a number of 96-well plates filled with HAT medium (Hypoxanthine-Aminopterin-Thymidine).

Selection of hybrid cells is performed in HAT medium. This medium allows the growth of only hybrid of lymphocyte and myeloma cells but does not allow the growth of myeloma fusion partner or lymphocyte. Myeloma cells are unable to synthesize hypoxanthine gaunine phosphoribosyl-transferase (HGPRT). This enzyme is useful for synthesizing nucleotide by using extra-cellular source of hypoxanthine as precursor. Hence, unfused myeloma cells can not survive in HAT medium. The unfused spleen cells from immunized animal eventually die in tissue culture as they have finite life. The only cells surviving and dividing in the HAT medium contain the tumour component (myeloma cells) and a component from spleen lymphocytes. These, hybrid cells are called as hybridoma (Fig. 11.1). The cell mixture is allowed to grow in HAT medium for 7 to 10 days. Most of the cells contain dead cells with a few small clusters of viable cells. Each cluster represents clonal expansion of a hybridoma.

Screening hybridomas for the desired antibodies is the important step in production of monoclonal antibodies. The supernatant of the cell cultures in each individual well are tested by Western blotting and ELISA on the presence of antigen-specific antibodies and hybridoma cells of each positive well frozen in liquid nitrogen. Non-electrophoretic blotting of antigens on nitrocellulose and passive binding on polystyrene or polyvinyl chloride 96-well plates are frequently used to screen large numbers of hybridomas. Once pure clones of antibody secreting hybridoma cells are obtained, they are transferred to HAT medium in tissue culture flasks. They are removed from the flasks and transferred to regular culture medium after appropriate incubation time. All aliquots are distributed into the well of 96-well plastic culture plates. The supernatant of each culture can be assayed for antigen specificity by ELISA, RIA or immunofluorcent techniques.

Single cells secreting the desired antibody are isolated from positive cultures and propagated into cell lines. Limiting dilution and soft agar are most widely used cloning techniques. In limiting dilution cloning, the cells in the culture are diluted and aliquoted into new wells, ideally to have one cell in each well. The resulting cell culture is obtained from only one 'mother cell' and therefore secrete only one unique antibody. In soft agar cloning, heterogeneous mixture of hybrid cells are separated by localising, growth of single cells in soft agar. The visible colonies (monoclonal) can be picked up from the agar with a Pasteur pipette and then grown in 24 well plates. Yield of monoclonal antibody in tissue culture flasks is 10 to 100 μg/ml. The yield is improved by propagating cells in the peritoneal cavity of histocompatible mice, where monoclonal antibodies are secreted into ascitie fluid in concentration of 1 to 25 mg/ml.

Antibodies obtained from the tissue culture fluids or the ascitic fluids from mouse can be purified by biochemical methods of salt precipitation. Purification is employed to remove contaminants such as proteins, nucleic acids, endotoxins and process additives. Immunological methods of affinity chromatography with protein A or antiimmunoglobulin columns can also be used. The choice of method for purification depends on the source, purity and stability of the antibody. Hybridoma cells are suspended containing 10% dimethyl sulphoxide in culture medium with serum for storage. Cells are frozen at – 80°C slowly by various methods and then transferred to liquid nitrogen having a temperature of – 197°C. Hybridoma cells are stored for long time by this process of cryopreservation without loss of viability.

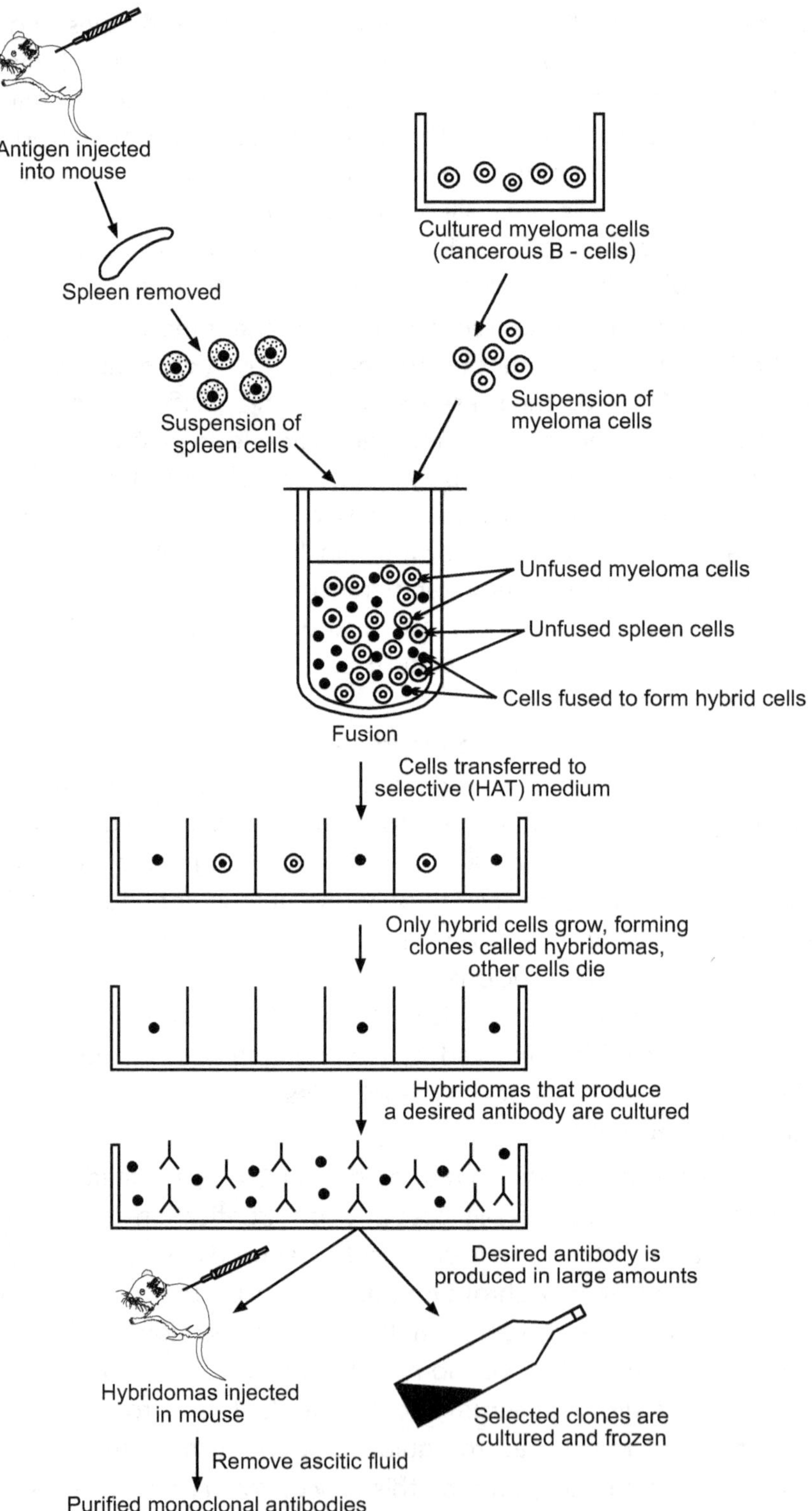

Fig. 11.1: Production of monoclonal antibody

The homogencity and specificity of monoclonal antibodies make them particularly suitable for *in-vivo* administration in humans for diagnostic or therapeutic purposes. The most common method of generation of human hybridomas secreting human monoclonal antibodies involves fusion of Epstein Barr Virus (EBV) transformed human B-lymphocytes with appropriate fusion partners. Lymphocytes are cultured with antigen in the presence of EBV to secrete desired antibody. The major difficulty in this method is to cause cancer (presence of EBV) and removal of Epstein Barr Virus (EBV) DNA is difficult and expensive. Vaccination of B-cell donor, prestimulation of B-cells to bring in appropriate growth phase and generation of a fusion partner are main requirements for generation of human hybridoma. Human myeloma cell fusion is another method for preparation of human hybridomas.

11.2.1 Large Scale Production of Monoclonal Antibodies

Commercially monoclonal antibodies are produced by mouse ascitic fluid (*in-vivo*) and tissue culture method (*in-vitro*).

Mouse ascitic fluid: In this method, hybridoma cells are injected into the peritoneal cavity of histocompatible mice. The peritoneal cavity of the mouse constitutes an ideal medium for the growth of hybridoma. The mice are pretreated by injection of pristane to irritate the peritoneal cavity and to establish a conditioned environment that facilitates the growth of ascitic tumor. The fluid can produce high concentration of secreted monoclonal antibodies in the range of 7 to 10 mg/ml. The main disadvantage of this production method is the animal suffer during the production and must be killed. The method is not reliable, costly and product may be contaminated with normal mouse antibodies and proteins.

Tissue culture method: The alternative method to produce monoclonal antibodies is by cell culture followed by purification of the secreted antibodies from the culture medium. Tissue culture scaling can be done by preparing many flasks of the antibody secreting clone. The culture volume can be increased by using spinner cultures or tissue culture trays. In case of human hybridoma usually tissue culture methods are used for scaling up.

11.2.2 Characterization and Quality Control of Monoclonal Antibodies

Analysis of potential monoclonal antibody producing hybridoma in terms of reactivity, specificity and cross reactivity can be performed using culture supernatant or a purified immunoglobulin preparation. Genetic stability of the cells lines may be determined by monitoring its properties during serial passage of the cells through culture. The properties includes size, shape and number of the chromosome, biochemical properties of the immunoglobin product and various growth and metabolic characteristics. The physical and chemical stability of the antibody can be determine during different conditions of storage and use. It is also characterized to define its affinity for antigen, immunoglobulin subclass, the epitopes for which it is specific and the effective number of binding site that it possesses by ELISA, Westeron blot and immuno-fluorescence. Characteristics of monoclonal antibodies are compared with polyclonal antibodies in several aspects. (Table 11.1)

Quality control tests are performed to assess residual impurities from the production sources and contamination with adventitious agents. Check the hybridoma cell lines for the stability, identity and absence of adventitious agents (viruses and mycoplasm). Testing of the final product of monoclonal antibodies is performed for its sterility, purity, potency, identity, apyrogenicity and safety.

Table 11.1: Comparisons of monoclonal antibodies with polyclonal antibodies

Sr. No.	Monoclonal antibodies	Polyclonal antibodies
1.	Specificity for only one antigenic determinant.	Specificity for all the determinants of an antigen.
2.	Composed of pure, single molecular species.	Composed of polyvalent antibodies.
3.	High reproducibility with respect to specificity and avidity.	Less reproducible for specificity and avidity.
4.	Antibody reactivity and titre is high.	Antibody reactivity and titre is low.
5.	Prepared by tissue cultures (*in-vitro*) and Ascites (*in-vivo*)	Prepared by using horses and human (*in-vivo*)
6.	Poor complement fixation and do not participates in standard double-immuno diffusion assay.	Better complement fixation and easily participates in standard double-immunodiffusion assay.
7.	Low cross-reactions are observed with monoclonal antibodies.	Polyclonal antibodies are easily cross reacts with other antigens.

11.3 APPLICATIONS OF MONOCLONAL ANTIBODY

Monoclonal antibodies have a remarkable range of applications in diagnostics, therapeutics, investigations and drug targeting (Table 11.2).

Table 11.2: Applications of monoclonal antibodies

Sr. No.	Main application	Examples
1.	Diagnosis	
	(a) Diagnostic reagents	Infectious diseases, pregnancy, tumours, HLA typing, diabetes.
	(b) Diagnostic imaging	Cardiovascular diseases, cell surface markers, detection of circulating antigens, cancer and hormones.
2.	Therapeutics	Autoimmune disease, cancer, cardiovascular diseases, bone marrow and organ transplant, toxin-drug conjugate, antidotes, enzymes and proteins.
3.	Investigations and Analytical	Radioimmunoassay, ELISA, lymphocyte phenotyping, autoantibody, finger printing, purification of proteins.
4.	Drug targeting	Antibody enzyme conjugates, immunotoxins, site specific modification.
5.	Miscellaneous	Autoantibody finger printing, catalytic monoclonal antibodies.

1. Diagnostic applications:

(a) Diagnostic reagents: Monoclonal antibody based diagnostic reagents are used for detecting pregnancy, diagnosing infectious organisms like bacteria, protozoa, viruses; monitoring therapeutic drug levels, matching histocompatibility antigens, detecting diabetes and tumor cells. All these test kits employ strips of paper impregnated with appropriate monoclonal antibodies.

(b) Diagnostic imaging: Radiolabelled monoclonal antibodies are employed in diagnostic imaging by using planner gamma camera (immuno-scintiography). Recently, camera utilizing single photon emission computed tomography (SPECT) has been used for three dimensional evaluations. Radioisotopes used in imaging are ^{123}I, ^{125}I, ^{131}I, ^{111}In and ^{99m}Tc. Various imaging applications of monoclonal antibodies are diagnosis of cardiovascular diseases like myocardial infarction and deep-vein thrombosis, sites of bacterial infections, sexually transmitted diseases and cancers.

In myocardial infarction, antimyosin MAb conjugated with chelator diethyl triamino penta acetic acid (DTPA), labelled with approximately 2 mCi of ^{111}In chloride. After incubation for about one minutes, the ^{111}In-labelled MAb is injected intravenously. Imaging is performed after 24 to 48 hours using a planner gamma camera or SPECT. Indium antimyosin is able to detect the location and extent of necrotic heart tissue. Deep vein thrombosis (DVT) is an ideal disease for imaging applications and in it labelled monoclonal antibodies are directed against platelets or fibrin. This technique is useful during the acute phase of thrombogenesis and ^{111}In-labelled Fab-DTPA is employed with imaging after 4 hours of injection.

Monoclonal antibodies have important applications in cell surface diagnosis. Anti-ABO, anti-rare blood groups and anti-HLA monoclonal antibodies are produced by immunizing mouse with corresponding antigen and are practically useful in blood group detection. The human major histocompatability complex, MHC (HLA antigen) is involved in important immunological processes, e.g. graft rejection, graft-versus-host reactions (GVH), cytotoxic reactions, cellular co-operation etc. The human leukocytes in the immunlogical processes are being detected using the antisera obtained from multiparous women. The process is called HLA tissue typing. Specific monoclonal antibodies against different cell surface antigenic determinants are employed in the study of different cells, e.g. rheumatoid arthritis, multiple sclerosis, systemic lupus erythroematosus (SLE) etc. Changes in the cell surfaces can be potentially monitored with the help of monoclonal antibodies and hence used in the study of cell-cell interactions.

Monoclonal antibodies can also be used in the detection of tumours which shed tumour specific antigens into the blood. Primary or metastatic tumours can be detected by radio-labelled monoclonal antibody specific to tumour associated membrane proteins e.g. breast cancer cells labelled with ^{131}I. Monoclonal antibody to breast cancer cells labelled with the metal gadolinium (Gd) can be detected by magnetic resonance imaging (MRI).

Tumour markers such as carcinoembryonic antigen (α-fetoprotein, ferritin, human chorionic gonadotropin, prostatic acid phosphatase etc.) and transferrin receptors (oncogene products, gangliosides, epidermal growth factor receptor, tumour-associated cells surface antigens) are used in monoclonal antibody imaging. Monoclonal antibodies have been tested experimentally as immunotherapeutic agents for cancer. **Levy** and co-workers successfully treated a patient with B-cell lymphomas with anti-idiotype monoclonal antibodies. Monoclonal antibodies have also been used to prepare tumour-specific immunotoxins and it consists of the inhibitor chain of a toxin linked to an antibody against a specific tumours.

Monoclonal antibodies against hormones are produced to study hormones and their pathophysiological role in the body. Monoclonal antibodies are prepared against different hormones such as insulin, human chorionic gonadotropin (hCG), human growth hormone (hGH), progesterone, renin, gastrin, human thyroid stimulating hormone (TSH) etc. Elevation in the levels of the human chorionic gonadotropin (hCG) hormone is detected in pregnancy testing kits. This hormone mainly occurs in the female urine and the blood in the early phase of pregnancy. Urine from the female containing hCG is mixed with anti-hCG antibodies. The mixture is mixed with latex microspheres coated with hCG. If sample contains hCG, it binds with anti-hCG antibodies and it prevent binding of anti-hCG antibodies with latex microspheres. There is no agglutination that indicates the positive test. In non-pregnant women urine, absence of hCG results into agglutination (negative test). Pregnant women bearing baby with some genetic defects is detected by various biotechnological techniques employing monoclonal antibodies (RFLP, probing, DNA analysis, ELISA etc.). Monoclonal antibody based latex-agglutination inhibition tests are employed in rapid detection of drugs in urine. Detection of drugs like cocaine, morphine, barbiturates, methadone, amphetamine etc. is possible by using monoclonal antibodies.

2. Therapeutic applications:

Monoclonal antibodies or its conjugates are employed to bind an antigen to neutralize its biological effects or block the activity of growth factor receptor. Radioisotope immunoconjugates are used to deliver cytotoxic doses of radioactivity to target cells. ^{125}I, ^{131}I, ^{186}Re, ^{188}Re and ^{90}Y isotopes are potential radioisotopes for therapy. Toxin and drug immunoconjugates are evaluated for the delivery of potent toxin and drugs to target cells. Abrin, ricin, gelonin, diphtheria toxin, pokeweed antiviral protein etc. are used as toxins. The therapeutic agents conjugated with monoclonal antibodies are chlorambucil, doxorubicin, methotrexate, melphanan, vinca alkaloids etc.

Orthrochroime OKT_3 and murine intact IgG antibody directed against CD_3 antigen or T lymphocytes are successfully evaluated for organ transplantation. Monoclonal antibodies are evaluated for graft versus host (GVH) disease in bone marrow transplantation. e.g. ricin toxin immunoconjugate. Monoclonal antibodies against endotoxin have been studied in antibiotic therapy of bacteria and sepsis HA-1A is the first human monoclonal antibodies used for clinical studies. Monoclonal antibodies against microorganisms are used in the isolation, identification, detection, genetic variation and classification of microbes. Monoclonal antibodies are under investigation to be used in autoimmune diseases like rheumatoid arithritis and multiple sclerosis, cardiovascular diseases, cancer and as antidotes.

3. Investigational and analytical applications:

Monoclonal antibodies for membrane proteins are used in identification, characterisation and separation of lymphocytes from cell population by using techniques like fluorescence activated cell sorter (FACS). It is also used for purification of proteins. **Secher** and **Burke** obtained highly purified sample of interferon from white blood cells. Monoclonal antibodies have the potential to supplement conventional antibodies in a series of immunoassays.

4. Drug targeting:

In this technique, drugs are coupled to an antibody to get a hybrid molecule with specificity of the immunological ligand as well as retaining the therapeutic activity of the drug. A novel method used in targeting antitumour enzymes at tumour site with conjugating their non-toxic pro-drug with monoclonal antibodies. This technque is called Antibody-Directed Enzyme Pro-Drug Therapy (ADEPT). The enzymes to be targeted are chosen for their ability to convert non-toxic pro-drug precursors into active form. The enzymes studied by this technique includes alkaline phosphatase, carboxypeptidase, glucoronidase, lactamase, nitroreductase, cytosine deaminase etc. In targeted immunotherapy (suppresser deletion therapy), it utilizes monoclonal antibody conjugated with hematoprophyrin by using carbodiimide to detect T-suppressor cells. The method is employed in immuno-modulation when tumour bearing animal rejects their own tissues. Microscopic spherical vesicles (liposomes) consisted of phospholipid have recently been reported as a new immunological technique. Liposomes based diagnostic kits are used for a group of streptococci and respiratory syncytial virus.

5. Miscellaneous applications:

Catalytic monoclonal antibodies (Abzymes) are antibodies with highly specific enzymatic activity towards substrate. Hapten, structurally resembling the transition state of substrate undergoing enzymatic activity is complexed with carrier to render it antigenic. **Lerner** studied the development of immunoglobulin-gene libraries to produce antibodies and screened for catalytic activity. Abzymes can be employed to cut peptides at specific amino acid residues. A new class of autoantibodies has been identified in blood, saliva, perspiration etc. in normal humans. The patients suffering from rheumatic diseases are found to have autoantibodies that react to cellular components. The autoantibodies are collected from blood or saliva and examined for crime detection. This technique is known as autoantibody fingerprinting using dipsticks. Some of the monoclonal antibodies, which are currently in clinical trial are given in Table 11.3.

Table 11.3: Monoclonal antibodies in clinical trial

Antibody	Indication	Company	Trial Status
Orthoclone	Allograft	Orthobiotech	FDA approved
Coresevin M	Anticoagulant	Centocor	I
Rhu MAb-E25	Allergy	Genetech/Norvartis	III
Smart anti-CD3	Autoimmune disease	Protein design lab	II
Antegren	Multiple Scelerosis	Elan	II
Antova	SLE	Biogen	II
Vitaxin	Sarcoma	Medimmune	II
ABX - 1L8	Psoriasis	Abgenix	II
Infliximab	Crohn's disease	Centocor	FDA approved
Ova Rex	Ovarian cancer	Altarex	III
BEC2	Lung cancer	Merck Lga A	FDA approved
Syngis	RSV virus	Medimmune	FDA approved
PRO542	HIV virus	Progeneics	II
Protoxir	CMV virus	Protein design lab/ Novartis	III

QUESTIONS

(A) Objective Type Questions:

1. Define 'Monoclonal antibodies'.
2. Write advantages and disadvantages of monoclonal antibodies.

(B) Short Answer Questions:

1. Write short about following applications of monoclonal antibodies:
   (a) Therapeutic use
   (b) Diagnostic imaging
2. Differentiate between monoclonal antibodies and polyclonal antibodies.

(C) Long Answer Questions:

1. Explain in detail about production and purification of monoclonal antibodies by hybridoma technology.
2. Write the applications of monoclonal antibodies.

(D) Multiple Choice Questions:

1. Most potent antigenic substance is _______.
   (a) Monosaccharides (b) Disaccharides
   (c) Protein (d) Lipid
2. Hybridoma cell technology is widely used for producing _______.
   (a) Organ culture (b) Tissue culture
   (c) Recombinant vaccines (d) Monoclonal antibodies
3. _______ medium is used for selection of hybrid cells in production of monoclonal antibody.
   (a) PEG (b) HGPRT
   (c) FTM (d) HAT

■■■

Chapter ... 12

IMMUNOBLOTTING TECHNIQUES

♦ LEARNING OBJECTIVES ♦

After completing this chapter, reader should be able to understand:

- *Introduction*
- *Blotting techniques*
    - *Southern Blotting*
    - *Northern Blotting*
    - *Western Blotting*
- *Elisa : Enzyme Linked Immunosorbent Assay*

12.1 INTRODUCTION

Blotting techniques are applied in the isolation and quantification of specific nucleic acid sequences and in the study of the organization, intracellular localization, expression and regulation. These techniques describe the immobilization of sample nucleic acids on a nylon or nitrocellulose membranes. The blotted nucleic acids are then used as 'targets' in subsequent hybridization experiments. DNA, RNA and proteins are easily separated by blotting method. The main blotting procedures are:

- Southern blotting
- Northern blotting
- Western blotting or protein blotting
- Dot and slot blotting.

Enzyme immunoassay includes all assays based on the measurement of enzyme labelled antigen, hapten or antibody. Enzyme immunoassys are classified into two types: homogenous and heterogenous. Homogenous enzyme immunoassays can be used only for assay of drugs and not for microbial antigens and antibodies. In this assay, there is no need to separate the bound and free fractions so that the test can be completed in one step with all reagents added simultaneously. Enzyme multiplied immunoassay technique (EMIT) is an example of homogenous enzyme immunoassay. This is a simple assay method used for detection of cocaine, opiates, barbiturates or amphetamine in serum. Heterogenous enzyme immunoassay requires the separation of the free and bound fractions either by centrifugation or by absorption on solid surfaces and washing. It is therefore, a multistep procedure, with reagents added sequentially. The major type of heterogenous enzyme immunoassay is Enzyme Linked Immunosorbent Assay (ELISA).

12.2 BLOTTING TECHNIQUES

Blotting techniques are widely used analytical tools for the specific identification of desired DNA or RNA fragments. Blotting refers to the process of immobilization of sample nucleic acids on solid support. The blotted nucleic acids are then used as targets in the hybridization experiments for their specific detection.

12.2.1 Southern Blotting

The original method of blotting was developed by E. M. Southern (1975) to identify the locations of genes and other DNA sequences on restriction fragments separated by gel electrophoresis. In Southern blotting technique, a sample of DNA containing fragments of different sizes are subjected to electrophoresis using either polyacrylamide or agarose gel.

DNA molecule is cut into small fragments by restriction enzyme and passed through agarose gel by electrophoresis method. It results into separation of DNA molecules based on their size. The DNA is then denatured into single strands by exposing the gel to alkaline solution. Gel is added on the top of the buffer saturated filter paper. It is covered with nitrocellulose filter overlayed with dry filter paper (Fig. 12.1). The buffer moves from the bottom of filter paper by the capillary action and DNA is trapped in the nitrocellulose membrane. This process is known as blotting. The nitrocellulose membrane is removed from the blotting stack and DNA is permanently immobilized on the membrane by baking at 80°C or ultraviolet induced cross-linking.

Single-stranded DNA has a high affinity for nitrocellular filter membrane. Hence, the membrane is treated with a solution containing 0.2% each of Ficoll, polyvinylpyrrolidone and bovine serum albumin. This treatment prevents non-specific binding of the radioactive probe. The membrane is placed in a solution of labelled RNA, single-stranded DNA or oligodeoxynucleotide (probe). These labelled nucleic acid is used to detect and locate the complementary sequence, it is called probe. The probe containing the sequence of interest is hybridized or annealed with the immbolized DNA on the membrane. After the hybridization reaction, the membrane is washed to remove the unbound probes. The washed membrane is exposed to X-ray film that detects the presence of the radioactivity in the bound probe. The film is developed to reveal bands indicating positions in the gel of the DNA fragments that are complementary to the radioactive probe.

The Southern blotting technique is very sensitive method and it is used to map the restriction sites around a single copy gene sequence in any genome. It is also used in preparation of restriction fragment length polymorphism (RFLP) maps, DNA finger printing, identification of the transferred genes etc. Nitrocellulose paper being very fragile is now replaced by nylon membrane.

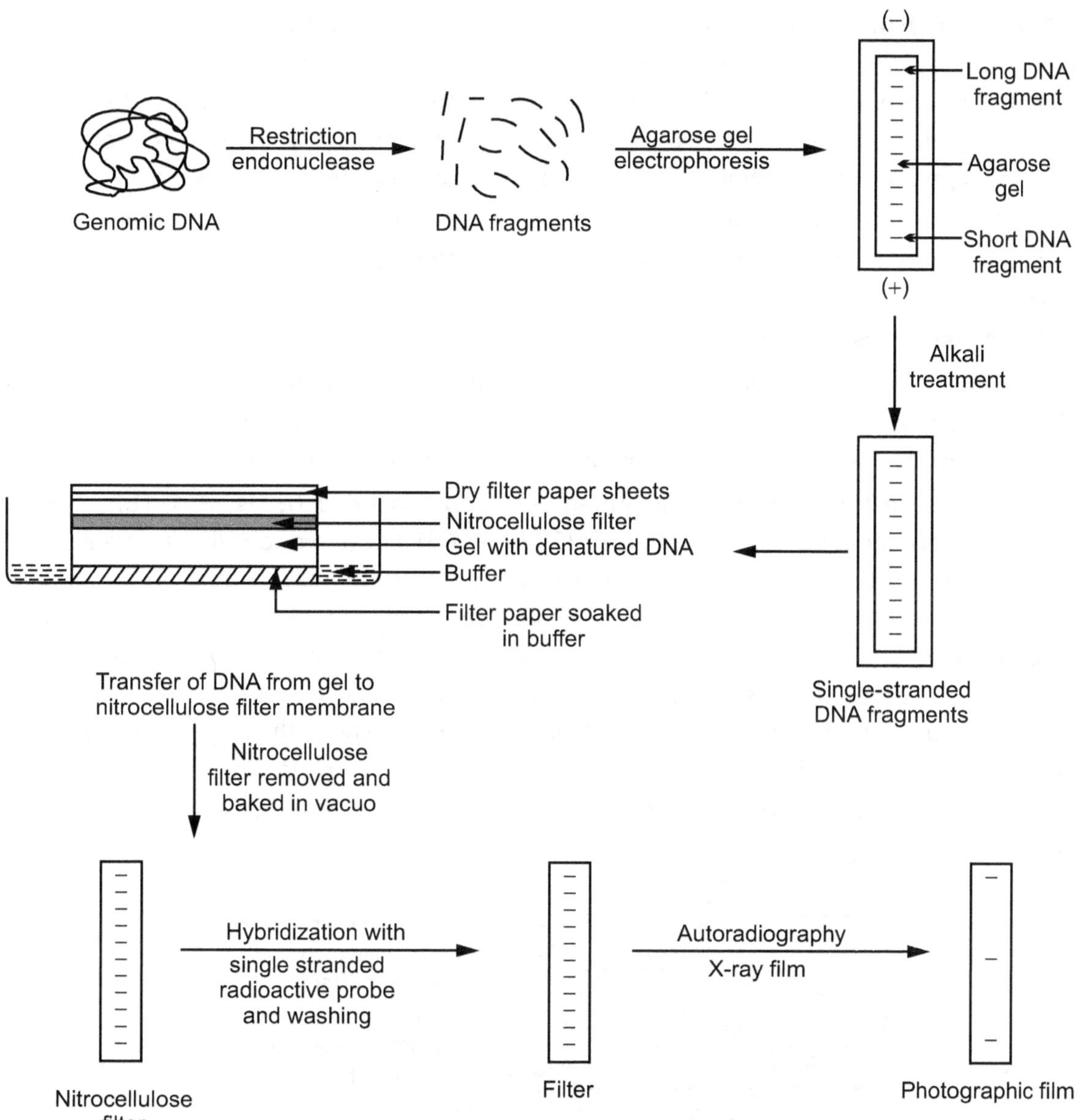

Fig. 12.1: Procedure of Southern blotting technique

12.2.2 Northern Blotting

Alwine et al (1979) devised a technique in which RNA bands are blot transferred from the gel onto chemically reactive paper. An aminobenzyloxymethyl cellulose paper prepared from Whatman paper 540 after a series of simple reactions. It is diazotised and rendered into the reactive paper. It becomes available for hybridization with radio-labelled DNA probes. The hybridized bands are found out by autoradiography. **Alwine's** method extends that of Southern method and hence, it has given the jargon term 'Northern blotting'.

Thomas (1980) found that mRNA bands can also be blotted directly on nitrocellulose paper under appropriate condition and it can be hybridized with a labeled DNA or RNA probe. Hybrids are treated with S-1 nuclease with RNAase which digests the single stranded RNA/DNA probe. Structure of mRNA is revealed to the extent to which mRNA protects the nucleic acid probe. In this technique, preparation of reactive paper is not required.

Northern blotting are mainly useful in studies of gene expression. It is also used to determine whether a particular gene is transcribed in all tissues of an microorganism or only certain tissues.

12.2.3 Western Blotting

Towbin et al (1979) developed the western blotting or protein blotting or electroblotting technique to find out the newly encoded protein by a transformed cell. Polyacrylamide gel electrophoresis is used for the separation and characterization of proteins.

Proteins are extracted from transformed cells and separated by using sodium dodecyl sulphate polyacrylamide gel electrophoresis (SDS – PAGE). Sodium dodecyl sulphate acts as a denaturant for proteins during electrophoresis. After electrophoresis, individual proteins are detected by using specific antibodies and polypeptides can also be transferred to a nitrocellulose membrane. The transfer of proteins from gels to nitrocellulose membranes is called western blotting. It is performed by using an electric current, hence, it is called electroblotting method (Fig. 12.2). Electric field is applied to cause the migration of proteins from the gel to nitrocellulose filter paper. Nitrocellulose membrane is used for probing with a specific labelled antibody. The antibody is labelled with ^{125}I and the signal is detected again with autoradiography.

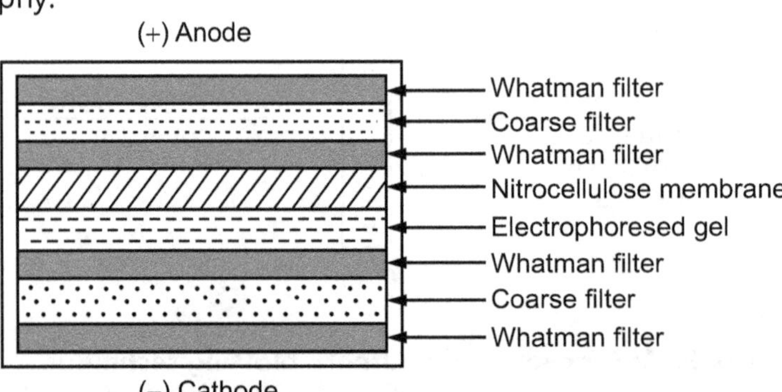

Fig. 12.2: Electroblotting or western blotting apparatus

12.3 ELISA: ENZYME LINKED IMMUNOSORBENT ASSAY

Enzyme linked immunoassay is an important immunological method for detecting and measuring antigens and antibodies. It is based on the same principle as that of radioimmunoassays. The main difference is that for enzyme immunoassays, the antigen or antibody is conjugated to an enzyme rather than a radioactive isotope. The enzyme is then detected by its ability to convert a colourless substance into a coloured one. Enzyme immunoassays have become very popular in view of their high sensitivity, safety, economy and the simple instrument requirements. The principle of ELISA (Fig. 12.3) is based on the following observations:

(i) Antigens and antibodies can attach to polystyrene plastic plates or other solid-phase support and maintain immunological capabilities.

(ii) Antigens and antibodies can be bonded to enzymes and the resulting complexes are fully functional both immunologically as well as enzymatically.

There are two important methods of enzyme immunoassay:

1. **Double-antibody-sandwich method:** Detection and measurement of antigen.
2. **Indirect ELISA method:** Detection and measurement of antibody.

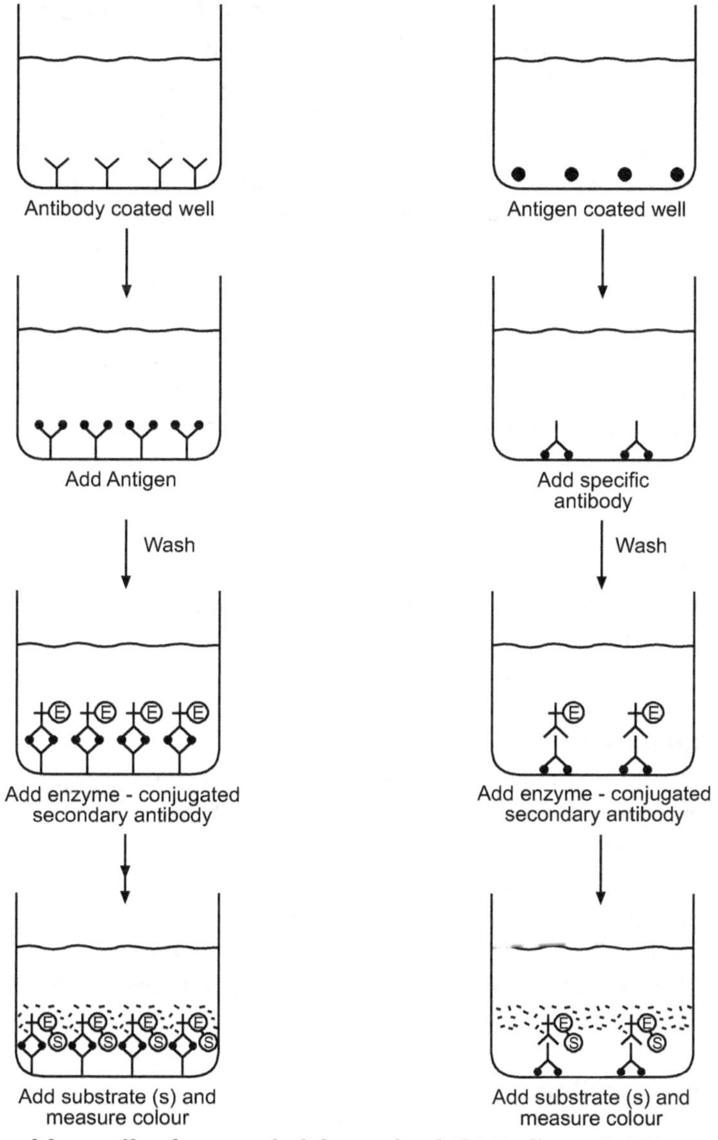

(a) Double-antibody - sandwich method (b) Indirect ELISA method

Fig. 12.3: ELISA

1. Double-antibody - sandwich method: In this technique, the wells or depressions in a polystyrene plate are first coated with an antibody and the sample containing antigen is then added and allowed to react with the bound antibody. The well is washed and the second enzyme linked specific antibody is added and allowed to react. This results in an antibody (with enzyme) – antigen-antibody sandwich. Finally, the enzyme substrate is added for reaction with the enzyme. The rate of enzyme action is directly proportional to the quantity of enzyme – labelled antibody present and that is proportional to the amount of test antigen (Fig. 12.3 (a)). Enzyme activity may be followed by a colour change which can be inspected visually or measured by a colourimeter. This method has been used to assay of hepatitis B-antigen.

2. Indirect ELISA method: The principle of this test can be illustrated by outlining its application for detection of anti-HIV–1 and anti-HIV–2 antibodies in the patient serum. The wells of the polystyrene microtitre plate are coated with antigen. Test antiserum is added and allowed to incubate. If the antibodies in the antiserum are homologous, they will bind to immobilized antigen. The well is then washed and enzyme - labelled antihuman antibodies are added to the system which link with the antibody-antigen complexes (Fig. 12.3 (b)). Finally, the enzyme substrate is added. The rate of its degradation (hydrolysis) is associated with a colour change proportional to the concentration of antibody present in the test sample. This colour change can be monitored visually or by a colourimeter.

ELISA is a simple and versatile technique. ELISA kits are commercially available for the detection of anti-HIV, hepatitis B surface antigen and rotavirus. ELISA kits have also been developed for detecting hepatitis - A - virus (from stools), *Haemophilus influenzae* antigens (from spinal fluid), *Toxoplasma* antigens (from serum), *Entamoeba histolytica* antigens (from faeces), *Escherichia coli* enterotoxin (from stools) etc.

QUESTIONS

(A) Objective Type Questions:

1. What is blotting? Explain.
2. List different blotting techniques with their applications.

(B) Short Answer Questions:

1. Explain the principle of ELISA.
2. Write the applications of ELISA test.

(C) Long Answer Questions:

1. Explain in detail principle and applications of Southern blotting.
2. Write the technique and importance of western blotting.

(D) Multiple Choice Questions:

1. ELISA test is used for detection of ______ .
   (a) Hepatitis B-antigen (b) Rotavirus
   (c) Antigen-HIV (d) All of the above
2. Southern blotting technique is commonly used for the specific identification of _____.
   (a) DNA (b) RNA
   (c) Protein (d) DNA and RNA
3. Western blotting method is used for identification of _____.
   (a) DNA (b) RNA
   (c) Protein (d) DNA and RNA

■■■

Chapter ... 13

EUKARYOTES AND PROKARYOTES

♦ LEARNING OBJECTIVES ♦

After completing this chapter, reader should be able to understand:

- *Introduction*
- *Microbial Genetics and Genome*
- *Genetic Organization of Prokaryotes*
- *Genetic Organization of Eukaryotes*

13.1 INTRODUCTION

Many biologists have accepted the system proposed by **Robert H. Whittaker** (1969) for the classification of living organisms. He proposed that all living beings can be classified under five kingdoms based on the nutrition and absorption of food materials. The prokaryotic organisms are included under the kingdom monera (lower protista). These organisms do not have the ingestive mode of nutrition. The unicellular eukaryotic microorganisms are placed in kingdom protista (higher protista). In microalgae it is photosynthetic, in protozoa it is ingestive and some other protista it is absorptive. Whittaker explained that some organisms assimilate carbon dioxide by means of photosynthesis while some obtaining through nutrients absorbed from other organisms and some obtaining organic nutrients by way of ingestion. He classified plants, fungi and animals in three separate kingdoms based on the mode of nutrition. In the scheme of Whittaker, microorganisms are accommodated in three of the five kingdoms.

This system places all living things (except viruses) into five kingdoms based on cellular organisation and nutritional patterns; the Monera, Protista, Fungi, Animalia and Plantae. Kingdom Monera includes all unicellular prokaryotes (e.g. bacteria, cyanobacteria) and Kingdom Protista includes unicellular eukaryotic cell (e.g. microalgae, protozoa). The multicellular and multinucleate eukaryotic organisms are found in the Kingdom Fungi, Kingdom Plantae and Kingdom Animalia which mainly utilize nutrients by absorption, photosynthesis and ingestion, respectively.

With the introduction of electron microscopy, it was made possible to observe internal cell structures. It was discovered (1940) that in some cells (e.g. typical bacteria), the genetic material was not enclosed by a nuclear membrane. In other cells (algae, fungi, protozoa), the nucleus was enclosed in a membrane. This resulted in the division of these organisms into Prokaryotes and Eukaryotes. Bacteria are prokaryotic (absence of nuclear membrane) microbes. Fungi, algae, protozoa, plant and animal cells are eukaryotic (presence of nuclear membrane) (Fig. 13.1). A comparison of prokaryotes and eukaryotes is given in Table 13.1.

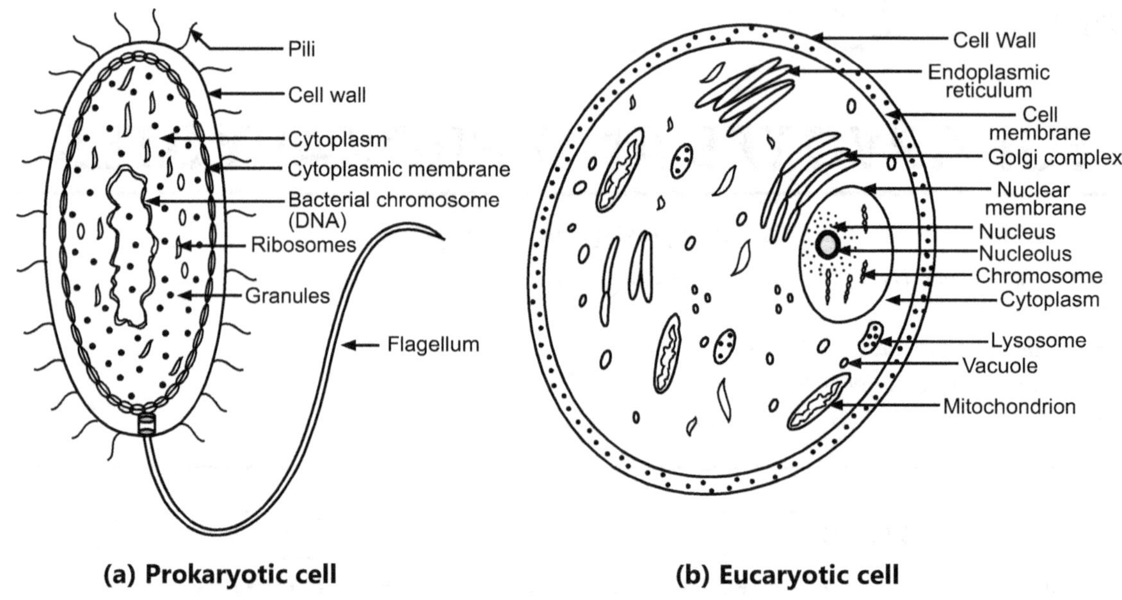

Fig. 13.1: Prokaryotic and Eukaryotic cell structures

The genome is the ultimate source of information about an organism. The word 'genome' coined by German botanist Hans Winkler (1920), was derived simply by combining 'gene' and 'chromosome'. Genome is all the DNA contained in an organism or a cell, which includes the chromosomes plus the DNA in mitochondria and DNA in the chloroplasts (plant cells). The first complete genome of bacterium *Haemophilus influenzae* was sequenced in 1995 and *Escherichia* coli in 1997. The first eukaryotic genome of *Saccharomyes cerevisiase* was sequenced in 1996. Prokaryotic genomes generally contain are large circular piece of DNA (chromosome) and eukaryotic DNA is divided between two are more chromosomes. The genome of *E. coli* contains 4×10^6 base pairs and genome of yeast cells contains 1.35×10^7 base pairs. The size of bacterial chromosomes ranges from 0.6-10 Mbp and eukaryotic chromosomes range from 2.9-4,000 Mbp.

Table 13.1: Comparison of Prokaryotes and Eukaryotes

Character	Prokaryotes	Eukaryotes
1. Nucleus:		
Nuclear membrane	Absent	Present
Nucleolus	Absent	Present
Chromosome	One (circular)	More than one (linear)
Mitotic division	Absent	Present
Deoxyribonucleoprotein	Absent	Present

contd. ...

2. Cytoplasm:		
Cytoplasmic streaming	Absent	Present
Pinocytosis	Absent	Present
Mitochondria	Absent	Present
Lysosomes	Absent	Present
Golgi apparatus	Absent	Present
Endoplasmic reticulum	Absent	Present
Chloroplasts	Absent	May be present
Membrane - bound (true) vacuoles	Absent	Present
Ribosomes	70S, distributed in the cytoplasm	80S arrayed one membranes as in endoplasmic reticulum, 70S in mitochondria and chloroplasts
Gas vacuoles	Can be present	Absent
Mesosomes	Present	Absent
3. Outer cell structures:		
Cytoplasmic membranes	Generally sterols absent	Sterols present
Cell wall	Peptidoglycan present	Peptidoglycan absent
Locomotor organelles	Simple fibril	Multifibirilled with 'g + z' microtubules.
Pseudopodia	Absent	Present in some.
4. Examples:	Bacteria, rickettsiae, chlamydiae, actinomycetes.	Fungi, protozoa, algae, plants, animals.

13.2 MICROBIAL GENETICS AND GENOME

Genome is the total genetic material of an organism. Living organisms classified into two categories as prokaryotes and eukaryotes. Prokaryotes are single celled organisms without membrane enclosed organelles. Hence, genetic material is present throughout the cell (cytoplasm). Prokaryotes have double stranded DNA molecules clustered into nucleoid. Prokaryotes often also have small circular pieces of DNA with only a small amount of genes called plasmids and can replicate independent of the chromosomal DNA. Eukaryotes have a specialized membrane enclosed organelle that contains the DNA (nucleus). Each nucleus contains multiple linear molecules of double stranded DNA, organized into 23 pairs of chromosomes. In eukaryote cell, mitochondria, chloroplasts contain their own DNA. Therefore, genome of eukaryote indicates entire genetic material contained within the cell.

The total amount of DNA (haploid content) in a genome is called C-value and this value is characteristic for a species. Genome size of some organisms are given in Table 13.2. The DNA of eukaryotes is tightly associated with specific proteins to form nucleoproteins whereas in the prokaryotes the DNA is mostly free of such structural proteins.

Table 13.2: Genome sizes of different organisms

Organism	Genome size (in base pairs)	Gene number
Hepatitis B virus	3.2×10^3	4
Vaccinia Virus	1.9×10^4	-
Bacteriophage	4.85×10^4	80
Escherichia coli	4.2×10^6	4400
Saccharomyces cerevisiae	12.15×10^6	6300
Drosophila	1.65×10^8	13600
Mammals	3×10^9	30,000
Mustard plant	1.25×10^8	25,500
Plasmodium falciparum	30×10^6	5,200
Homo sapiens (human)	32×10^8	22,000

Prokaryotes and eukaryotes are also significantly different in their structural organization. Most prokaryotes reproduce asexually and are haploid (single copy of each gene) but eukaryotes reproduce sexually containing multiple chromosomes and diploid (two copies of each gene). The organization of prokaryotic DNA differs from that of eukaryotes in several important ways (Table 13.3).

Table 13.3: Differences in prokaryotic and eukaryotic chromosomes

Prokaryotic	Eukaryotic
1. Many prokaryotes contain a single circular chromosome.	1. Eukaryotes contain multiple linear chromosomes.
2. Most prokaryotes contain only one copy of each gene (haploid).	2. Most eukaryotes contain two copies of each gene (diploid).
3. Prokaryotic genome are small in size.	3. Eukaryotic genome are larger than prokaryotic genome.
4. DNA found in cytoplasm (nucleiod).	4. DNA found in nucleus.
5. Genes do not contain introns.	5. Genes may contain introns.
6. Non-essential prokaryotic genes are commonly encoded on extra- chromosomal plasmids.	6. Extrachromosomal plasmids are not commonly present in eukaryotes.

contd. ...

7. Prokaryotic chromosomes are condensed in the nucleoid via DNA supercoiling and the binding of various architectural proteins.	7. Eukaryotic chromosomes are condensed in a membrane-bound nucleus via histones.
8. Prokaryotic genomes are efficient and compact containing little repetitive DNA.	8. Eukaryotes contain large amounts of non-coding and repetitive DNA.
9. Prokaryotic DNA can interact with the cytoplasm, transcription and translation occur simultaneously.	9. In eukaryotes, transcription occurs in the nucleus and translation occurs in the cytoplasm.

13.3 GENETIC ORGANIZATION OF PROKARYOTES

Most of well characterized prokaryotic genomes consist of circular, double-stranded DNA organized as a single chromosome (haploid) 0.6-10 Mb in length and one or more circular plasmid species of 2Kb-1.7 Mb. Prokaryotic DNA is supercoiled, requiring ATP and enzyme topoisomerase to uncoil DNA. Plasmids allow the cell to infect other surrounding cells and they are unlimited in bacteria. Prokaryotes do not contain histones, as they are not needed in binary fission (prokaryotic process) but they are needed in mitosis (eukaryotic process). Prokaryotic DNA is circular because there is only one strand of DNA and it is unprotected by nucleus. Prokaryotic cells do not contain introns, which are segments of DNA or RNA that do not code for proteins in a continuous genetic sequence.

DNA replication occurs in the cytoplasm of the cell and there is only one point of replication per DNA molecule. These are formed of about 100-200 nucleotides and two replication forks are used. DNA supercoiling is necessary for the genome to fit within the prokaryotic cell (Fig. 13.2). The DNA in the bacterial chromosome is arranged in several supercoiled domains. As with eukaryotes, topoisomerases are involved in supercoiling DNA. DNA gyrase (type of topoisomerase) found in bacteria and some archaea that helps to prevent the overwinding of DNA.

Transcription in prokaryotic cells occurs in the cytoplasm of the cells and there is no specific stage of the cell cycle in which it occurs. Single RNA polymerase synthesized the three types of RNA. There is no RNA processing and no initiation factors are needed for transcription. Gene expression refers to genotypes being exhibited by the phenotypes of organisms. It is the process from DNA to RNA to protein. In prokaryotic cell, genes are usually clustered onto the chromosome and it make use of operons to control gene expression. These operons can regulate transcription in response to environmental changes.

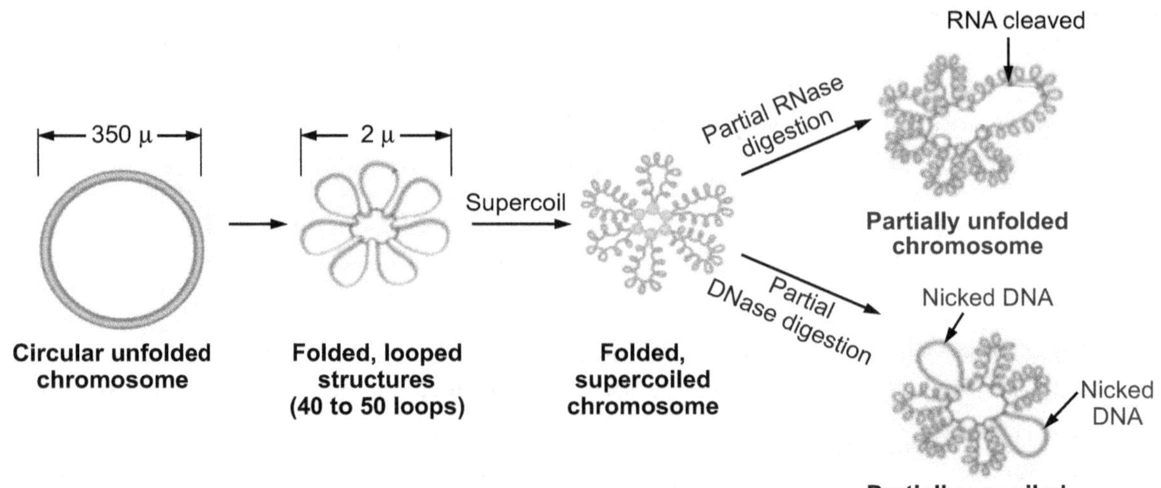

Fig 13.2: DNA supercoiling of Prokaryotic cell

Prokaryotic cells divided by the process of binary fission. In this process, the cell replicates its DNA and sequesters these copies to opposite ends of the cell without the help of spindle fibres. Then the cytoplasm is split and a new cell wall is formed.

13.4 GENETIC ORGANIZATION OF EUKARYOTES

Eukaryotic chromosomes are linear and it contains multiple distinct chromosomes. Many eukaryotic cells contain two copies of each chromosome (diploid). In addition of nucleus, mitochondria in animal and plant cells and chloroplasts in plant cells contain their own DNA. Eukaryotic chromosomes are comprised of linear DNA strands that are tightly coiled to form the condensed chromosomes. All DNA strands are tightly protected by proteins (histones) that allow the chromosomes to condense to develop the cell for the prophase stage is mitosis and meiosis. DNA-binding proteins (histones) perform various levels of DNA wrapping and attachment to scaffolding proteins. The combination of DNA with these attached proteins is referred as chromatin. The packaging of DNA by histones may be influenced by environmental factors that affect the presence of methyl groups on certain cytosine nucleotides of DNA. The influence of environmental factors or DNA packaging is called epigenetics. Eukaryotic DNA also contains introns, which are segments of genetic material that do not code for specific proteins. Introns are present in the initial RNA transcript (pre-mRNA) and they must be removed before mRNA transcription may occur in the cell. Eukaryotic cells contain chromatin DNA instead of coiled DNA. They are made of complex macromolecules of DNA, RNA and proteins.

The process by which DNA is twisted to fit inside the cell is called DNA supercoiling (Fig. 13.3). Supercoiling may result in DNA that is either underwound or overwound from its normal relaxed state. Protein involved in supercoiling is topoisomerases which helps to maintain the structure of supercoiled chromosomes, preventing overwinding of DNA during certain cellular processes.

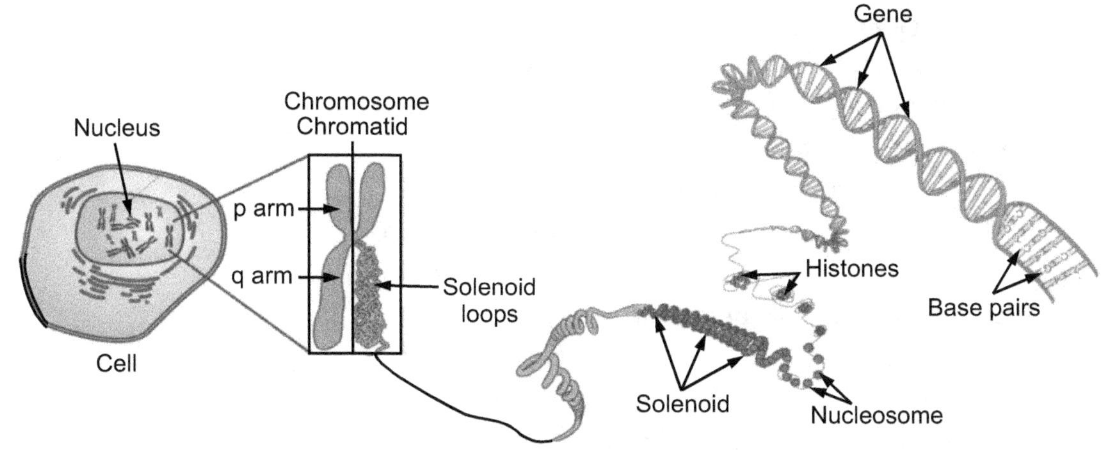

Fig 13.3: Genetic organization of Eukaryotic cell

DNA replication in eukaryotic cells occurs inside the nucleus as it also occurs in mitochondria and chloroplasts with their own DNA. In each eukaryotic chromosome, there are approx. 1000 origins of replication in which each consisting of about 150 nucleotides. Several replication forks are simultaneously formed in each replicating DNA molecule.

Transcription in eukaryotic cells occur in the nucleus as well as the mitochondria and chloroplasts and it takes place during the G_1 and G_2 phases of the cell cycle. RNA polymerase II and III synthesize three kinds of RNA (mRNA, rRNA, and tRNA). The mRNA has a primary transcript with surplus nucleotides. Gene expression can not occur where the DNA is too compact, which is controlled by histones. Epigenetics is another mechanism for regulating gene expression without altering the sequence of nucleotides. Enhancers and silencers control the rate of transcription within the cell.

Eukaryotic cells divide by mitosis and meiosis process. These are two complex processes that systematically replicate and condense chromosomes for replication. In mitosis and meiosis processes, use spindle fibers to transfer genetic material on the same chromosome to opposite ends of the cell.

QUESTIONS

(A) Objective Type Questions:

1. Draw the structure of Prokaryotic cell
2. Define the term with suitable examples:
   (a) Taxonomy
   (b) Prokaryotes

(B) Short Answer Questions:

1. Differentiate between Prokaryotic cell and Eukaryotic cell.
2. Write note on Eukaryotic cell.

(C) Long Answer Questions:

1. Write in detail genetic organization of Eukaryotes.
2. Explain in detail genetic organization of Prokaryotes.

(D) Multiple Choice Questions:

1. ______ is Prokaryotic microorganism.
   (a) Fungi (b) Rickettsiae
   (c) Algae (d) Viruses
2. Chloroplasts are mainly present in ______
   (a) Animal cell (b) Plant cell
   (c) Bacterial cell (d) Fungal cell
3. ______ is mainly present in prokaryotic cell.
   (a) Mitochondria (b) Endoplasmic reticulum
   (c) Golgi apparatus (d) Mesosomes
4. Where does energy production occur in prokaryotes?
   (a) Mitochondria (b) Endoplasmic reticulum
   (c) Cytoplasmic membrane (d) Golgi apparatus
5. Prokaryotic genome contains ______
   (a) Linear chromosomes (b) Plasmids
   (c) Chloroplast DNA (d) Mitochondrial DNA
6. The structure of the typical eukaryotic genome describes as ______
   (a) Singular (b) Linear
   (c) Diploid (d) Double stranded
7. Histones are DNA binding proteins that are important for DNA packaging in ______
   (a) Eukaryotes and bacteria (b) Eukaryotes and archaea
   (c) Bacteria and archaea (d) Bacteria and viruses.
8. The proteins associated with DNA is ______
   (a) Glycoprotein (b) Histone
   (c) Lipoprotein (d) None of above
9. The prokaryotic chromosome is a single circle of ______
   (a) ss DNA (b) ss RNA
   (c) ds DNA (d) ds RNA

■■■

Chapter ... 14

MICROBIAL GENETICS

♦ LEARNING OBJECTIVES ♦

After completing this chapter, reader should be able to understand:

- *Introduction*
- *Transformation*
- *Transduction*
  - o *Generalised Transduction*
  - o *Specialised Transduction*
- *Conjugation*
- *Plasmids*
- *Transposons*
- *Mutation*
  - o *Types of Mutation*
  - o *Mutagenic Agents*
  - o *Spontaneous Mutation*

14.1 INTRODUCTION

Genetics is the study of inheritance (heredity) and the variability of the characteristics of an organism. Heredity concerns the exact transmission of genetic information from parents to their progeny. Variability of the inherited characteristics can be accounted for a change either in the genetic makeup of a cell or in the environmental conditions. Genes comprise the genome of cell which may consist of a single DNA molecule or some other small DNA molecules (plasmids). The genotypic variation brought about by changes in genetic information can be due to mutation or loss of plasmids. Each bacterium contains about 1000 genes which are located in its circular chromosome. If the book of information contained is a genome, then paragraph is a loci, the sentences are genes, words are codons and letters are nucleotides.

The 'Central dogma' of molecular biology is that deoxyribonucleic acid (DNA) carries genetic information, which is transcribed onto ribonucleic acid (RNA) and then translated, by ribosomes into particular polypeptide (DNA $\rightarrow$ RNA $\rightarrow$ Polypeptide). The essential material of heredity is DNA which is the storehouse of all information for protein synthesis. However, RNA viruses are an important exception in which the genetic material is RNA instead of DNA.

Genetic recombination is the formation of a new genotype by exchange of genetic material between two different chromosomes which have similar genes at corresponding sites (homologous chromosomes).

In bacterial recombination, usually only a portion of the chromosome from the donor cell (male) is transferred to the recipient cell (female). The recipient cell thus forms a merozygote and recombination can take place. Bacterial recombination may occur by direct or indirect gene transfer method or sexual or asexual process. Genetic recombination can occur by different types of gene transfer techniques i.e. conjugation, transduction, transformation, protoplast fusion etc.

14.2 TRANSFORMATION

Transformation is the process whereby cell free or naked DNA containing a limited amount of genetic information is transferred from one bacterial cell to another. The DNA is obtained from the donor cell by natural cell lysis or by chemical extraction. Donor DNA passes into recipient through the cell wall and cell membrane of the recipient cell. DNA having molecular weight from 3,00,000 to 8 million daltons is most suitable for transformation. Once DNA enters into a cell, it integrates into chromosome of recipient cell. One strand is degraded by deoxyribonucleases while other strand undergoes base pairing with a homologous part of the recipient cell chromosome and then becomes integrated into the recipient DNA (Fig. 14.1).

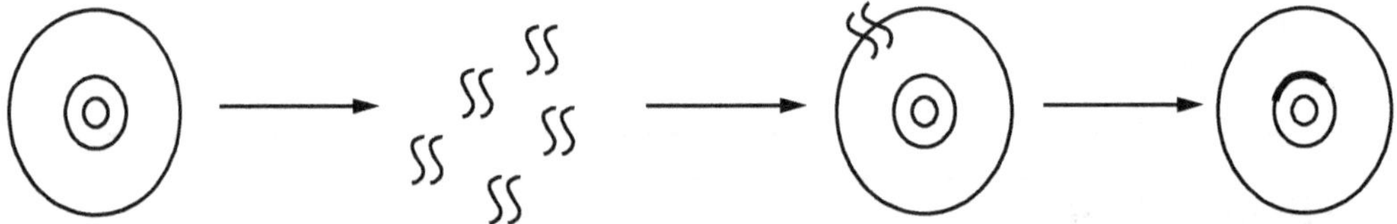

(a) Donor cell **(b) Donor DNA fragments** **(c) Binding of donor DNA fragments to recipient cell** **(d) Integration of single strand of donor DNA (Transformed cell)**

Fig. 14.1: Bacterial transformation

Bacterial transformation was first discovered by **F. Griffith** (1928) during his investigations of pneumococcal infections in mice. He had found that in *Streptococcus pneumonia*, virulence to mice was related to the presence of a capsular material and the absence of capsule made the bacteria avirulent. The wild type strain is surrounded by a polysaccharide capsule and forms a colony with a smooth (s) surface. This strain is pathogenic (virulent) and causes severe infection of pneumonia. A mutant strain does not have the capsule and it forms a colony with a rough (R) surface. The mutant (R) strain is non-pathogenic (avirulent). Griffith's experiments involved the infection of mice with heat killed and living preparations from two strains of *Streptococcus pneumoniae.* Injection of avirulent mutant 'R' bacteria or heat killed virulent 'S' bacteria did not cause any harm to mice. Injection of a mixture of the two bacterial types [R and S (heat-killed)] killed some mice and live, virulent 'S' bacteria recovered from these animals (Fig. 14.2). The strain 'R' type acquired the ability to produce capsules and become virulent. This induction in change of 'R' strain was called transformation. **Griffith** thought that the transferring agent was a protein.

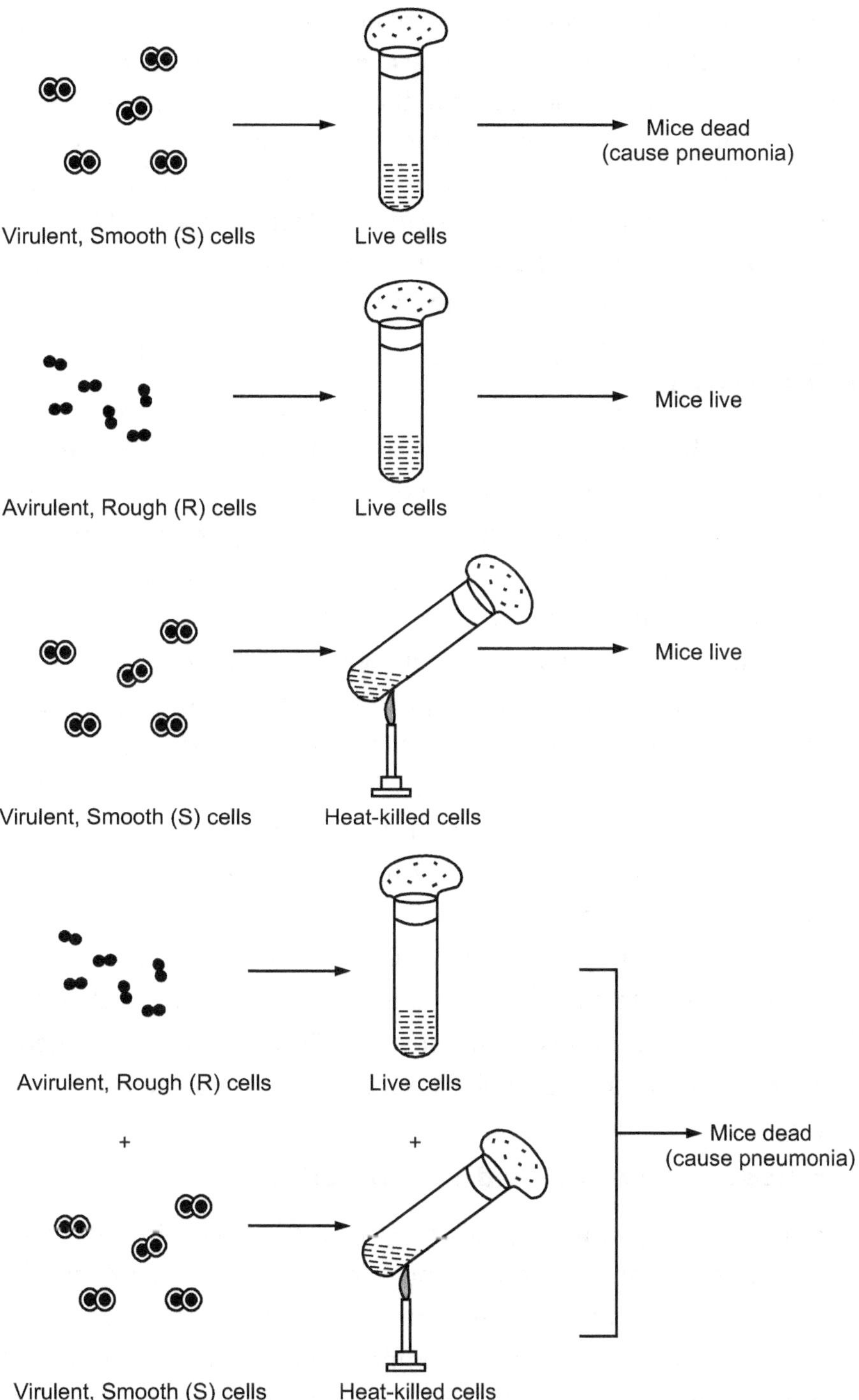

Fig. 14.2: Griffith's transformation experiment with *Streptococcus pneumonia*

Avery, **Macleod** and **McCarty** (1944) showed that the substance responsible for transformation was DNA. Their studies with purified DNA from the smooth (S) cells and its ability to transform rough cells in a test tube explained the observations made by **Griffith**. From this experiment, it was concluded that the heat killed capsulated cells carried the information for the synthesis of the capsule which was transferred to the live non-capsulated cells. Transformation has now been demonstrated in *Streptococcus, Bacillus, Escherichia, Neisseria, Hemophilus, Salmonella, Rhizobium, Xanthomonas, Staphylococcus* and *Streptomyces*. It is now possible to introduce intact plasmids by artificial transformation into bacteria, yeast, plants and animals. The development of artificial transformation is important for recombinant DNA technology.

14.3 TRANSDUCTION

The transfer of genetic material from one cell to another by a bacteriophage is called transduction. Bacterial genes may be transferred from strain to strain using bacteriophages as vectors. This genetic transfer technique was discovered by **Norman Zinder** and **Joshua Lederberg** (1952) while searching for sexual conjugation in *Salmonella* species. They mixed auxotrophic mutants together and isolated prototrophic recombinant colonies from selective nutritional media by using **Davis** U-tube experiment (Refer Fig. 14.3). Auxotrophic strains were added in each arm of U-tube and separated by a microporous sintered glass filter. The prototrophs were found in one arm of the tube that indicated some phenomenon other than conjugation was involved. It was subsequently observed that the active component was a bacteriophage which was carried by one of the strains in the prophage condition. Some bacterial cells have the ability to carry phage DNA within their own DNA and such cells are called as lysogenic bacteria. In such bacteria, the prophage, under certain conditions multiplies and destroys the host cell with the release of a number of phage particles. These phages can infect other bacteria and carry the bacterial DNA to the recipient cells. Such phages are called as 'transducing phages'. These are two fundamentally different transduction processes such as generalized (unrestricted) transduction and specialized (restricted) transduction.

14.3.1 Generalised or Unrestricted Transduction

Transduction mediated by virulent phages is called generalized transduction because it transfers any portion of the bacterial chromosome from one cell to another. Virulent phages infect bacteria by adhering to the surface of the host cell and inject the DNA into it. The phage DNA directs the cell to make phage components as DNA and protein. These phage components assemble into mature phage particles that are released from the cell after cell lysis. These particles may subsequently infect other susceptible cells, completing the lytic cycle (Fig. 14.3).

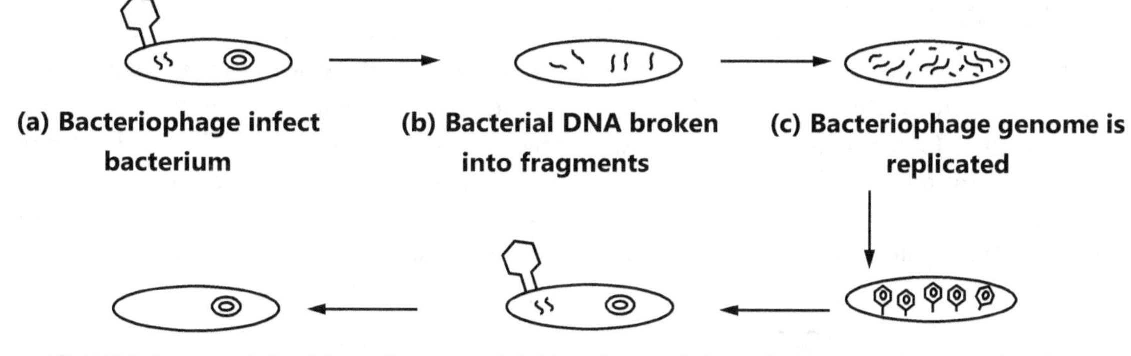

(f) DNA from original host is inserted into genome of its new host

(e) New bacterial strain is infected by bacteriophage

(d) Bacteriophage particles are formed

Fig. 14.3: Process of generalised transduction (lytic cycle)

14.3.2 Specialised or Restricted Transduction

Some temperate phages can transfer only a few restricted genes of the bacterial chromosome to the receipient bacterial cell. This transfer of bacterial genes adjacent to prophage only to the recipient chromosome is called specialised transduction.

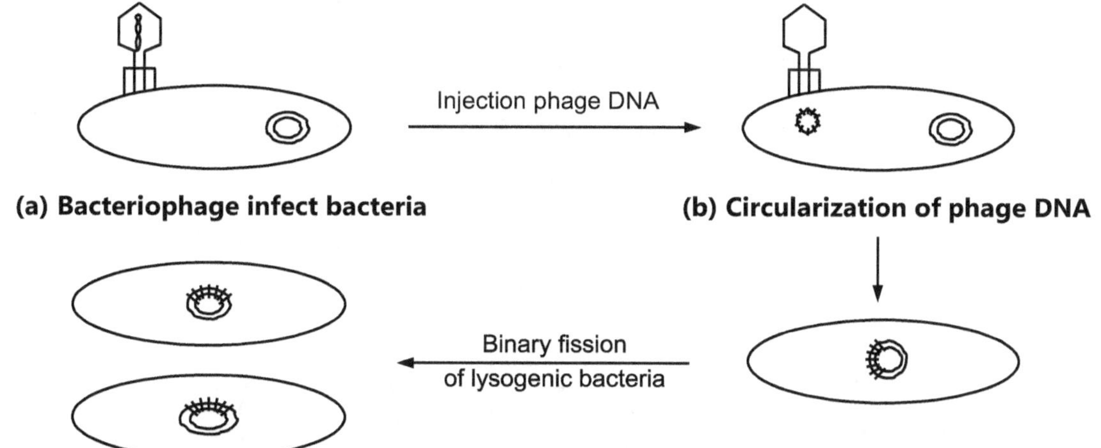

(d) New bacteria with prophage

(c) Integration of phage DNA with host chromosome

Fig. 14.4: Process of specialised transduction (lysogeny)

Morse and **Lederberg** (1956) found that in the lambda (λ) phage the transducing activity was restricted to the galactose locus. Temperate phages have two types of life cycles such as lytic cycle and lysogenic cycle. When a phage genome is introduced in the bacterial cell, it becomes integrated with bacterial chromosome as prophage. The prophage behaves like a segment of the host chromosome and replicates synchronously in bacterial cell. This is called lysogeny (Fig. 14.4). Under certain conditions (e.g. UV light or chemicals), the prophages enter the lytic cycle and kill the hosts.

14.4 CONJUGATION

Bacterial conjugation was first reported by **Joshua Lederberg** and **Edward Tatum** (1946) who proved the process of transfer of genetic material by cell to cell contact. **Lederberg** and **Tatum** produced two auxotrophic strains (58-161 and W677) of *Escherichia coli* K12 by mutation. The strain 58-16 was found unable to synthesize, amino acid methionine and vitamin biotin and hence, genotype of this strain is represented as: thr$^+$ len$^+$ meth$^-$ bio$^-$. The strain W677 cannot produce amino acids like threonine and leucine.

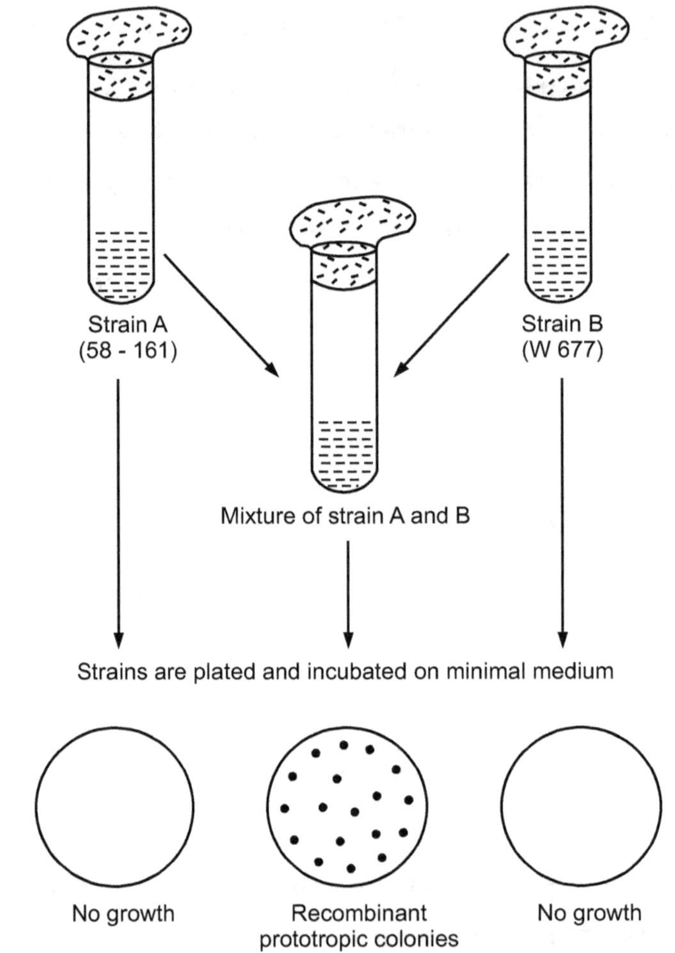

Fig. 14.5: The Lederberg and Tatum experiment of bacterial conjugation

The genotype of this strain (W677) is meth$^+$ bio$^+$ thr – len$^-$. These mutant strains cannot grow on the minimal medium. These mutant strains are called the auxotrophic and the wild strain is called as prototroph (Fig. 14.5). Mixing of two auxotrophs and plating on minimal medium (absence of growth factors) produce the prototroph (i.e. thr$^+$ len$^+$ meth$^+$ bio$^+$). These prototroph cells have the capacity to synthesize all four growth factors. This experiment indicates that recombination was brought by direct cell contact or process of conjugation.

The evidence for cell-to-cell contact was provided by **Bernard Davis** (1950) by using U-shaped tube (Fig. 14.6). Two separate pieces of curved glass tubes were prepared and fused at the base to form a U-shape with a sintered glass filter which permitted the passage of the nutrient medium. The filter did not allow bacteria to pass from both the ends of U tube. Nutrient medium was inoculated with different auxotrophic strain of *Escherichia coli*. The culture medium was made to pass through the filter from one arm to the other by altering pressure. The strains from both the arms of U-tube were plated on minimal medium and incubated for growth. The bacterial colonies or prototrophs did not appear on medium which indicates the contact between the two auxotrophs cells was essential for the formation of recombinant prototrophs.

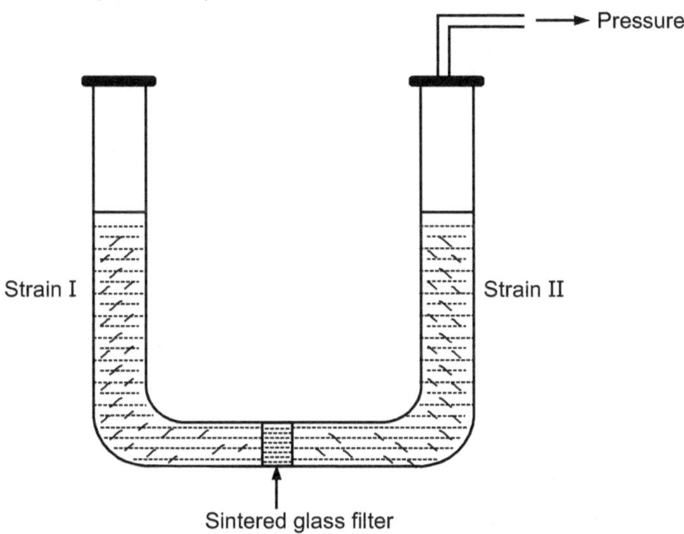

Fig. 14.6: Bernard Davis U-tube experiment

Conjugation is a natural process found in certain bacterial species involves the active passage of genetic material from one cell to another cell by means of the sex pili. Male cells contain in a small circular piece of DNA (plasmid), which is in the cytoplasm called the sex factor of F-factor (fertility factor). These donor cells are referred as F^+ cells and recipient cells are referred as F^- cells (absence of fertility factor). However, in $F^+ \times F^-$ crosses, the male replicates its sex factor and one copy is transferred to the female recipient. The F^- cell is converted to an F^+ cell and it itself acts as donor cell (Fig. 14.7). Therefore, as long as the cell grow, the conjugation process can continue in an infectious way with repeated transfer for the sex factor. The presence of F-factor in a bacterial cell determines its autonomous replication and sex pili formation. The F-factor remains in two stages as plasmid and as episome. The F-plasmid replicates independently but sometimes it is integrated with the normal chromosome of the bacterium. Therefore, it is referred as episome. The bacterial conjugation process is commonly observed in *Escherichia, Shigella, Pseudomonas* and *Vibrio* species.

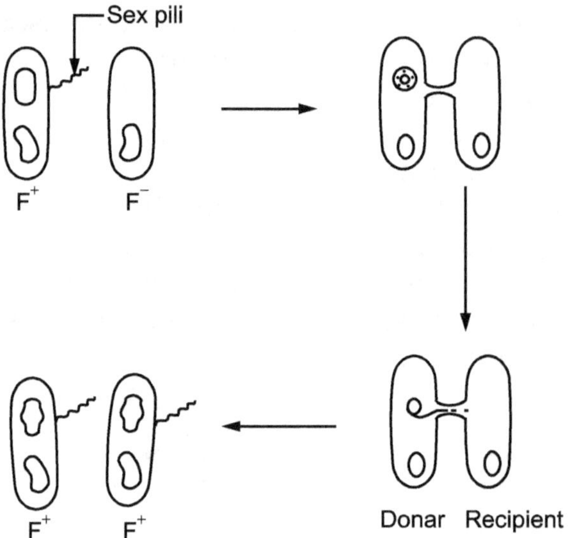

Fig. 14.7: Process of conjugation

The chromosomes of F^+ cell integrates with F-plasmid then these cells are called high frequency recombination (Hfr) cells. High frequency recombination cells arise from F^+ cells in which F-factor becomes integrated into the bacterial chromosme (Fig. 14.8). They differ from F^+ cells in that the F-factor of the Hfr is rarely transferred during recombination. Thus, in Hfr $\times$ F^- cross, the frequency of recombination is high and the transfer of F-factor is low and in $F^+ \times F^-$ cross, the frequency of recombination is low and the transfer of F-factor is high. When F-factor is excised from the chromosome of an Hfr strain with some chromosomal genes then these cells are called F' cells. The plasmid in an F' cells is self-replicating. The excision of an F' plasmid from an Hfr strain occurs about once for every 10 cells divisions.

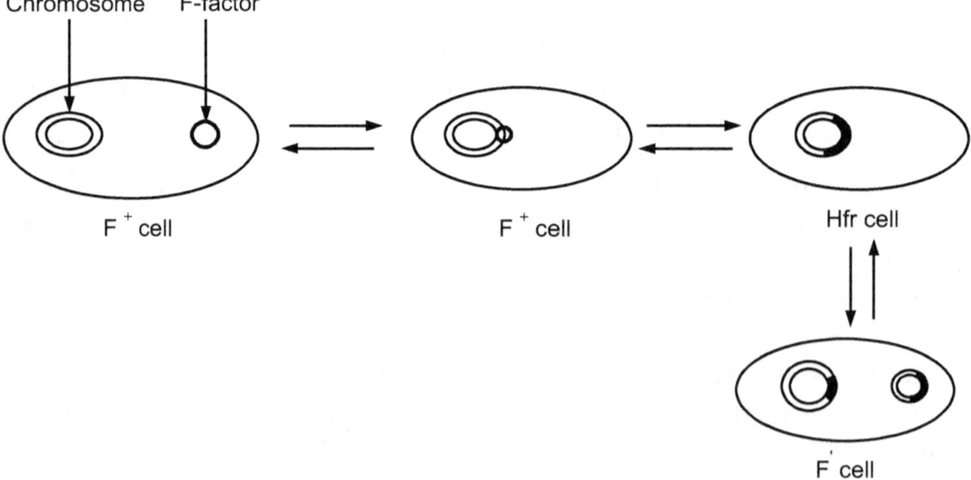

Fig. 14.8: Formation of high frequency recombination (Hfr) and F' cell

14.5 PLASMIDS

In addition to chromosomal DNA, most bacteria possess extra-chromosomal genetic materials. These materials are known as plasmid. The general properties of plasmids are as follows:

(i) They are small extrachromosomal piece of genetic material that can replicate autonomously within the host cell.

(ii) They consist of a circular piece of double stranded DNA.

(iii) They can integrate with each other and with the host chromosome which may lead to exchange of genetic material (episome).

(iv) They are not essential for the normal life and cell survival.

(v) They may contain genetic information for controlling their own replication.

(vi) Plasmids may be lost spontaneously or by curing agents.

(vii) They can promote their own transfer by host cell conjugation.

(viii) Plasmids may have some additional properties such as drug or heavy metal resistance, bacteriocin production, toxigenicity etc.

Plasmids (Fig. 14.9) vary both in numbers per cell and in size. Each contains 50 to 100 genes. Plasmids can be classified as conjugative or self-transmissible and non-conjugative or non-self transmissible or determinants. The conjugative plasmids are large and self transmissible. They have an apparatus through which they can mediate their own transfer to another cell, e.g. R, F and bacteriocinogen plasmids. Those plasmids which do not possess information for self transfer to another cell are known as non-conjugative plasmids. They can be transferred with the help of transfer factor such as colicin plasmid (Col I) and through the agency of bacteriophages (transduction). A number of properties of bacteria are attributed to extra chromosomal DNA.

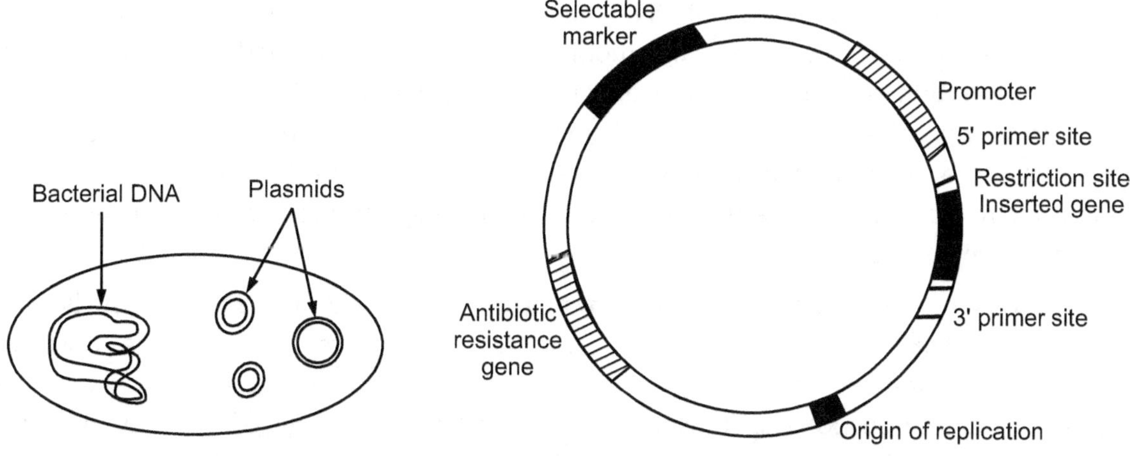

(a) Bacterial DNA and plasmids **(b) Structural features of plasmids**

Fig. 14.9: Plasmids and their structural features

Many plants have received attention for DNA cloning and expression of foreign DNA in plant cells. Major work is done on soil-borne bacteria such as *Agrobacterium tumefaciens* causing crown gall disease and *Agrobacteirum rhizogenes* causing hairy root disease on the stems of numerous plants. *Agrobacterium* plasmids (Ti and Ri) have been used for introduction of genes of desirable traits into plants. Explants are commonly used for gene transfer. These explants are co-cultured with *Agrobacterium* containing vector with modified foreign gene. The transformed colonies are selected and used for regeneration of whole plant. These plants are tested for the transfer of gene with the help of screenable markers (reporter genes). The reporter genes are also transferred along with desired genes.

Agrobacterium tumefaciens contains plasmid which induces tumour in plants (For detail, please refer Chapter 18), these plasmid is called as Ti-plasmid (180 to 250 Kb). Ti-plasmid contains T-DNA region of about 23 to 25 Kb which is transferred into plant cells. *Agrobacterium tumefaciens* mainly present in soil and cause infection to dicotyledonous plants. Bacterial species secrete lipopolysaccharide which help in attachment with polygalacturonic acid fractions of plant cell wall. Phenolic compound (acetosyringone) is secreted from the wounded cell walls of plants which induces the vir genes of Ti-plasmids. Vir genes encode an enzyme which nick the double stranded T-DNA on the same strand at two points. It produces single stranded DNA molecules and are carried into plant cells. A desired DNA fragment can be cloned in the region of Ti plasmid which will introduce the DNA fragment into plant genome. *Agrobacterium rhizogenes* causes formation of adventitious roots and this rhizogenicity has been correlated with the presence of a large plasmid (Ri-plasmid). Plasmid of this species also contains a T-DNA which causes the development of hairy roots. Ri-plasmid of *Agrobacterium rhizogenes* is useful for production of secondary root systems for ability to resist anoxia from flooding of the soil and better anchorage of plants.

14.6 TRANSPOSONS

Transposons are a sequence of DNA that can move from one location or position to another location in the genome. These mobile elements are also called as 'jumping genes', cassettes, insertion sequences or transposons. The formal name for this family of mobile genes is transposable elements and their movement is called transposition. Transposable elements are a small, mobile DNA sequences that move around chromosomes with no regard for homology and insertion of these elements may produce deletions, inversions or chromosomal fusions.

Transposons were first discovered in maize (corn) by American scientist Barbara McClintock (1948) for which she was awarded Noble prize in 1983. She observed chromosome mutations caused by these transposons and about 50% of total genome of maize consists of transposons. Transposons are found in many forms of life. They may have arisen independently many times or perhaps just once and then spread to other kingdoms by horizontal gene transfer.

Transposons are classified into two basic types such as class I transposons (retrotransposons) and class II transposons (DNA transposons). According to their mechanism, transposons may be classified as copy and paste (class I) and cut and paste (class II). Retrotransposons represent a highly unique group of transposable elements and form large portions of the genomes of many eukaryotes. They generate second copy of transposable elements and inserted in the genome. This process (copy and paste) results in the insertion of repetitive sequences of DNA throughout the genome. The first step of retrotransposition occurs when the transposable DNA is copied into RNA by transcription. The RNA segment then jumps to another location in the genome. The RNA must be copied back into DNA by an enzyme reverse transcriptase. The newly formed DNA which is a copy of the transposon gets intergrated into the genome. This integration may occur randomly on the same chromosome or a different chromosome.

Retrotransposons also classified as long interspersed nuclear elements (LINEs) and short interspersed nuclear elements (SINEs). A class I element (clade LINE-1) consist of a 5'-UTR with internal promoter activity and two open reading frames (ORFs). ORF1 encodes a nucleic acid binding protein and ORF2 encodes a protein with endonuclease (EN) and reverse transcriptase (RT) activity (Fig. 14.10 (a)). It lacks long terminal repeats (LTR) and ends in a poly (A) tail.

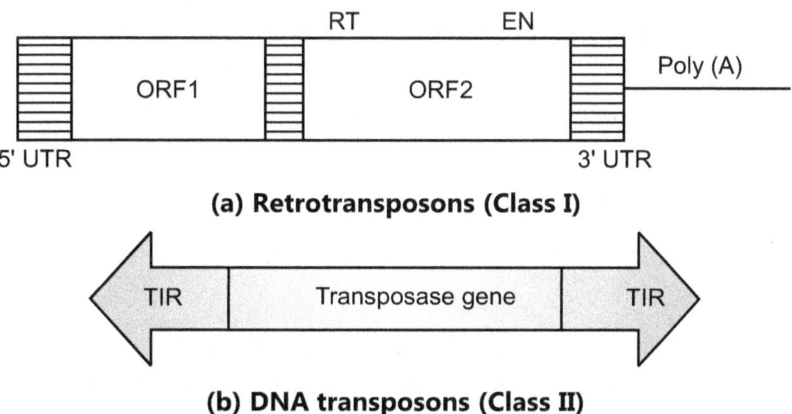

(a) Retrotransposons (Class I)

(b) DNA transposons (Class II)

Fig. 14.10: Types of transposable elements (TEs)

DNA transposons (class II) generally move by a 'cut and paste mechanism in which the transposon is excised from one location and reintegrated in another location. DNA transposons consist of a transposase gene that is flanked by two terminal inverted repeats (TIRs). The transposase recognizes these TIRs (Fig. 14.10 (b)) to perform the excision of the transposon DNA body, which is inserted into a new genomic location.

Miniature inverted repeat transposable elements (MITEs) are non-autonomous, short (100 to 600 bp) DNA transposon-like elements present in large numbers in many eukaryotes. They have TIRs and are flanked by TSDs. They lack transposase coding potential and are presumably dependent on autonomous DNA transposons for their mobilization. MITEs have been identified in the genomes of *Oryza sativa, Caenorhabditis elegans* and other organisms. Mariner-like elements are another prominent class of transposons found in multiple species including humans. The mariner transposon was first discovered by Jacobson and Hartl in *Drosophila*. This class transposable element is known for its uncanny ability to be transmitted horizontally in many species.

Transposabale elements also contains additional genes as a antibiotic resistance factors. Antibiotic resistance typically occurs when an infecting bacterium acquires a plasmid that carries a gene encoding resistance to one or more antibiotics. These resistance genes are carried on transposable elements that have moved into plasmids and are easily transferred from one organism to another. Some of diseases caused by mutations are due to insertion of transposons into a genes. Diseases are mainly cause due to insertion of transposons into particular regions of genes that are involved in regulating gene activity.

14.7 MUTATION

Mutation is a random undirected, heritable variation caused by an alteration in the nucleotide sequence at some point of the DNA of the cell. A cell or an organism which shows the effects of mutation is called a mutant. The different form of gene produced by mutation is called alleles. Each gene undergoes mutation with a fixed frequency. Mutation rates of individual genes in bacteria range from 10^{-2} to 10^{-4} per bacterium per division. Alterations in DNA can be caused by chemical or physical means or they can occur spontaneously.

14.7.1 Types of Mutation

Mutation can be divided conveniently into point mutation, frame shift mutation and multistage mutation.

The substitution of one nucleotide for another in the specific nucleotide sequence of a gene is called point mutation. The substitution of one purine for another purine or one pyrimidine for another pyrimidine is termed a transition type of point mutation. A transversion is the replacement of a purine by a pyrimidine or vice-versa. The base-pair substitution may result in one of the three kinds of mutations affecting the translation process. A missense mutation is one in which the triplet code is altered so as to specify an amino acid different from that normally located at a particular position in the protein. Deletion of a nucleotide within a gene may cause premature polypeptides chain termination by generating a non-sense codon and is called non-sense mutation. The altered gene triplet produces a mRNA codon and which specifies the same amino acid because the codon resulting from mutation is a synonym for the original codon and this is called neutral mutation.

Frame shift mutations result from an addition or loss of one or more nucleotides in a gene and are termed insertion or deletion (Fig. 14.11) mutations, respectively. This results in a shift of the reading frame. In frame shift mutations, new sequence of amino acids is synthesised from a frameshift reading of the nucleotide sequences of mRNA.

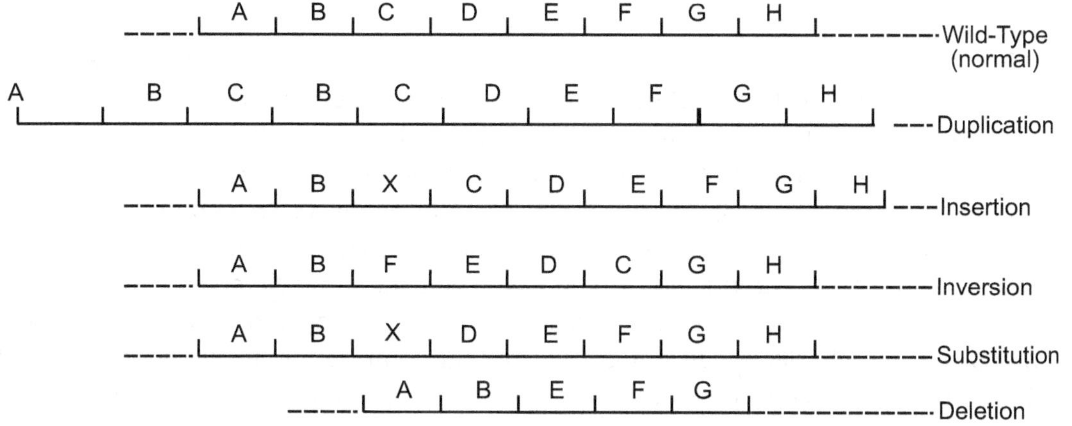

Fig. 14.11: Types of mutations

Multisite mutation is called macrolesion. There are extensive chromosomal rearrangements such as inversions, duplications and deletions.

Mutations are also classified as induced mutation and spontaneous mutation.

14.7.2 Mutagenic Agents or Mutagens

Mutagens are chemical or physical agents that increase the rate of mutation and these mutations are called 'induced mutations'. Mutation of an individual gene occurs independently of mutation in other genes. The mutation rate is generally defined as the average number of mutations per cell per division. It is expressed as a negative exponent per cell division. If a mutation occurs once in 1 million divisions, the rate of mutation is 10^{-6}. Generally, the mutation rate for any single gene ranges between 10^{-3} and 10^{-9} per cell division. A variety of mutagens are known to increase the rate of mutation in micro-organisms. These include both physical and chemical agents.

Physical agents: Physical agents commonly used to induce mutations are ultraviolet (UV) light, X-rays, γ-radiations, heat etc. All these agents can cause non-selective mutations. Irradiation of DNA with UV rays generally results in the formation of covalent bonds between thymine molecules on the same strand of DNA yielding thymine-thymine dimers (Fig. 14.12). Most UV mutations are non-sense type of mutations and are the result of a change in one or few bases in the DNA. Many micro-organisms have enzymes that can repair this damage in the dark (dark repair). The light repair system involves a photoactivated enzyme that breaks the bonds between the thymine dimers. This protective mechanism is active only in visible light. X-rays and γ-rays are ionizing radiations and they can cause damage to the DNA but no dimer formation occurs.

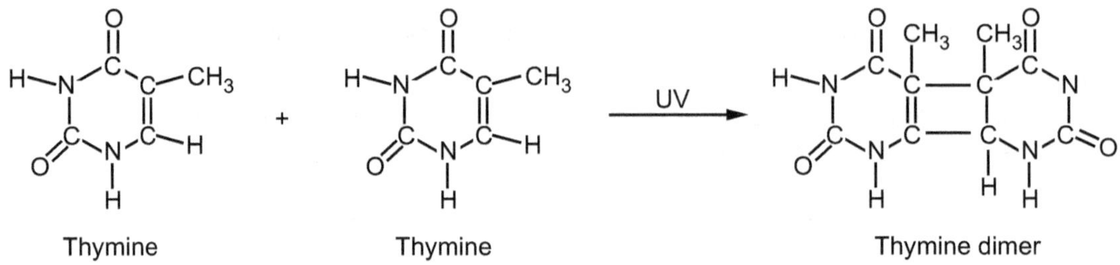

Thymine + Thymine —UV→ Thymine dimer

Fig. 14.12: Effect of ultraviolet irradiation on thymine

Chemical agents: Chemical agents used to induce mutations are nitrous acid, hydroxylamine, base analogues (2-amino purine, 5-Bromouracil) alkylating agents such as ethyl ethane sulphonate (EES), ethyl methane sulphonate (EMS), sulfur mustard and nitrosoguanidine. Nitrous acid oxidatively deaminates cytosine to uracil and adenine to hypoxanthine (Fig. 14.13). During subsequent DNA replication, uracil recognises adenine and hypoxanthine pairs with guanine resulting in a AT to GC transition. Base analogues are compounds that are chemically similar to the natural compounds used to synthesize DNA. When base analogous are incorporated into DNA, they do not base pair correctly like the natural bases and cause mispairing and mutations. Alkylating agents are the most potent group of chemical mutagens and they transfer the alkyl group to the carbonyl oxygen of a base. Ethyl methyl sulfonate chemically alters thymine to make it pair with guanine instead of adenine.

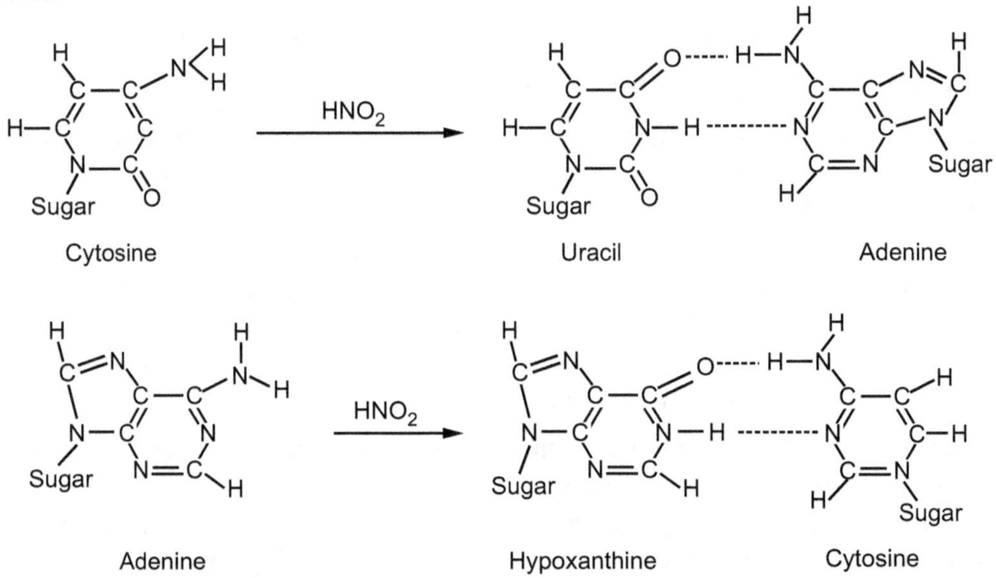

Cytosine —HNO_2→ Uracil ··· Adenine

Adenine —HNO_2→ Hypoxanthine ··· Cytosine

Fig. 14.13: Effect of nitrous acid on cytosine and adenine

14.7.3 Spontaneous Mutation

Mutations that occur in the absence of all mutagenic agents are called spontaneous mutations. Spontaneous mutation, independent of the environment was first produced by **Salvador Luria** and **Max Delbruck** (1943) by the 'fluctuation test'. They found very wide fluctuations occurring in the numbers of bacteriophage resistant *Escherichia coli* colonies when samples are plated from several separate small volume cultures as compared to samples tested from a single large volume culture (Fig. 14.14).

In fluctuation test, a series of tubes containing 0.5 ml of cells are incubated without phage until a certain population size (10^8 cells/ml) is reached. The cultures are then exposed to phage by pouring the contents of each tube into an agar plate containing phage. The colony counts (phage resistant mutant) from series of similar cultures are then compared with the results of a series of samples taken from one culture (10 ml test tube) started with a similar density of cells/ml and allowed to reach a similar population number (1 ml). The results showed that resistant bacteria arise spontaneously prior to the exposure to phage. A series of similar cultures yielded results different from those obtained with a series of samples from one culture. Luria and Delbruck found that the number of resistant mutants fluctuated from sample to sample indicating that mutants existed in the population prior to exposure to the phage. They concluded that mutations in bacteria occur spontaneously.

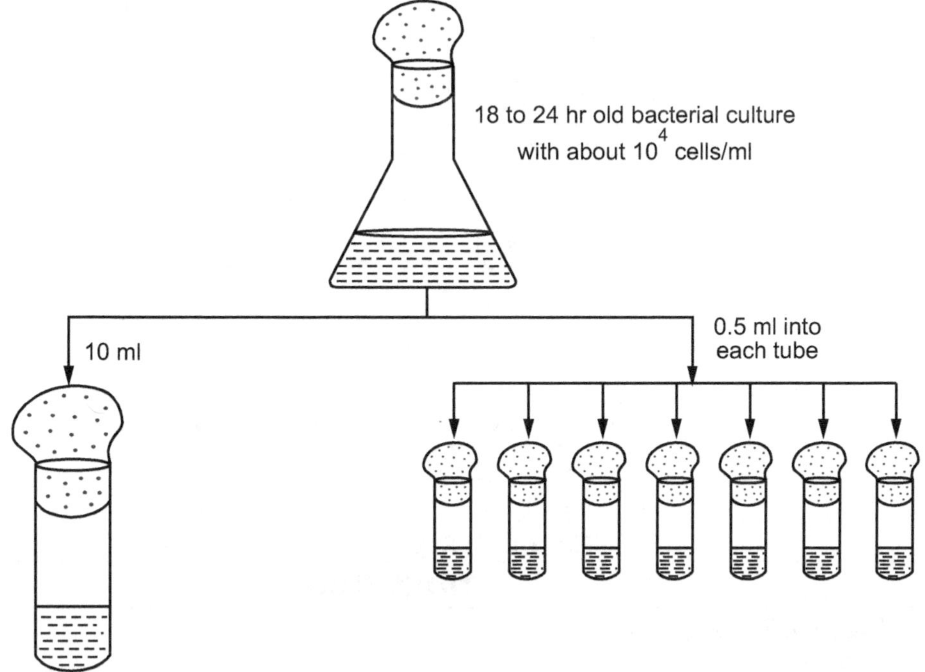

Incubate all test tubes till population reached to 10^8 cells/ml and then exposed to the phage

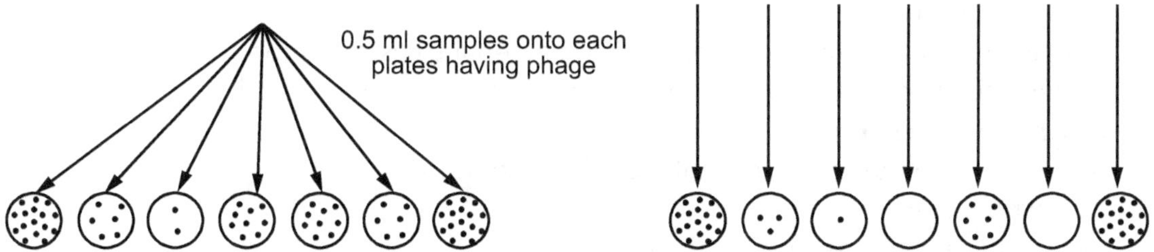

Fig. 14.14: The fluctuation test

These results are further elaborated by **Josua Lederberg** and **Esther Lederberg** by the use of the replica plate technique. The technique consists of first plating a small number of test bacteria on a master plate and incubating it until growth occurred. A sterile velvet pad on a transfer block is then used to inoculate each of the colonies from the master plate onto a plate containing an inhibitor or a selective agent to detect resistant mutants (Fig. 14.15). If resistant mutants are developed on the master plate before exposure to the inhibitor, then such resistant colonies should be located at exactly the same position on each of the replica plates, while if mutation occurred as a consequence of exposure to the inhibitor then the resistant colonies should be at different locations on different replica plates. **Josua** and **Esther Lederberg** found that spontaneous mutations occur in bacteria in the absence of a selective agent. After this conclusion, the replica plate technique has been extensively used as a basic technique for mutant detection.

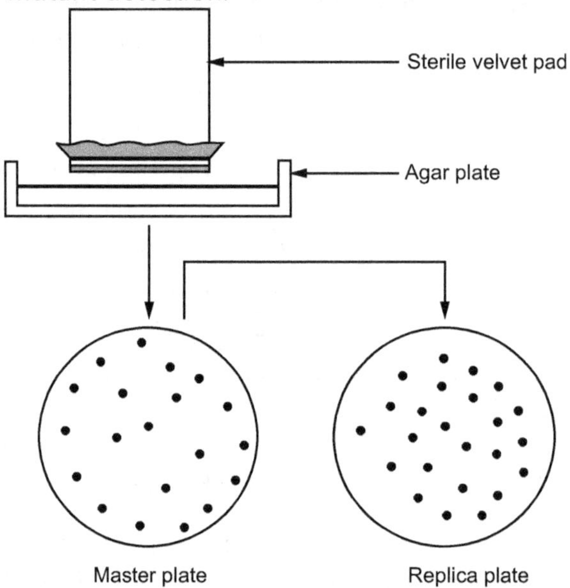

Fig. 14.15: Replica plate technique

QUESTIONS

(A) Objective Type Questions:

1. Define the terms:
   (a) Conjugation
   (b) Specialised transduction
   (c) Mutation
2. Explain in short Griffith's experiment for bacterial transformation.
3. Differentiate between induced mutation and spontaneous mutation

(B) Short Answer Questions:

1. What are transposons? Explain its role in gene transfer.
2. Write notes on:
   (a) Replica Plate method
   (b) Davis U-tube experiment.

(C) Long Answer Questions:

1. What is bacterial recombination? Explain bacterial transduction technique used in gene transfer.
2. Explain the role of plasmids in gene transfer.

(D) Multiple Choice Questions:

1. The process in which temperate virus can transfer specific bacterial genes that are located near the viral integration site is called ______.
   (a) Generalised transduction (b) Specialised transduction
   (c) Conjugation (d) Transformation
2. Drug resistance in tuberculosis is due to ______.
   (a) Transformation (b) Transduction
   (c) Conjugation (d) Mutation
3. The transfer of foreign gene into another cell is done by the following method ______.
   (a) Transduction (b) Microinjection
   (c) Transformation (d) All of the above
4. The highest rate of conjugation and recombination is associated with the ______.
   (a) F-plasmid (b) R-plasmid
   (c) C-plasmid (d) M-plasmid
5. Microbial cells produce a pink pigment at room temperature. The pink colour of the colonies is example of ______.
   (a) Change in DNA base (b) Adaptation of the environment
   (c) Genotype (d) Phenotype
6. A sequence of DNA that can move from one location or position to another location in the genome is called ______.
   (a) Transposons (b) Plasmids
   (c) Spontaneous mutation (d) Specialized transduction
7. ______ gene incorporated into plasmids to detect recombinant cells.
   (a) Antibiotic resistance (b) Antibiotic susceptible
   (c) Reverse transcriptase (d) Virus receptors
8. ______ is used for formation of dimers of purine and pyrimidine.
   (a) Cathode rays (b) X-rays
   (c) Gamma rays (d) UV-rays

■■■

Chapter ... 15

MICROBIAL BIOTRANSFORMATION

♦ LEARNING OBJECTIVES ♦

After completing this chapter, reader should be able to understand:

- *Introduction*
- *Methods used in Biotransformation*
- *Microbial Bioconversion and Applications*
  - *Oxidation*
  - *Reduction*
  - *Hydrolysis*
  - *Esterification*
  - *Isomerization*
  - *Amide formation*
  - *Halogenation*
  - *Decarboxylation*
  - *Condensation*

15.1 INTRODUCTION

Microbial transformation is a biological process in which organic compounds are modified into reversible products. These biotransformation reactions are catalysed by purified enzymes present in microbial cells or pure cultures of microorganisms. Microbial enzymes are highly versatile in nature. Microorganisms are more adoptogenic and they can develop new enzymes for metabolism. Microbial bioconversions are routinely used in the commercial production of steroids, antibiotics, vitamins, prostaglandins, citric acid and many other therapeutic molecules.

Steroids can be produced by chemical synthesis or by microbiological transformations. Steroids are physiologically active compounds which include progesterone, testosterone, cholesterol, ergosterol, corticosterone etc. Steroidal hormones are known to be regulators of metabolism in the animal or human body. Prednisone and prednisolone are effective in the treatment of rheumatoid arthritis and progestogens and oestrogens are used as oral contraceptives. **Mamoli** and **Vercellone** (1937) made the first successful microbial transformation of steroids. **Peterson** and **Murray** (1952) reported the 11-hydroxylation of progesterone using a fungi *Rhizopus arrhizus*. Steroidal transformations are mainly affected by bacteria, actinomycetes and fungi. The structure of a basic steroid is shown in

Fig. 15.1 (a). Prostaglandins are naturally occurring hormone-like substances derived biosynthetically from C-20 polyunsaturated fatty acids containing three or four double bonds. They are potent vasoactive substances that play a key role in regulating cellular metabolism. Structurally, prostaglandins are derivatives of prostanoic acid [Fig. 15.1 (b)] and have a cyclopentane ring with two side-chains attached to adjacent carbon atoms. The microbial transformations are commonly reported in different antibiotic classes such as β-lactam, peptide, macrolide, actinomycin, chloramphenicol, novobiocin, griseofulvin, anthracycline, lincomycin etc.

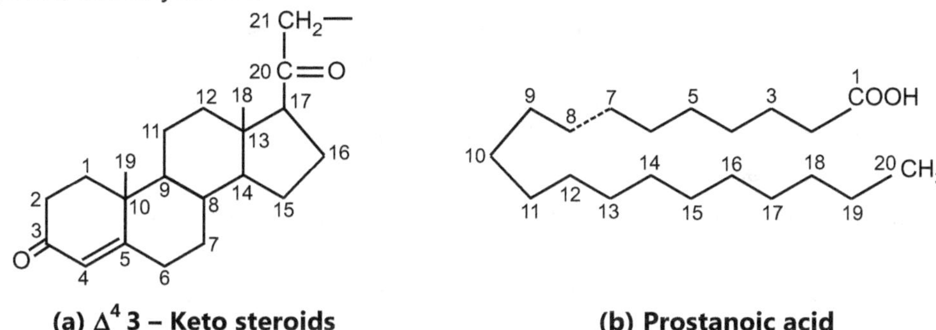

(a) Δ^4 3 – Keto steroids **(b) Prostanoic acid**

Fig. 15.1: Basic structure of (a) Steroid and (b) Prostaglandins

Microbial transformations are brought about by enzymes secreted by selected strains of microorganisms. These reactions are essentially detoxifying mechanisms employed by the microorganisms. Some of the other advantages are listed below:

1. The microbial transformations react specifically. Side reactions do not occur if one enzyme is involved in a biotransformation. The catalytic activity is usually restricted to a single reaction type.
2. Microorganism catalysing bioconversions act a stereospecific catalysts i.e. specific microorganisms must be used to carry out a specific type of transformation.
3. The substrate molecule is usually attacked at the same site, even if several groups of similar reactivity are present (regiospecificity).
4. Microbial bioconversion reactions can be carried out under mild conditions such as neutral pH, room temperature and at normal pressure.
5. Biotransformation reactions can reduce the multistep chemical reaction to a single step.
6. As compared to chemical reactions, microbial transformations require less chemicals, labour, time and money, and release good yield.
7. Microbial transformation can selectively introduce functional groups at certain non-activated positions in a molecule, which can not be attracted by chemical reagents.

15.2 METHODS USED IN BIOTRANSFORMATION

Microbial cells serve as a major tool for biotransformation. The main process used for biotransformation is fermentation. Fermentation is carried out in the following phases:

(i) Phase – I: Growth phase: In the growth phase, a culture is grown in a nutritionally rich medium. The medium for the growth is simple or of complex type. Aeration and agitation are provided during growth and optimum temperature is maintained. The time of incubation period depends on the type of culture and environmental conditions.

(ii) Phase – II: Transformation phase: Transformation phase begins with the addition of steroids at the end of the growth phase. Steroids may be added simultaneously with the inoculation. Amount of steroid to be added depends on the transforming capacity of the culture, toxicity of substrate or type of product.

An enzyme secreted by the microbial cells acts on the steroid. The desired transformation occurrs under controlled conditions of temperature, pH, agitation, aeration and time.

Steroidal bioconversion is performed by using submerged aeration technique in stainless steel tanks. The media employed are prepared at minimal nutritional levels to allow greater ease of extraction and purification of the transformation product. The selection of medium depends on the type of microorganisms. Glucose or molasses are commonly used as a carbon source for growth of different microorganisms. Microbial transformation requires 24 to 48 hours. After the transformation, microbial growth is separated from the fermentation liquor and extracted with a suitable solvent. Methylene chloride, chloroform, methyl isobutylketone and ethyl acetate solvents are commonly used for extraction of steroids. Products obtained from cells or substrates should be extracted separately. The extracted samples are analysed by using thin layer chromatography, paper chromatography, gas chromatography or high pressure liquid chromatography. The structure of the new product is elucidated by different analytical techniques (IR, NMR, mass, elemental analysis).

15.3 MICROBIAL BIOCONVERSION AND APPLICATIONS

Microorganisms may perform different types of simple or mixed reactions. The bioconversion reactions are classified as follows:

(A) Oxidation:

1. Hydroxylation
2. Dehydrogenation
3. Epoxidation
4. Aromatization

(B) Reduction:

1. Reduction of double bond
2. Reduction of ketones, aldehydes and acids

(C) Hydrolysis

(D) Esterification

(E) Isomerization

(F) Amide formation

(G) Halogenation

(H) Decarboxylation

(I) Condensation

These reactions are described as follows:

15.3.1 Oxidation

These are the most important reactions of microbial transformations.

1. **Hydroxylation:** Filamentous bacteria and fungi are generally used for their versatile hydroxylation at non-activated carbons in a variety of substrates like steroids, prostaglandins, alkaloids and hydrocarbons. Microbial hydroxylation is the involvement of direct replacement of the hydrogen atom on a given carbon. Microbial hydroxylation of steroids at C-11 helps to meet the increased demand for cortisone and hydrocortisone. 11α-hydroxylation, 11β-hydroxylation, 16α-hydroxylation and 21-hydroxylation of steroids are important industrial reactions. Some of the hydroxylation reactions are shown in Fig. 15.2.

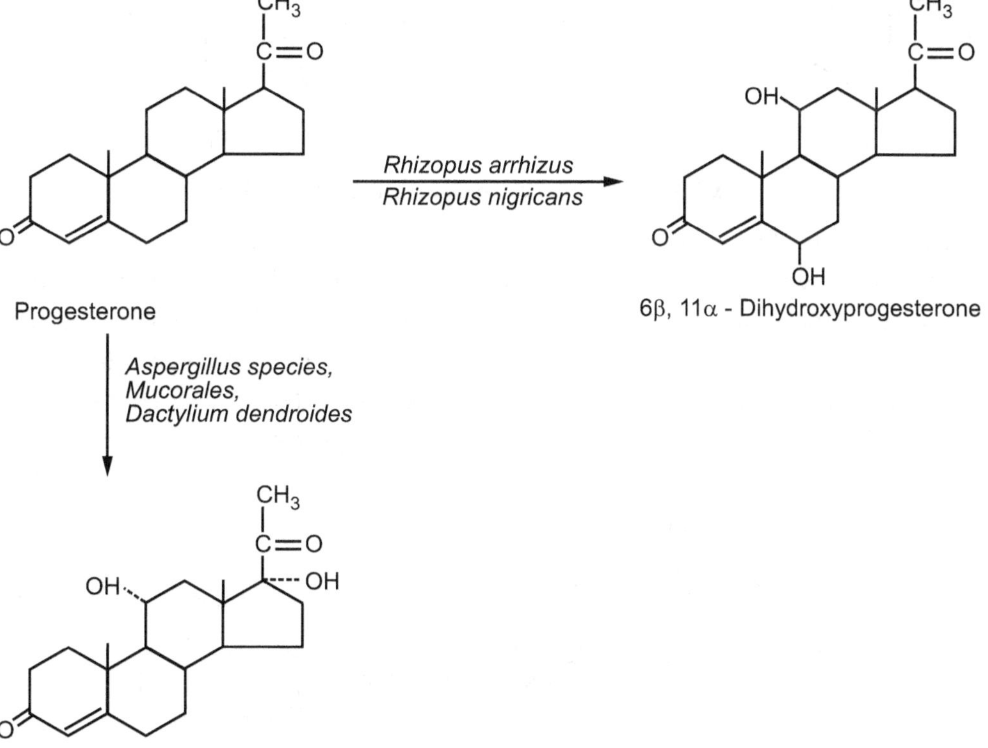

Fig. 15.2: Microbial hydroxylation reactions

2. **Dehydrogenation:** Bacterial and fungal species are capable of dehydrogenation of steroids. Addition of a double bond has been reported for all the four rings of steroid nucleus but majority of microbes attack the ring 'A'. Conversion of cortisone to prednisone and cortisol to prednisolone are shown in Fig. 15.3.

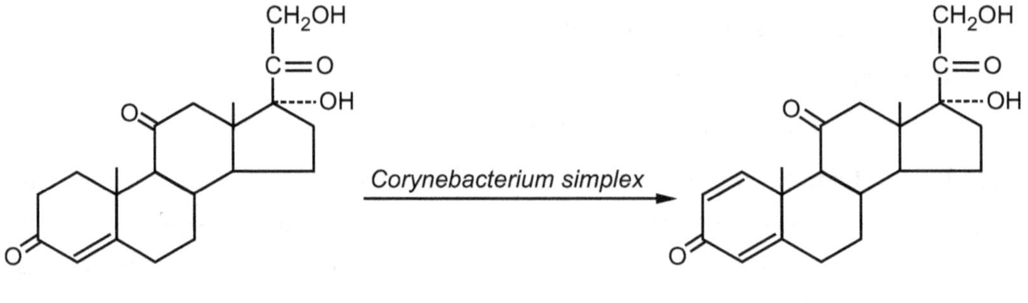

Corynebacterium simplex

Cortisone Predisone

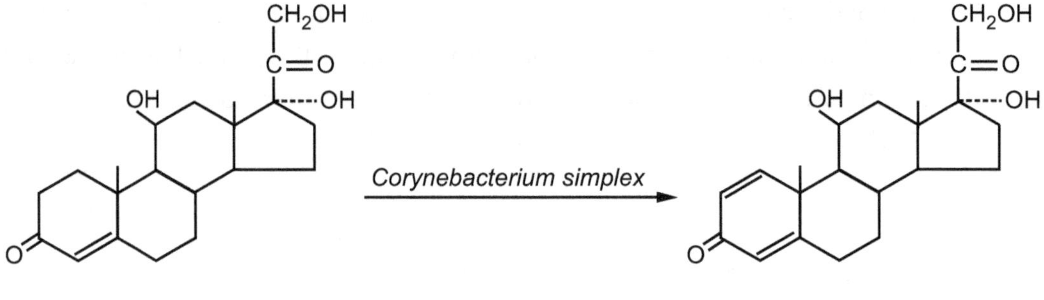

Corynebacterium simplex

Cortisol Predisolone

Fig. 15.3: Microbial dehydrogenation reactions

3. **Epoxidation:** Epoxidation is a very rare transformation. The microorganisms which normally hydroxylate saturated steroid will epoxidize the unsaturated analog provided the newly introduced hydroxyl function should be axial in nature. **Bloom** and associates (1956) demonstrated the examples of epoxidation by using *Curvalaria lunata* and *Cunninghamella blakesleena* (Fig. 15.4). These microbial cells normally introduce the 11β–hydroxyl and 14 α–hydroxyl into compound 'S'.

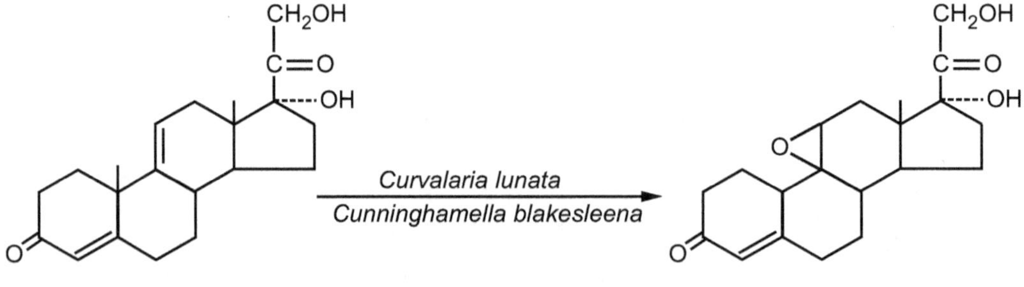

Curvalaria lunata
Cunninghamella blakesleena

$\Delta^{9(11)}$ - Dehydro - compound - 'S' 9β, 11β - epoxido - compound - 'S'

Fig. 15.4: Microbial epoxidation reaction

4. **Aromatization:** 19-Hydroxyl cholesterol and 19-hydroxyl-β-sitosterol are converted to estrone with *Nocardia restricta* by aromatisation (Fig. 15.5). C–1–Dehydrogeneration with substrate lacking methyl group at carbon 10 or suitably substituted at carbon 19 results into aromatization.

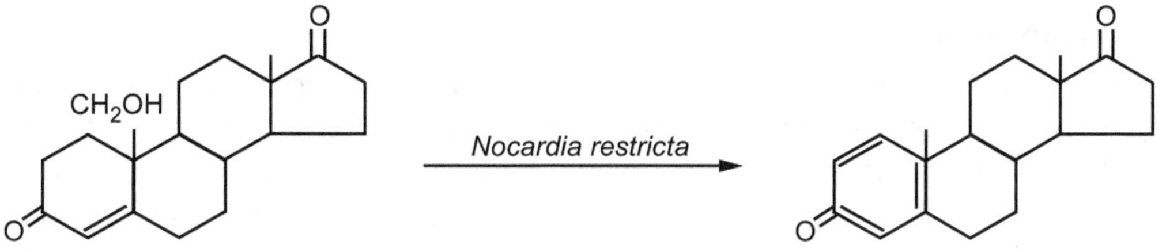

19 - Hydroxy - 4 - androstene 3,17 - dione Estrone

Fig. 15.5: Formation of estrone by aromatization

15.3.2 Reduction

1. Reduction of double bond (–C=C–): The enzymes oxido-reductases catalyse both dehydrogenation and reduction reactions. Ring hydrogenation (reduction) mainly occurs in steroids at Δ^1, Δ^4 and Δ^{16}, Δ^1. The conversion of prednisone to cortisone and prednisolone to cortisol with *Bacillus megatherium* is reported by reduction. The conversion of 4-androstane-3, 17-dione to androsane-3, 17 dione with *Bacillus putrificus* is reported for Δ^4 hydrogenation. (Fig. 15.6).

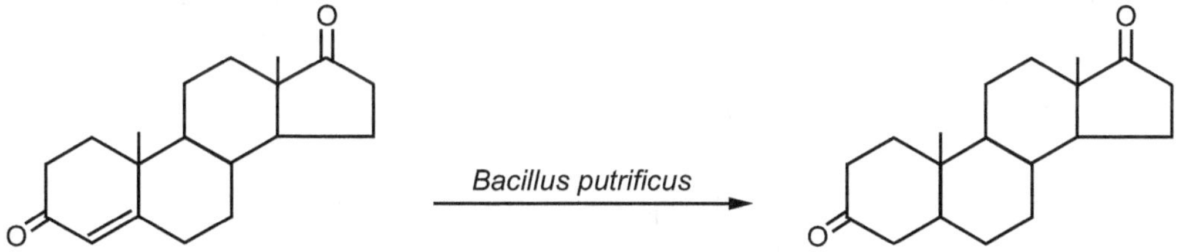

4 - androstene - 3,17 - dione Androst - 3,17 - dione

Fig. 15.6: Microbial reduction of steroid (double bond)

2. Reduction of ketones, aldehydes and acids: Hydroxyl groups at C_6, C_{11} and C_{17}, α-methyl group at C_{16} and Δ' unsaturation lead to decrease in the reduction rate in steroids. The presence of electron withdrawing groups at the C-6 in 3 keto-Δ^4 substrate, shift the direction from oxidation to reduction. Reduction of C-20 ketone occurs in presence of *Streptomyces lavendulae* (Fig. 15.7).

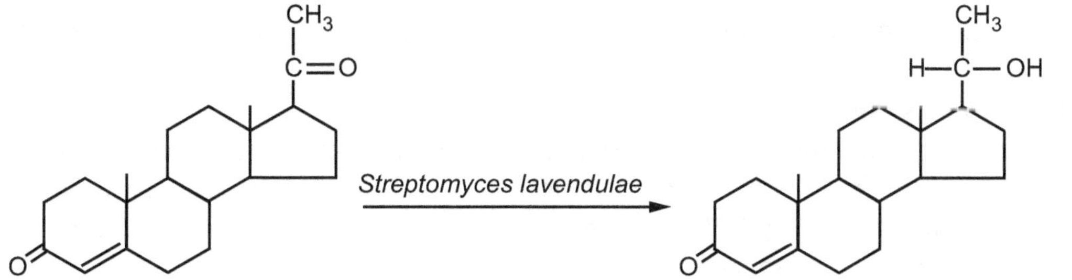

Progesterone 20 β - hydroxy - 4 - pregnane - 3 - one

Fig. 15.7: Reduction of C-20 ketones

15.3.3 Hydrolysis

A large number of esters, lactones, β-lactams, glycosides, epoxides and amides can be hydrolysed by a number of microorganisms. Tartaric acid is prepared from maleic anhydride by hydrolysis of the intermediary cis-epoxy-succinic acid with *Achromobacter tartarogenes.* The 6-aminopenicillanic acid (6-APA) is the intermediate in the preparation of semisynthetic penicillins. Bacterial hydrolysis of benzyl penicillin to 6-aminopenicillanic acid has become an essential step in the manufacturing of semisynthetic derivatives.

The hydrolytic cleavage of prostaglandin esters has been demonstrated by using microbial enzyme systems. *Saccharomyces* species, *Cladosporium resinae, Rhizopus oryzae, Corynespora cassicola* and Baker's yeast have been reported for hydrolysis of prostaglandins. *Corynespora cassicola* is used to hydrolyze 15-epi PGA_2 acetate methyl ester. In steroid hydrolysis, 3 and 21-acetates are generally hydrolysed prior to hydroxylation or dehydrogenation. Ester hydrolysis is also frequently accompanied by dehydrogenation (Fig. 15.8.)

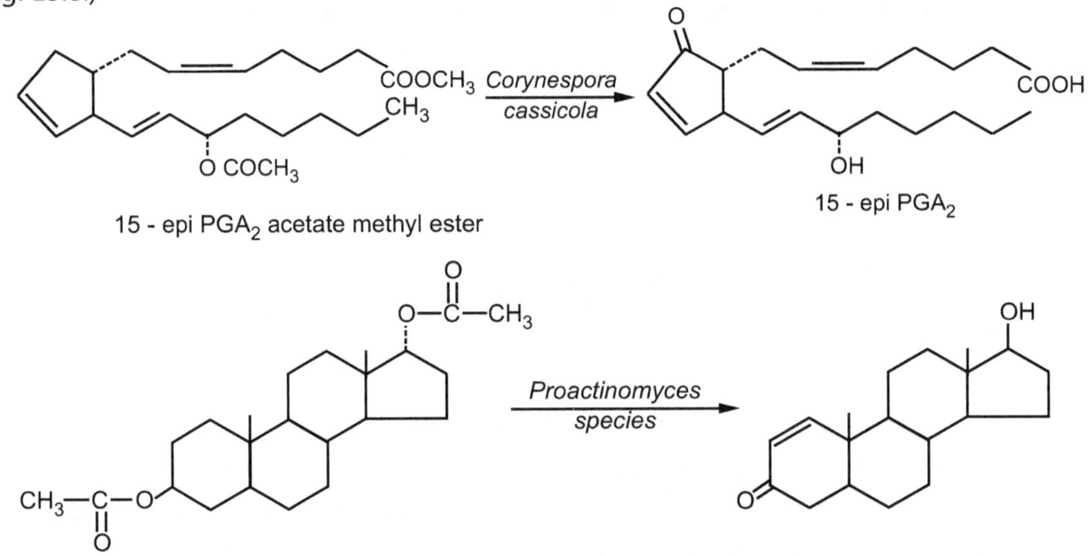

COOCH$_3$ CH$_3$ O COCH$_3$ — *Corynespora cassicola* → COOH OH

15 - epi PGA_2 acetate methyl ester → 15 - epi PGA_2

O—C(=O)—CH$_3$ CH$_3$—C(=O)—O — *Proactinomyces species* → OH O

Fig. 15.8: Hydrolysis of prostaglandins and steroids

15.3.4 Esterification

Microbial transformation by esterification is rarely reported in literature. Different steroids are prepared by esterification using *Sacchromyces fragilis* and *Trichodermaglauca* (Fig. 15.9).

15.3.5 Isomerisation

Isomerisation is an important process mainly useful for the preparation of high fructose syrup (food sweetener). Microbial isomerisation of prostaglandins is not very important but under basic conditions, PGA (10, 11 double bond) is converted into PGB (8, 12 double bond) without the aid of microorganisms.

Isomerisation of steroids is very common. Deoxycorticosterone is prepared by isomerisation of the double bond from Δ^5 to Δ^4 with *Corynebacterium mediolanum*.

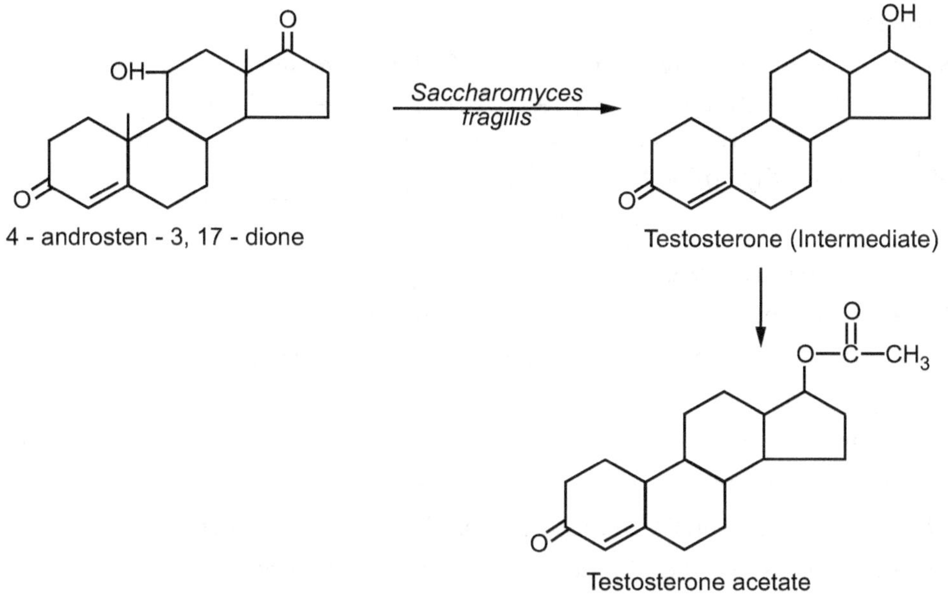

Fig. 15.9: Esterification of steroids

15.3.6 Amide Formation

Amide formation is a relatively rare microbial transformation. **Smith** and his coworkers reported the transformations of steroids with *Streptomyces roseochromogenus.*

15.3.7 Halogenation

Halogenation reactions are carried out at pH 3. Haloperoxidase enzymes from *Caldariomyces fumago* catalyse the halogenation reactions of steroids (Fig. 15.10).

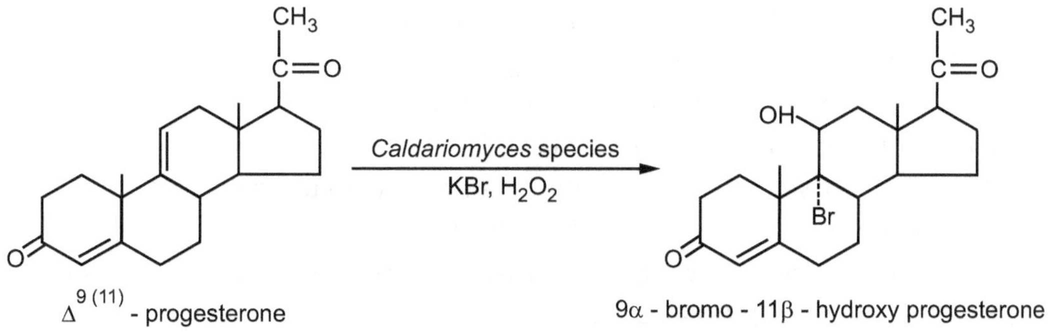

Fig. 15.10: Halogenation of steroids

15.3.8 Decarboxylation

Decarboxylation of aromatic and linear carboxylic acids is very common and of practical importance. L-lysine can be synthesised by stereospecific decarboxylation of meso-α,–α'–diaminopimelic acid (DAP) to L-lysine. The reaction is catalysed by *Bacillus sphaericus.*

15.3.9 Condensation

Microbial condensation was utilised in 1934 in the synthesis of natural ephedrine. Acetaldehyde reacts with benzaldehyde in the presence of fermenting yeast and gives (R) – 1 – phenyl – 1 – hydroxy – 2 – propanone. The propanone undergoes reductive condensation with methylamine to yield (1R, 2S) – ephedrine.

QUESTIONS

(A) Objective Type Questions:

1. Write the advantages of microbial transformations.
2. Write one example of the following types of bioconversions:
   (i) Hydrolysis
   (ii) Esterification

(B) Short Answer Questions:

1. What is microbial transformation? Explain Microbial transformation by reduction.
2. Write short note on Microbial transformation by oxidation.

(C) Long Answer Questions:

1. Explain in detail different biotransformation reactions with special reference to steroids.
2. Write the applications of microbial biotransformation in synthesis of active molecules.

(D) Multiple Choice Questions:

1. Microbial transformations have the following advantages except ______ .
   (a) It can reduce multistep reactions to a single step.
   (b) Reactions can be carried out under mild conditions.
   (c) Reactions are stereospecific and regiospecific.
   (d) It require more chemicals, labour and time.
2. Steroidal transformation mainly occurs at ______ .
   (a) Growth phase (b) Transformation phase
   (c) Death phase (d) None of the above
3. Prednisone is produced from cortisone with *Corynebacterium simplex* by dehydrogenation at position ______ .
   (a) Δ^1 (b) Δ^7
   (b) Δ^{13} (d) Δ^{16}
4. Estrone is produced from 19-hydroxy-4-androstene-3, 17-dione with *Nocardia restricta* by aromatization of ring ______ .
   (a) A (b) B
   (c) C (d) D

■■■

Chapter ... 16

FERMENTATION

♦ LEARNING OBJECTIVES ♦

After completing this chapter, reader should be able to understand:

- *Introduction*
- *Inoculum Development*
- *Fermentation Media*
- *Fermenter*
  - *Types of Fermenter*
    - *Submerged Fermenters*
    - *Surface Fermenters*
- *Large Scale Production Fermentor Design*

16.1 INTRODUCTION

Fermentation may be defined as the process of growing microorganisms in a nutrient media by maintaining physicochemical conditions and thereby converting feed into a desired end product. Fermentation is a biochemical reaction in which micro-organisms serve as biocatalysts. Microorganisms are designed to produce different pharmaceuticals such as antibiotics, enzymes, amino acids, insulin, vitamins etc. Microorganisms useful in fermentation are bacteria, actinomycetes, viruses and fungi. The vessels or containers in which fermentation processes are carried out are called as fermenters. A fermenter is frequently confused with a bioreactor. Fermenters are mainly used for growth of prokaryotic cells such as bacteria, actinomycetes etc. and bioreactors are used as for growth of eukaryotic cells such as insects mammalian cells etc. Fermenters also differ from bioreactors In their parts such as agitators and mixers. The selection of a good medium is very important to the success of an industrial fermentation. The medium supplies nutrients for cell growth and biosynthesis of fermentation products. The fermenter is designed and operated for production of different pharmaceuticals under conditions of constant temperature, pH, dissolved oxygen and substrate concentration. The complete fermentation process is represented in Fig. 16.1. A list of major industrial products prepared from fermentation is given in Table 16.1.

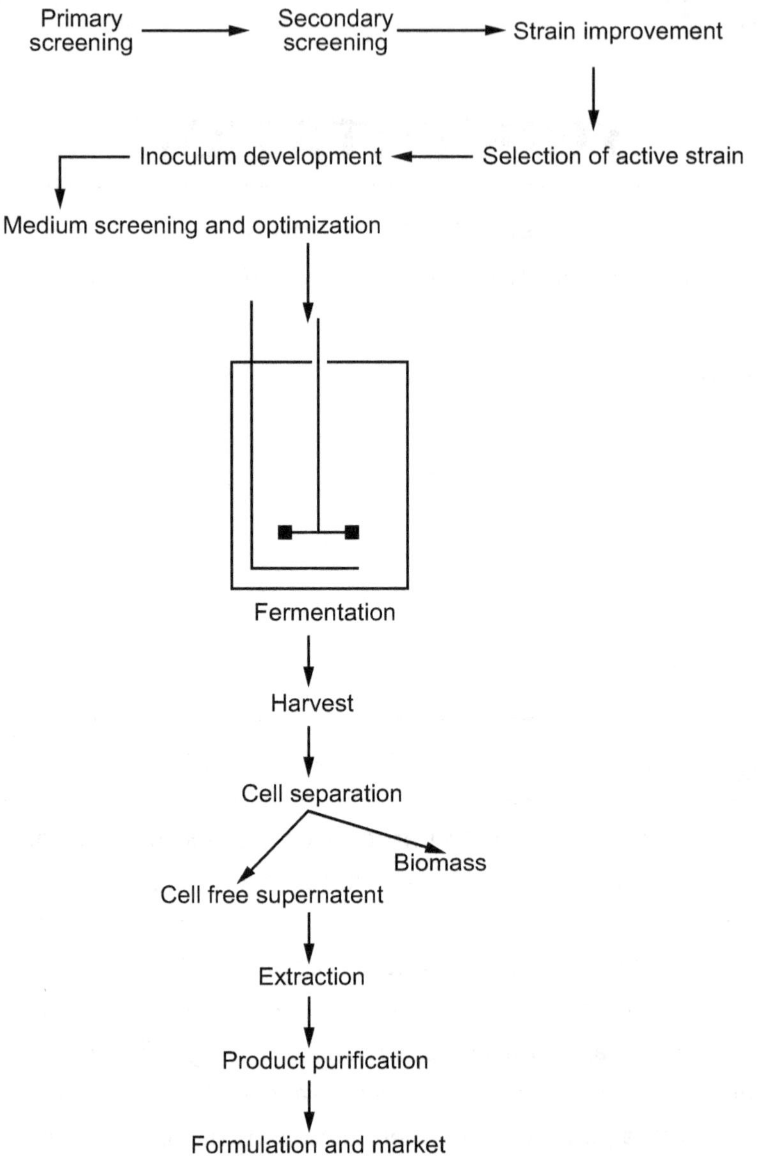

Fig. 16.1: Flow sheet of typical fermentation process

Table 16.1: Major fermentation products

Group	Product	Producing micro-organism
Antibiotics	Penicillin Streptomycin Chlorampenicol Polymyxin	*Penicillium chrysogenum* *Streptomyces griseus* *Streptomyces venezuelae* *Bacillus polymyxa*

contd. …

Enzymes	Amylases	*Aspergillus oryzae*
	Proteases	*Bacillus* species
	Lipases	*Saccharomycess lipolytica*
Amino acids	L-lysine	*Corynebacterium glutamicium*
	Glutamic acid	*Corynebacterium glutamicium*
Polysaccarides	Dextran	*Leuconostic mesenteroids*
	Xanthan gum	*Xanthomones compestris.*
Vitamins	Riboflavin	*Ashbya gossypi*
	Vitamin B_{12}	*Pseudomonas dentrificans*
Industrial chemicals	Ethanol (from glucose)	*Saccharomyces cerevisiae*
	Citric acid	*Aspergillus niger*
	Lactic acid	*Lactobacillus delbrueckii*
Food and beverages	Beer or bread	*Saccharomyces cerevisiae*
	Cheese	*Streptococcus* species.

16.2 INOCULUM DEVELOPMENT

The microbial cells are required to inoculate large quantities of production medium in a larger fermenter. A single loopful of culture can not meet the requirement of complete fermentation. Hence, inoculum is prepared as a stepwise sequence employing increasing volume of media (Fig. 16.2). The fermenter can be inoculated with a large quantity of actively growing microbial cells. The size of the inoculum is normally between 1 to 10 per cent by volume. The chemical composition of the inoculum medium may be different from the production medium. The main objective of inoculum medium is to produce active biomass of cells and that of production medium is to produce the required fermentation product. The inoculum must be available as actively growing cells and must be free from contaminants.

Microbial cells must pass through many generations during inoculum production. It is possible for microbial cells to undergo mutation during inoculum development. Mutation does not poses a serious problem if the strain used in fermentation is not a mutant. These cells mutation is generally infrequent and if occurs it does not interfere with the growth of non-mutated cells. It becomes a serious problem if mutated strain is used for the fermentation process. These mutated strains have high frequency of the occurrence of a back mutation. This may be overcome by employing media and incubation conditions which tend to select the growth of the mutant strain.

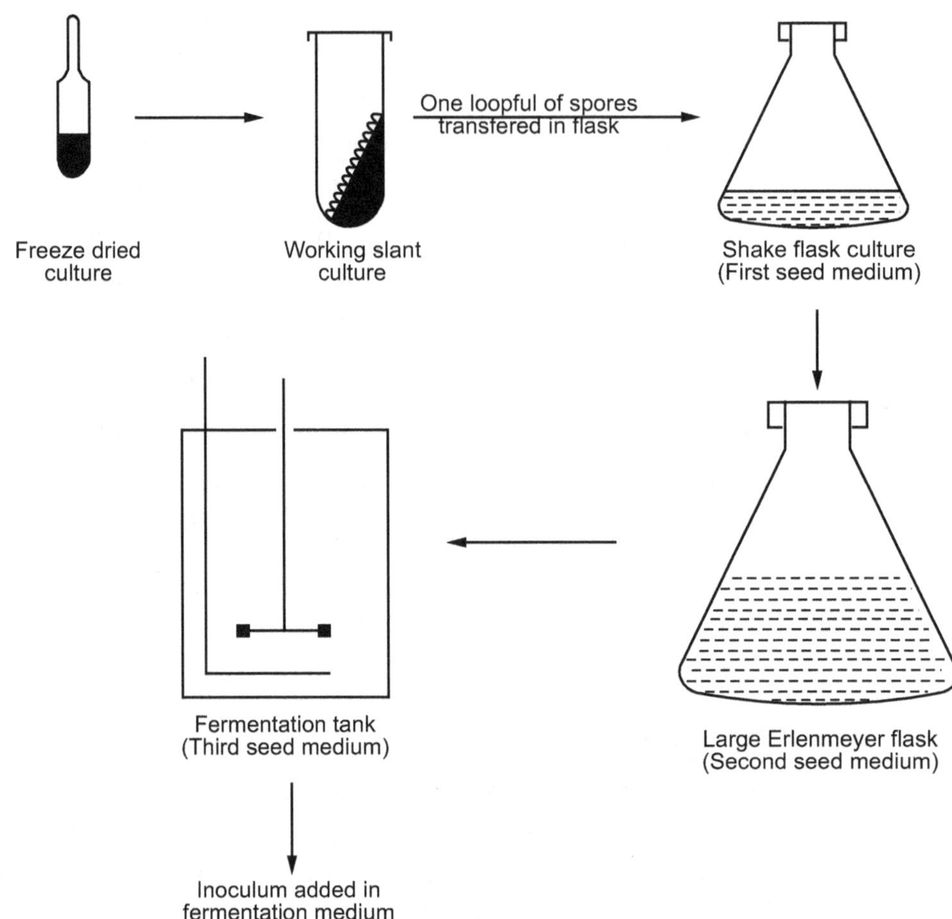

Fig. 16.2: Inoculum development technique of spore forming micro-organisms

Industrially important micro-organisms are filamentous and are capable of producing spores (fungi, actinomycetes, bacteria). The initiation of growth in the liquid inoculum media depends upon the nature of micro-organisms. Bacterial cells or spores are suspended in a sterile diluents for transfer in the liquid inoculcum medium. *Clostridium* species often require heat treatment to induce germination of spores. Spores of fungi and actinomycetes are germinated by using special medium. Then these germinated spores are transferred to the normal inoculum medium. One example of inoculum development technique is given in Fig. 16.2. The preparation of spore suspensions (e.g. actinomycetes) is done by adding a suitable diluent to sporulated agar growth. The spores must be loosened from the surface with a sterile wire loop. It is also required to add a non-toxic wetting agent (e.g. sodium lauryl sulfonate) in the diluent to make the distribution of spores uniform in the dilution fluid. In contrast, some stationary fungal fermentation (e.g. *Aspergillus niger* citric acid fermentation) require the spores to be floated on the surface of the liquid medium. In case of poorly sporulating fungi or actinomycetes, fragmented hyphae are transferred to the broth medium.

16.3 FERMENTATION MEDIA

The choice of a good medium is very important for the success of industrial fermentation. All microorganisms require water and sources of nitrogen, carbon, mineral elements, vitamins amino acids etc. for growth. The microbial cells also require different growth factors, precursors of fermentation products, dissolved gases, buffers, antifoaming agents for the synthesis of specific fermentation products. One of the major problems for the fermentation industry is to design a suitable production medium. This is only done by a trial and error method.

The ideal characteristics of fermentation medium should meet the following criteria:

- Production of the maximum yield of product or biomass in short duration.
- A minimum yield of undersized other products.
- A simple, suitable chemical composition of production medium.
- Free from any toxic effect on culture or product.
- Low cost, good quality and easily available.
- Raw materials required for production medium are easily available at a low cost.
- Most suitable for production process such as agitation, extraction, purification, waste treatment etc.
- Production medium must be suitable for adjustment pH, consistency and composition.
- Inhibition or slowing of the growth of contaminating micro-organisms.
- Allowing the proper growth and maintenance of the genetic stability of active microorganisms.
- Foaming must be minimum.
- Media components must not interfere with the extraction and purification of desired product.

The composition of a fermentation medium may be simple or complex depending on the particular micro-organism, its nutritional needs and the product required. A synthetic medium contains known components and these media components are easily redesigned to increase possible yield of the product. Foaming is not a problem of fermentation which contains synthetic media because these media do not contain any high molecular weight peptides and proteins. The purification of fermentation products is also simple with the synthetic media. The synthetic media may be expensive because of the high cost of pure ingredients and the yields obtained from these media are low. Crude or non-synthetic medium mainly produce higher yield of fermentation products. Crude medium mainly contains soyabean meal, black strap molasses and corn steep liquor as a source of carbon and nitrogen.

Carbon sources:

The common carbon sources used in pharmaceutical fermentation processes are glucose, fructose, sucrose, molasses, hydrolyzed starch, organic acids, hydrocarbons plant oils etc. Beet and cane molasses are the concentrated syrups formed in the sugar-refining process as by-products of sugar industry. Blackstrap molasses is the cheapest and most useful sugar source for industrial fermentation. In addition to sucrose, blackstrap molasses also contain small amounts of complex polysaccharides and invert sugars. Glucose, sucrose and fructose are more expensive as compared to molasses but it gives more clean medium. Complex starch-containing substrates such as cornmeal are widely used in secondary metabolite fermentation. Plant oils are a rich source of carbon than carbohydrates.

Cellulose materials are complex carbohydrates made up of repeating units of β-glucose. Sulfite waste liquor is the spent sulfite liquor obtained from the paper-pulping industry. It is a dilute sugar solution having approximately 2% sugar content. Hexoses (D-glucose, D-galactose, D-mannose) and pentoses (D-xylose, L-arabinose) are mainly present in sulfite waste liquor as monosaccharides.

Nitrogen sources:

The most common nitrogen sources are yeast extract, peptone, ammonia, distillers solubles, soyabean meal, corn steep liquor, fish meal, cottonseed meal etc. Distillers solubles are prepared from fermented grain or maize by distillation using alcohol. Effluent is concentrated to reach the solid content 35% w/v (evaporator syrup). This syrup is then dried to yield 'distillers solubles'. It is used as a production medium and it supplies nitrogen with many accessory food factors. Corn-steep liquor is the water extract by-product resulting from the steeping of corn during the production of starch, gluten and other corn products. The spent steep waters are concentrated to approximately 50% solids and this concentrate is called corn-steep liquor. It was first extensively used in fermentation media for the production of penicillin. Corn-steep liquor mainly contains lactic acid, amino acids, glucose, salts and vitamins. Soyabean meal is the components left after deoiling of soyabean seeds and it contains approximately 8% w/v nitrogen.

Buffers:

Buffers are generally added in the production medium for their buffering capacity. During microbial growth in the fermentation, pH may be changed by acidic or alkaline products. Decarboxylation of organic acids among the medium constituents may raise the pH and deamination of strongly basic organic amines lower the pH of fermentation media. Calcium carbonate is generally added in fermentation media to provide neutralization of acidic fermentation products. Media containing proteins, peptides and amino acids possess good buffer capacity in the pH range near neutrality.

Antifoaming agent:

Fermentation media containing proteins or peptides can produce foam in the process of agitation and aeration. Proteolytic bacteria mainly produce high levels of foam. If this foam is not controlled, it may rise in the head space of the tank. This condition is mainly responsible for causing contamination of the fermenter. In high levels of foam, medium may be forced out from the tank as foam. Therefore, antifoam agents are added in the media to control the foam. These antifoam agents can lower the surface tension and decrease the stability of the foam bubbles. Two types of antifoam agents are commonly used in fermentation i.e. crude organic materials and inert antifoams. Antifoams made from crude organic materials are sterilized separately and then added in the fermentation. Corn oil, soyabean oil, lavd oil, octadecanol and other fatty acids are commonly used as antifoam agents. These antifoam agents may be toxic or lower the pH of media or provide specific nutrients to cultures. Silicon compounds are mainly used as inert antifoam agents. These agents are not utilized by the micro-organisms and they are also non-toxic.

Minerals:

Most fermentation process requires minerals for the growth of micro-organisms. Minerals such as potassium, phosphorus, sulfur, copper, chloride, cobalt, iron, manganese and zinc are frequently added in the media. These compounds are mainly present in complex nitrogen or carbon sources.

Precursors:

Precursors are added prior to or simultaneously with the fermentation. These substances are used to increase the yield or improve the quality of the product. Phenylacetic acid is added in the fermentation medium of penicillin G and inorganic cobalt in the medium of vitamin B_{12} as a precursor.

All fermentation media are generally sterilized by boiling or passing steam through the medium or steam under pressure i. e. autoclaving. In a small-scale laboratory fermenter, the medium is directly placed in the fermenter and then the fermenter is sterilized by autoclave. Large-scale medium is sterilized by passing it through heated retention tubes containing steam jet heaters. The medium constituents at double to triple strength are mixed with water in a mixing tank. The final medium is then passed through retention tubes and heat exchangers. Retention tubes contain steam jet heaters that inject high pressure steam into the medium to sterilize it. The rate of passage of steam is adjusted to provide proper sterilization without over cooking. Sterilizing synthetic media requires less time than the crude media. Media containing vitamins and enzymes cannot be sterilized by the heat method. These sensitive components are sterilized separately by a bacteriological filter and then added into the sterilized media.

16.4 FERMENTER

The industrial microorganisms require to grow in a large vessel containing considerable quantities of nutrient media by maintaining favorable conditions. These containers are called as fermenters. These fermenters provide optimum growth and metabolism to microbial strains for production of the desired product. The term 'bioreactor' is often used synonymously for fermenter. Generally, fermenters are used for growth of prokaryotic cells while bioreactors are used for growth of eukaryotic cells. The design of the fermenter depends upon the purpose for which it is to be used. An ideal fermenter should possess the following characteristics.

(i) It should provide the best possible growth conditions to industrial strains.

(ii) It must make some provision for the control of contaminating microorganisms during fermentation.

(iii) It should have the provision and control over various operations like pH, temperature, agitation, aeration etc. It may have facilities for monitoring all conditions.

(iv) The fermenter should provide all aseptic conditions at the time of sample withdrawal and addition of inoculum.

(v) The fermenter vessels must be strong enough to withstand the pressures and toxicity of media.

(vi) Fermenter must have the facility of incorporation of sterile air and stirring.

(vii) It should provide all facilities for intermittent addition of antifoam agents, alkali or acid and other nutrients.

(viii) Fermenter should have additional inoculum, seed or media tanks.

(ix) It should be designed in such a way that it consumes less power, has less evaporation, can be used for long periods of operation and has proper sampling facilities.

(x) It should have the facility for complete removal of broth from the tank and should be easy to clean.

Types of fermenter:

Fermenters are available in various sizes and their sizes are defined on the total volume capacity of the fermenter. According to size, fermenters are classified as follows:

(i) Small laboratory and research fermenter: 1 to 50 litre

(ii) Pilot plant fermenter: 50 to 1000 litre

(iii) Large size industrial production scale fermenter: more than 1000 litre.

Small scale fermenters are autoclavable while large scale fermenters are sterilized by in-situ sterilization. The small laboratory fermenters are designed to provide varying conditions for the growth of micro-organisms and are adjusted to provide similiar growth conditions mainly found in the largest industrial production tanks. Broadly, the fermenters are also classified as submerged fermenters and surface fermenters (Fig. 16.3).

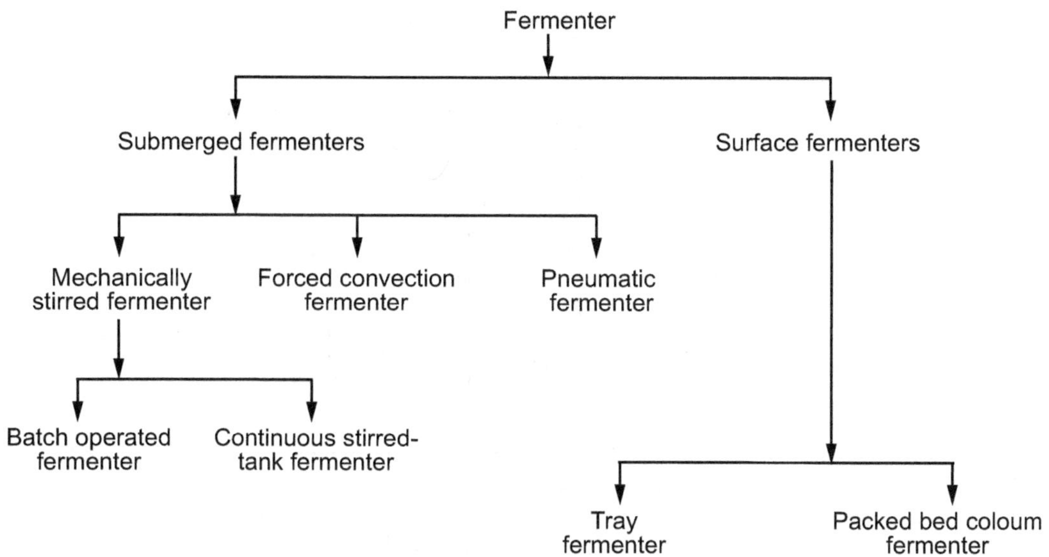

Fig. 16.3: Types of fermenters

16.4.1 Submerged Fermenters

In submerged fermenters (suspended-growth system), the micro-organisms are dispersed in nutrient medium (liquid) at maintained environmental conditions. On the basis of mechanism of agitation, fermenters are further classified as follows.

1. **Mechanically stirred fermenters:** These fermenters are equipped with a mechanical agitator so as to maintain homogencity and rapid dispersion and mixing of materials. Mechanically stirred fermenters are stirred tank fermenter, stirred multistage fermenter (continuous process), paddle wheel reactor and stirred loop reactor. Stirred tank fermenter is the most applicable fermenter in fermentation industry for the batch process. The main advantage of this fermenter is the flexibility in design and is used in the range of 1 litre to 100 ton capacity sizes. The agitators consist of one or more impellers mounted on a shaft. Different types of blades are used according to the requirements. It is rotated with the help of an electric motor. A basic computer controlled stirred tank fermenter is shown in Fig. 16.4.

A continuous stirred-tank fermenter (CSTF) is basically the same as a batch fermenter. However, in addition of feed and overflow devices, steady-state condition can be achieved by 'chemostatic' or 'turbidostatic ' principles. In continuous fermentation, fresh medium is added continuously in the fermentation vessel and in other end medium is withdrawn for recovery of fermentation products. A continuous fermenter can be conducted in various techniques. It can be performed as a 'single stage' in which single fermenter is inoculated and then kept in continuous operation by balancing the input and output culture media [Fig. 16.5 (a)]. In a 'recycle' continuous fermentation, a portion of the withdrawn culture or residual unused substrate plus the withdrawn culture is recycled to the fermentation vessel [Fig. 16.5. (b)]. The 'multiple-stage' continuous fermentation, involves two or more stages with the fermenters being operated in sequence [Fig. 16.5 (c)].

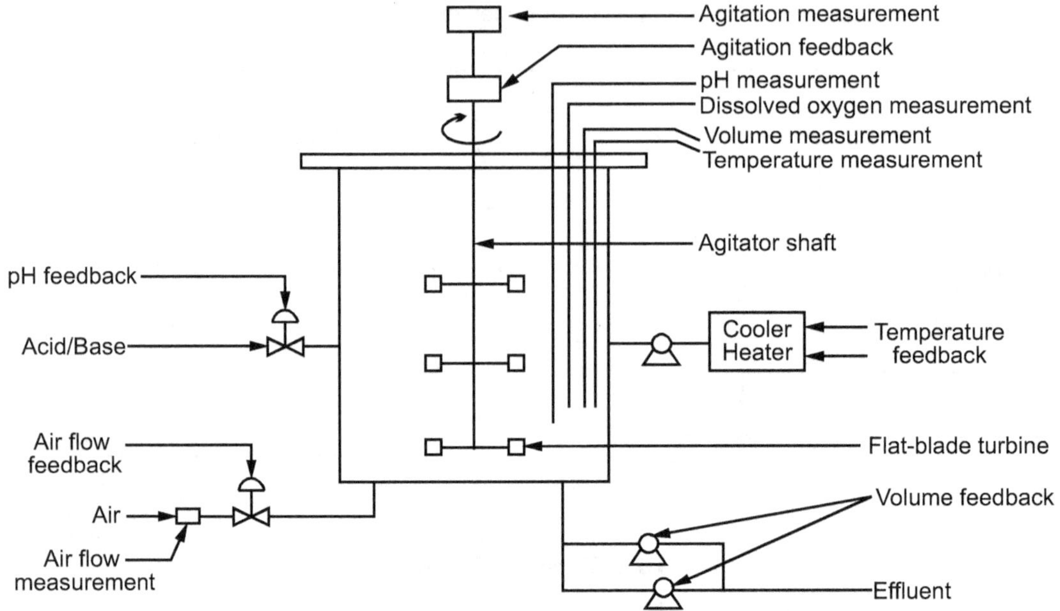

Fig. 16.4: A computer controlled stirred-tank batch fermenter

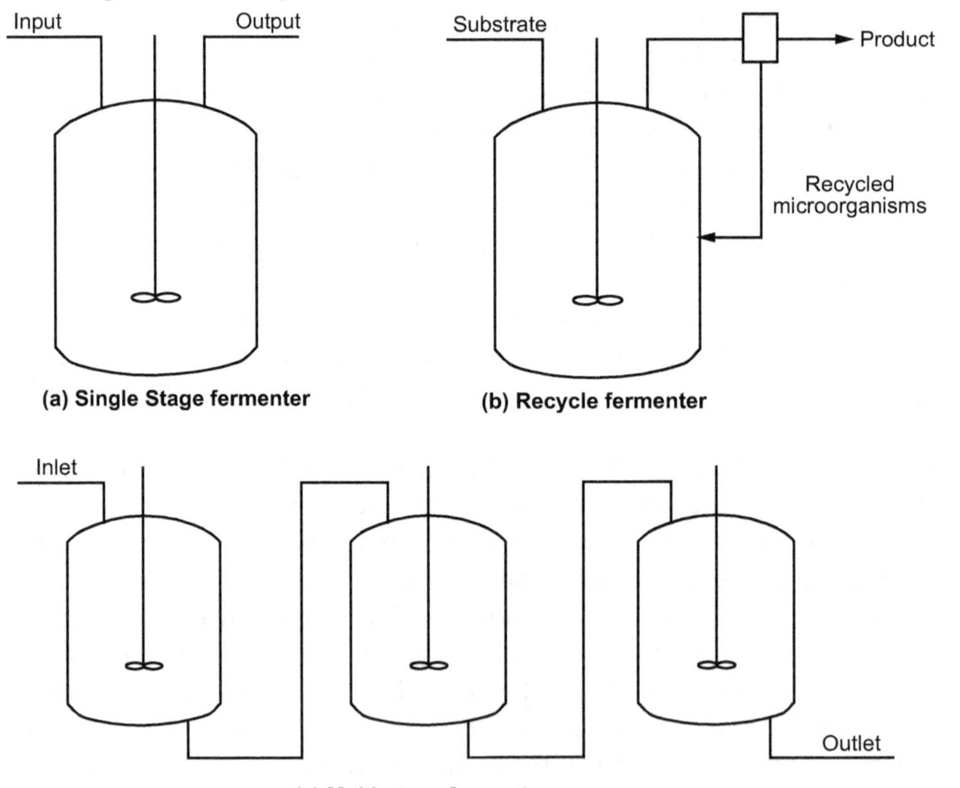

(a) Single Stage fermenter

(b) Recycle fermenter

(c) Multi-stage fermenter

Fig. 16.5: Types of continuous fermentation

Advantages of batch fermentation:

- Less risk of contamination or cell mutation because of short growth period.
- More flexibility with different product and biological systems.
- Process is more economical and simple.
- Raw material conversion level is more.

Disadvantages of batch fermentation:

- Low productivity due to the time required for sterilizing, filling, cooling, emptying, cleaning etc.
- More expenses are required for subcultures for inoculation, labour and process control.
- More focus on instrumentation due to frequent sterilization
- Larger industrial hygiene risks due to potential contact with pathogenic micro-organisms.

Advantages of continuous fermentation:

- Less labor expense due to automation of fermentation process.
- Less toxicity risks to operator by any toxins producing by micro-organisms.
- High yield and good quality product due to invariable operating parameters and automation of the process.
- Less stress on fermenter as sterilization is not very frequent.

Disadvantages of continuous fermentation:

- Uniformity in media quality is necessary to ensure that the process remains continuous.
- Higher investment cost in control and automation equipment.
- More risk of contamination and cell mutation.
- Slight variation only is possible in the continuous process.

2. Forced convection fermenters: In forced convection fermenters, the agitation is affected by using a pump, instead of a mechanical stirrer. 'Loop fermenter' and deep jet fermenter are available involving liquid movement and gas entertainer. In the loop fermenter, gas distribution device is a subsidiary vessel, where a liquid saturated with gas is circulated by forced convection into the fermenter vessel. In deep jet fermenter, gas is entertained into a high power jet of liquid into the liquid of the fermenter. Two different types of forced convection fermenters are available i.e. gas-lift or air-lift fermenter and bubble column or sparged tank fermenter. Different forced convection fermenters are shown in Fig. 16.6 and Fig. 16.7.

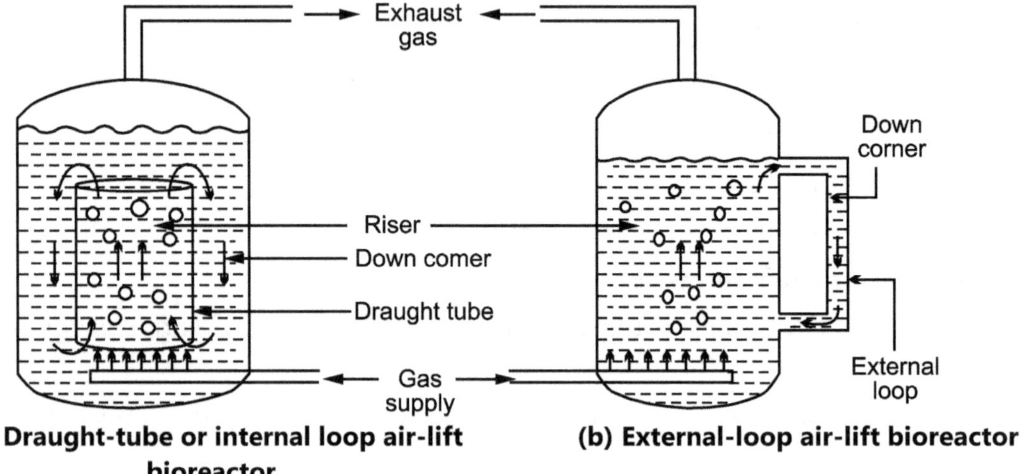

(a) Draught-tube or internal loop air-lift bioreactor

(b) External-loop air-lift bioreactor

Fig. 16.6: Air-lift bioreactors

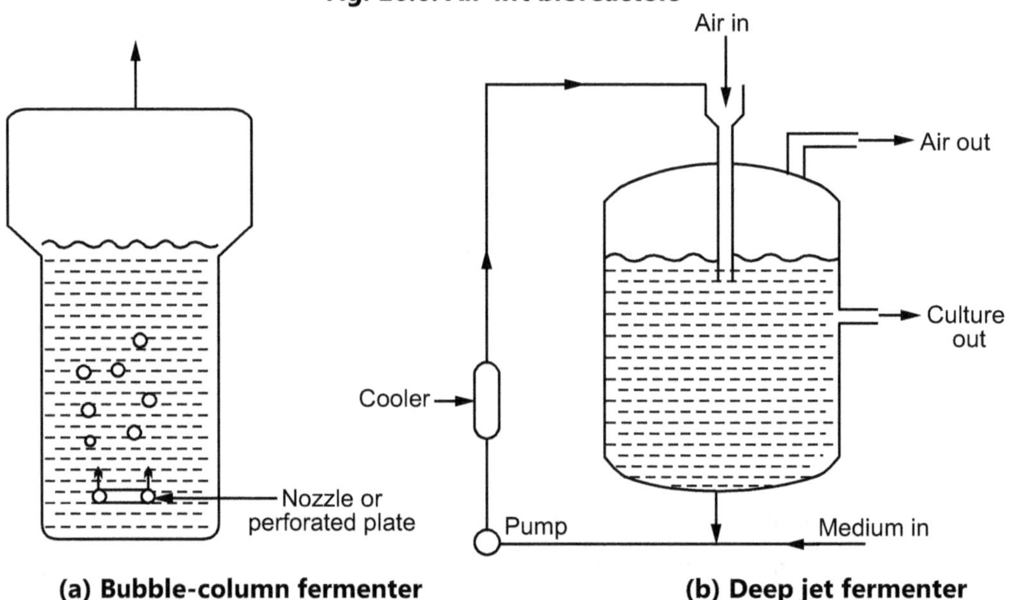

(a) Bubble-column fermenter

(b) Deep jet fermenter

Fig. 16.7: Bubble-column and Deep jet fermenter

Air-lift fermenters are classified as draught tube or internal loop fermenter and external loop fermenter. In the gas-lift fermenters, internal liquid circulation in the vessel is achieved by sparging the vessel with gas. Fluid volume of the vessel is divided into two interconnected zones by draught tube. Air is typically fed through a sparger ring into the bottom of a central draught tube that controls the circulation of air and the medium. The airlift external-loop reactor system is used for circulation of direct air and liquid throughout the vessel. This system consists of a riser and an external down comer, which are connected at the bottom and the top respectively. The injected air at the bottom of the riser creates gas bubbles that rise through the fermentation tank and the heavier solution descends through the down comer. The external-loop airlift reach system has some advantages as compared to standard airlifts (Internal-loop reactors). These are:

- Easy measurement and control in the riser and the down comer.
- Efficient temperature control and heat-transfer.
- Low friction with an optimal hydraulic diameter for riser and down comer.
- Specific residence time in the individual section.

Bubble column reactor is a cylindrical column, in which the gas is sparged at the bottom through nozzles on a perforated or porous distributor plates. The gas bubbles rise through the liquid in the vessel and may be redispersed by a succession of horizontal perforated baffle plates. Temperature controls are maintained by the temperature jacket or the internal coils.

Air-lift fermenters provide many advantages as compare to the standard fermenter.

- High flexibility, less shear rate.
- Controlled flow and efficient mixing.
- Simple design without any moving parts like agitator.
- Easy maintenance, less risk of defects and easy sterilization.
- Specific defined residence time for all phases.
- Large volume tanks, possible specific interfacial contact-area with low energy input.
- Higher mass-transfer due to enhanced oxygen solubility achieved in larger tank with greater pressure.

3. **Pneumatic fermenter:** Fluidized bed bioreactor is an example of pneumatic bioreactor used in fermentation involving fluid with suspended particulate biocatalyst (enzyme) or cell particles or microbial flocs (Fig. 16.8). The cell particles are fluidized with up-coming stream of liquids. Top part of the fluidized fermenter is expanded to reduce superficial velocity of fluidized bed. Solids set easily in setting zone and then dropped into fluidized zone.

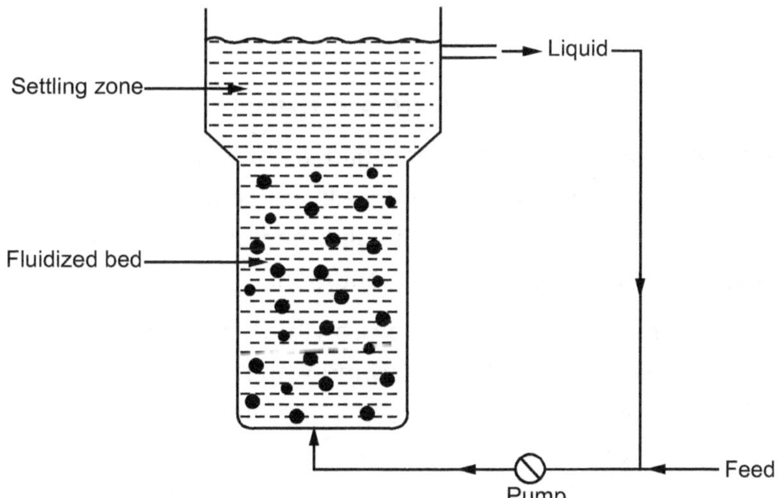

Fig. 16.8: Fluidized bed bioreactor

16.4.2 Surface Fermenters

Microbial cells are cultured on the surface layer of the nutrient medium (solid/ liquid) held in a dish or a tray and is generally called as surface culture system or supported growth system. This technique is commonly used for production of citric acid from *Aspergillus niger* and nicotanic acid from *Aspergillus terrus*. Microbial films can be developed on the surfaces of suitable packing medium. This may be in the form of a fixed bed, stones or plastic sheets. This system is commonly used in biological waste water treatment. Packed bed column fermenter and tray fermenter are the example of surface fermenters.

1. **Packed bed column fermenter:** This is type of surface culture bioreactor in which solid particles form the packed bed on which enzymes are immobilized. A liquid nutrient is allowed to flow continuously through the packed bed. Metabolic products are released in the fluid and removed in the outflow (Fig. 16.9). When the film of micro-organisms is formed on the surface of packing material then this is called as film bioreactor.

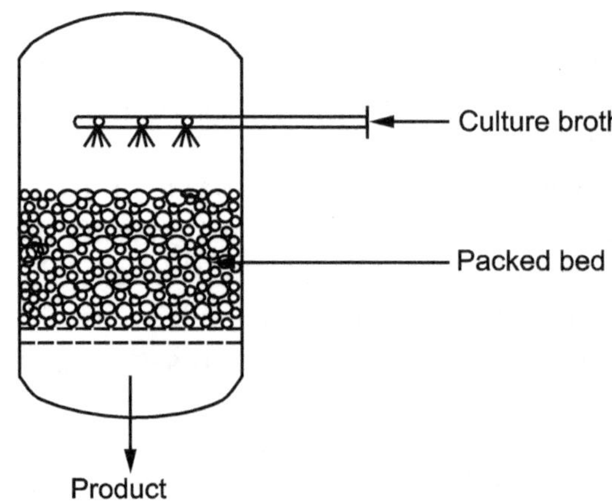

Fig. 16.9: Packed bed fermenter

2. **Tray fermenter:** In tray fermenter, solid as well as liquid media are used for fermentation. If liquid medium is used, cells are allowed to float easily and to make the process continuous (Fig. 16.10). If solid medium is used for tray fermenter then the process is called as solid state fermentation.

Solid state fermentation is defined as the growth of microorganisms (mainly fungi) on moist solid materials in the absence of free-flowing water. These processes have been used for the production of antibiotics, alkaloids, enzymes, organic acids, and also for bioremediation of hazardous compounds, biological detoxification of agro-industrial residues, nutritional enrichment, biopharmaceutical products etc. Solid state fermentation (SSF) has become a more attractive alternative to liquid fermentation for many productions.

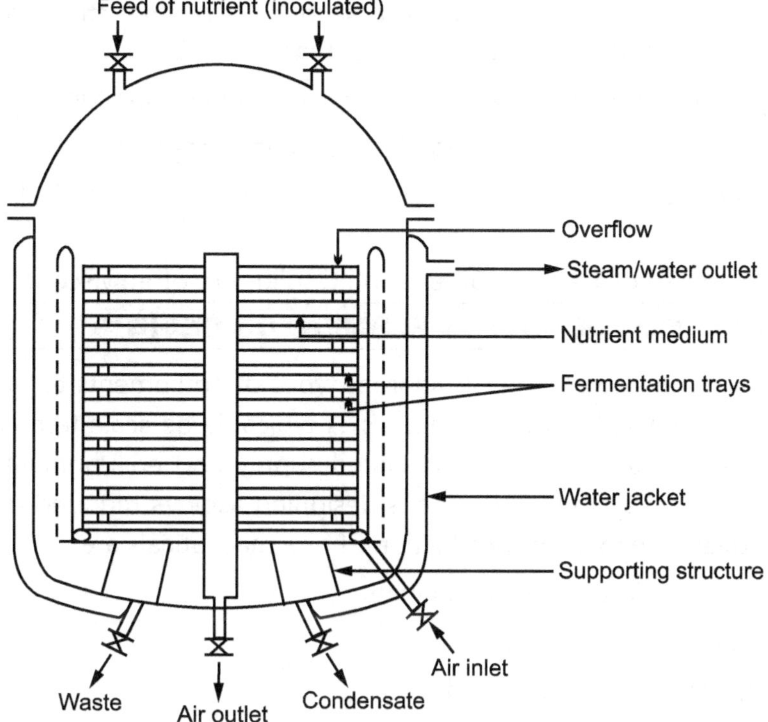

Fig. 16.10: Tray fermenter as a continuous process

Advantages of solid state fermentation:

- Solid state fermentation produce higher yields than submerged liquid fermentation.
- The possibilities of contamination by bacteria and yeast are very less because of low availability of water.
- All natural habitats for fungi are easily maintained in solid state fermentation.
- Culture media are very simple and it provides all the nutrients for growth of microorganisms.
- Simple design of fermenter and low energy requirements.
- Small reactors are used due to concentrated nature of the substrate.
- Low moisture availability may favor the production of specific compounds.
- Inoculations with spores (fungi) facilitate its uniform dispersion through the medium.

Disadvantages of solid state fermentation:

- The solid nature of the substrate causes problems in the monitoring of the process parameters (pH, moisture content, substrate and oxygen concentration).
- Agitation and biomass determination is very difficult.
- Solid state fermentation is only suitable for microorganisms that can grow at low moisture levels.

- The substrates require pre-treatment such as size reduction, homogenisation, chemical or enzymatic hydrolysis, vapours treatment etc.
- Possibility of contamination by different types of undesirable fungi.
- Aeration may be difficult due to high level of solid contents.
- Spores have larger lag times due to need for germination and also require more cultivation times.
- Products obtained by leaching of fermented solids are often viscous.

16.5 LARGE SCALE PRODUCTION FERMENTOR DESIGN

Fermenter is a system consisting of different types of equipments to provide microbial growth by controlling environmental conditions. A typical large scale fermenter consists of three parts such as the culture vessel, associated supply and environmental systems and measurement and control system. The various designing aspects required to be considered in constructing a ideal fermenter for production of pharmaceuticals are:

- Provide operation free from contamination.
- Adequate mixing and aeration.
- Maintain specific temperature and pH.
- Access points for inoculation and sampling.
- Non-toxic to microorganisms and safety.
- Minimize liquid loss from the fermenter.
- Monitoring and control of dissolved oxygen.
- Allow feeding of nutrient solution and reagent.
- Suitability for wide range of microbial cultures.
- Minimal use of labour and finances.
- Cheapest materials and smooth internal surfaces for vessel.

The fermenter is made up of stainless steel or borosilicate glass. They are non-corrosive, non-toxic and easily cleanable. The head plates provide parts for nutrient medium probes, gas input and waste product removal. Head plates and other accessories are fitted to the vessel by making use of gaskets, lip-seal and silicon rubber o-rings. Aeration and agitation are achieved by using stirrers, baffles, agitators (impeller), paddles and aeration system (sparger). Agitation and aeration system is one of the major requirements of aerobic fermentation.

Aeration of the fermentation medium is required to supply oxygen to the production of microorganisms and remove carbon dioxide from the fermenter. Air contains microorganisms, hence, it is sterilized before addition into the fermeter. Air is sterilized by heat treatment at 250 to 300°C or ultraviolet light or cellulose filter or porcelain filter or cotton wool packed filters or fibre glass wool filters. Filters are used, which have the effective porosity to filter microorganisms larger than 0.25 μ in size. Filters used for aeration are made up of metal or plastic or glass. Oxygen is introduced at the bottom of the fermenter through a sparger. Spargers are situated at the bottom of the fermentation tank below the impeller. Spargers are prepared from non-corrosive metal, rubber, porous carbon, sintered glass or ceramic substance. Fine bubbles are produced with the help of sparger to dissolve maximum oxygen. Aeration is required to produce larger amount of biomass and growth of culture. Rate of airflow is measured in terms of volume of air/volume or medium/min or cubic ft. / sq. ft. of bottom of fermenter. The aeration capacity of the medium can be enhanced by stirring. The aeration capacity of the stirred fermenter is proportional to the stirring speed, rate of air flow and the internal pressure.

Agitation in fermenter is most important for oxygen transfer, develop larger interface for oxygen dissolution, mixing of media contents and maintains uniform environment inside the production tank. Fermenters have impellers (Fig. 16.11) present to bring about agitaton in the medium. Position and number of impellers are dependent on size, volume and height of fermenter. Stirrer shaft can enter the vessel from the top (normal case) or from side or from the bottom. Stirrer is rotated by the motor through adjustable pulley and belt or through direct drive. Proper sealing is required at the entry point of shaft into fermenters to prevent contamination. Agitation results into vertex formation and escape the bubbles into hollow cone. Impeller action causes spinning of liquid as a mass. Vertical plates or baffles are present on inside wall of fermenter to correct situation. Speed of impeller depends on size of the fermenter vessel and nature of microorganisms.

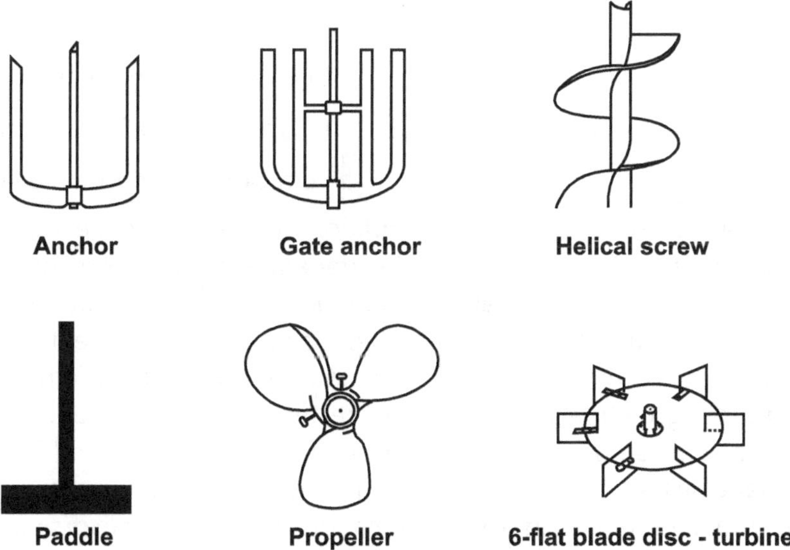

Fig. 16.11: Types of Impellers

Fermentation Monitoring and Control

Measurement and control of environmental conditions and biological variable is called fermentation monitoring. The process monitoring parameters are listed in Table 16.2. New developments in digital electronics have permitted a high level of monitoring and control of fermentation processes. The computer can be a vital instrument for process optimization and control.

Table 16.2: Controlled parameters and monitoring devices in fermentation

Sr. No	Process control	Monitoring device
1.	Air flow (0 to 6 lit/ min)	Flow meter
2.	Water flow	Rota meter.
3.	Temperature (8 to 60°C)	Thermometer/ thermistor/ thermocouple
4.	pH (2 to 12)	pH meter
5.	Agitator speed (0 to 1000 rpm)	Tachometer
6.	Pressure (2000 m bar)	Pressure gauze.
7.	DO_2 (0 to 100%)	DO_2 analyzer
8 .	Power input	Vom, target
9.	Foam	Foam, sensing and control unit.
10.	Rheology	Tube or cone-plate viscometer
11.	Cell concentration	Gravimetric dry weight or turbidimetry.
12.	State of culture	Enzyme probes, substrate concentration.
13.	Gas analysis	CO_2 analyzers, gas chromatography.
14.	Redox potential	DO_2 analyzer, DCO_2 analyzer, Polarographic probes, Galvanic probes.

Process parameters are the optimum conditions which are to be maintained for the production organism. These conditions may be dependent on type of organisms such as bacteria, actinomycetes, yeast, mould etc. It also depends on fermentation process such as aerobic or anaerobic, surface fermentation or submerged fermentation and batch fermentation or continuous fermentation. The most important part in fermentation process is to maintain optimal growth environment in the fermenter for production of maximum product. Maximum efficiency of the fermentation can be achieved by continuously monitoring the variables such as temperature, pH, dissolved oxygen, pressure, adequate mixing, nutrient concentration and foam formation. Improved sensors are available for continuous and automated monitoring of these variables.

Temperature control: The temperature control in the fermenter or pipe is an important parameter for a good fermentation process. Lower temperature causes reduced product formation, while higher temperature adversely affects the growth of microorganisms. The bioreactors are normally equipped with heating and cooling systems that can be used to maintain the optimal temperature. Temperature may be measured by mercury in glass thermometers, pressure bulb thermometers, bimetallic thermometers, thermocouples, metal-resistant thermometers or thermistors. Metal resistant thermometers and thermistors are used in most fermentation applications.

pH monitoring and control: Many microbial cells growth optimally between pH 5.5 and 8.5. Microbial cells grow rapidly in fermentation medium and release the metabolites which are responsible for change in pH. Hence, the pH of the medium should be continuously monitored and maintained at the optimal level. Rapid changes in pH can often be reduced by careful design of production medium with respect to carbon and nitrogen sources. The pH of fermentation medium is also controlled by addition of acid or alkali base. Combined glass electrode is routinely used for pH measurement. Other electrodes such as silver chloride, calomel, mercury etc. are commonly used for pH measurements with connection to pH meter.

Dissovled oxygen: In most aerobic fermentations, it is essential to ensure that the dissolved oxygen concentration does not fall below a specified minimal level. Oxygen is sparingly soluble in water and it is continuously supply to the culture medium in the form of sterilized air. Continuous monitoring of dissolved oxygen concentration is most important for optimal product formation. In small fermenters, the component electrodes are galvanic and have a lead anode, silver cathode and employ potassium hydroxide, chloride, bicarbonate or acetate as electrolyte. The sensing tip of electrode is a Teflon, polyethylene or polystyrene membrane which allows passage of the gas phase. These electrodes are suitable for monitoring very slow changes in oxygen concentration. Polarographic electrodes are commonly used in pilot and production fermenter with gold using aqueous potassium chloride as the electrolyte. Dissolved oxygen concentrations may be determined by a tubing method. The oxygen which diffuses from the fermentation medium through the tubing wall into the inert gas stream and then determined using a paramagnetic gas analyzer.

Pressure measurement: Positive pressure is maintained in fermentation vessel and it may differ from process to process. Positive pressure helps to dissolve the oxygen into medium. It does not allow external organisms to enter from any gaps which may be present at joints or valves. Positive pressure in the fermenter vessel in controlled by adjustment of pneumatic control valve in the exhaust line. The pressure maintained is 12 to 15 lb per sq. inch.

Foam formation and control: Foam formation is dependent on composition of media, type of microorganisms, aeration, agitation and type of metabolic product. Foam formation can cause serious problems in fermentation. Antifoaming agents are added in fermentation, when the culture starts foaming above certain predetermined level. Mineral oils based on silicone or vegetable oils are commonly used as antifoaming agents. Antifoaming agents may be added slowly at a predetermined rate by small pump so that foaming never occurs and there is no need to foam sensing system. A foam sensing and control unit is often used and it is a probe inserted through the top plate of the fermenter. Mechanical antifoaming devices may be used such as disc, propellers, brushes or hollow cones attached to the agitator shaft above the surface of the broth. The foam is broken down when it is thrown against the walls of the fermenter.

QUESTIONS

(A) Objective Type Questions:

1. Draw a neat labelled diagram of a fermenter.
2. How will you regulate concentration of gases in fermentation?
3. Draw a complete typical flow sheet of fermentation process.
4. Write advantages and disadvantages of air-lift fermenter.
5. Differentiate between internal loop air-lift fermenter and external loop airlift fermenter.

(B) Short Answer Questions:

1. Discuss the different factors for designing of a fermenter.
2. How will you develop inoculum of spores forming microorganisms for fermentation process?
3. Write a short note on:
   (a) Continuous fermentation
   (c) Fluidized bed bioreactor

(C) Long Answer Questions:

1. List different types of fermenters. Explain any one surface fermenter.
2. How will you monitor and control different parameters in large scale fermentation?
3. What is submerged fermentation? Explain any one submerged fermenter.

(D) Multiple Choice Questions:

1. Air-lift bioreactors contain draught tube which is situated in to the fermenter.
   (a) Internal (b) External
   (c) Both of the above (d) None of the above
2. External loop reactor system is a type of ________ fermenter.
   (a) Air-lift (b) Stirred-tank
   (c) Tray (d) Packed-bed

3. Sparger is used in fermenter for a addition of ______.
   (a) Antifoaming agent (b) Antimicrobial agent
   (c) Sterile medium (d) Sterile air
4. The size of the inoculum is normally _______ % added into a production tank.
   (a) 0.1 – 1 (b) 1 – 10
   (c) 10 – 20 (c) 20 – 30
5. Antibiotics are mainly produced by microorganisms in ______ phase.
   (a) Lag (b) Log
   (c) Stationary (d) Death
6. In fermentation process, impellers are used for ______.
   (a) Aeration (b) Antifoaming
   (c) Centrifugation (d) Agitation

■■■

Chapter ... 17

PRODUCTION OF PHARMACEUTICALS

♦ LEARNING OBJECTIVES ♦

After completing this chapter, reader should be able to understand:

- *Introduction*
- *Penicillin*
- *Citric Acid*
- *Vitamin B_{12}*
- *Glutamic Acid*
- *Griseofulvin*

17.1 INTRODUCTION

Production of antibiotics, vitamins, enzymes and alcoholic products is the main aim of the fermentation industry. Most pharmaceuticals are produced by the process of fermentation using specific microbial strains. Interest in utilization of antibiotics for therapy began in 1929 when **Alexander Fleming** found that a mould *Penicillium* had an effect against *Staphylococcus aureus*. Penicillin was the first antibiotic commercially produced from the *Penicillium* species by the process of fermentation. Its use in treatment of infections, led to the invention of thousands of antibiotics. These antibiotics are mainly produced from fungi, actinomycetes and bacteria. These substances have wide applications in medical, veterinary and agriculture practices.

Antibiotics are the most important class of pharmaceuticals produced by microbial biotechnological processes as a secondary metabolites. Antibiotics are most important as antimicrobial agents for chemotherapy. These antibiotics produced by microbial fermentation or chemical synthesis or a combination of both. The basic molecules of antibiotic may be produced by fermentation and its therapeutic value can be increased by chemical modifications.

Microorganisms can be successfully used for the commercial production of vitamins. Vitamins are organic compounds that are used for normal maintenance and optimal growth of organisms e.g. thiamine, riboflavin, vitamin B_{12}, ascorbic acid, provitamin A etc.

17.2 PENICILLIN

Production of penicillin began in the United States (1941) by surface culture fermentation of *Penicillium notatum*. During World War II, penicillin producing fungi were studied extensively to increase yields of penicillin. Now-a-day, penicillin is produced from

Penicillium chrysogenum by submerged culture techniques. Penicillin is effective against Gram-positive bacteria and also some large viruses and *Rickettsia*. Natural pencillins (penicillins V and G) are effective against several Gram-positive bacteria. They inhibit the bacterial cell wall synthesis and destroy the cell. Penicillin is easily hydrolyse by enzyme β-lactamase. Hence, natural penicillins are ineffective against microorganisms that produce β-lactamase. Semi-synthetic penicillins that are resistant to β-lactamase have been successfully used against a Gram-negative bacteria. Penicillin is a generic term applied to an entire group of antibiotics.

The basic structure of penicillins is 6-amino-penicillanic acid (6 - APA) which consists of a thiazolidine ring with a condensed β-lactum ring. The β-lactum ring - thiazolidine ring of penicillin contains two amino acids such as L-cysteine and D-valine. Penicillins are N-acyl derivatives of 6-amino penicillanic acid (6-APA). If penicillin fermentation is carried out without addition of any side-chain precursors then the active compounds are called as natural penicillins. In commercial process, only penicillins G, penicillin V (Fig. 17.1) and very limited amount of penicillin O have been produced. Penicillin X, do not have any therapeutic value but benzyl penicillin has therapeutic value. The fermentation can be controlled by addition of side-chain precursor so that only desired penicillin is produced.

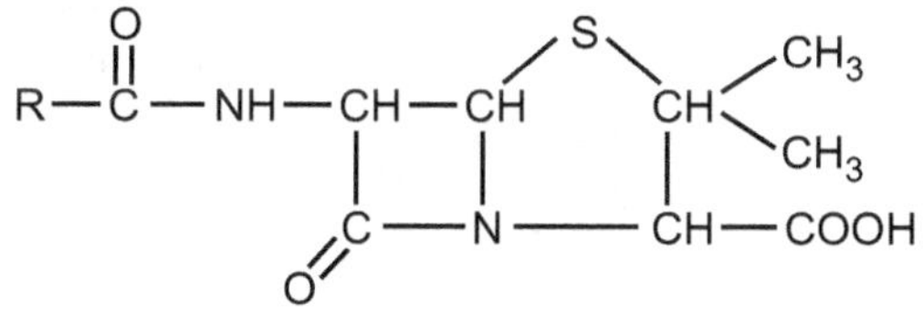

```
     O               S
     ||            /   \        CH3
R—C—NH—CH—CH       CH<
            |    |        |     CH3
           C——N———CH—COOH
          //
         O
```

R – $C_6H_5CH_2$ – Penicillin G (Benzyl penicillin)

R – $HOC_6H_4CH_2$ – Penicillin X (Hydroxy benzyl penicillin)

R – $C_6H_5OCH_2$ – Penicillin V (Phenoxy methyl penicillin)

R – $CH_3CH_2CH = CHCH_2$ – Penicillin F (2-Pentenyl penicillin)

R – $CH_3(CH_2)_3CH$ – Dihydropenicillin F (n-Pentyl penicillin)

R – $CH_3(CH_2)_5CH_2$ – Penicillin K (n-Heptyl penicillin)

Fig. 17.1: Types of penicillin

The penicillin G or penicillin V is mostly used as the starting materials for the production of several semi-synthetic penicillins. Natural penicillins are chemically or enzymatically split to first obtain 6-APA, which is then reacylated to synthesis desired derivative of penicillins. Semisynthetic penicillins are more stable, resistance to β-lactamase enzymes and expanded antimicrobial spectrum. Penicillin G is also produced as poorly soluble procaine salt of penicillin which is used as long-lasting injectable.

Production of 6-APA:

Penicillin G can be produced with good yields economically by using *Penicillium chrysogenum* and adding phenyl acetic acid precursor during fermentation. Acyl group from position 6 can be removed from penicillin G by deacylation to obtain 6 APA. Semisynthetic penicillins are produced by carrying out acylation reaction to introduce new acyl group at position 6 to 6 APA (Fig. 17.2). Penicillin acylase is used for production of 6-APA isolated from *Escherichia coli. E. coli* slurry is added as crude enzyme source directly to a penicillin solution in a batch process at 37°C temperature and pH 8.0. Bacterial cells are removed by filtration after the end of process. The filtrate is adjusted to pH 2.0 and 6-APA is separated from phenyl acetic acid and non-converted penicillin by extraction with methylisobutyl ketone. Precipitate the 6-APA at its isoelectric point (pH 4.3) and the crystals are washed and dried.

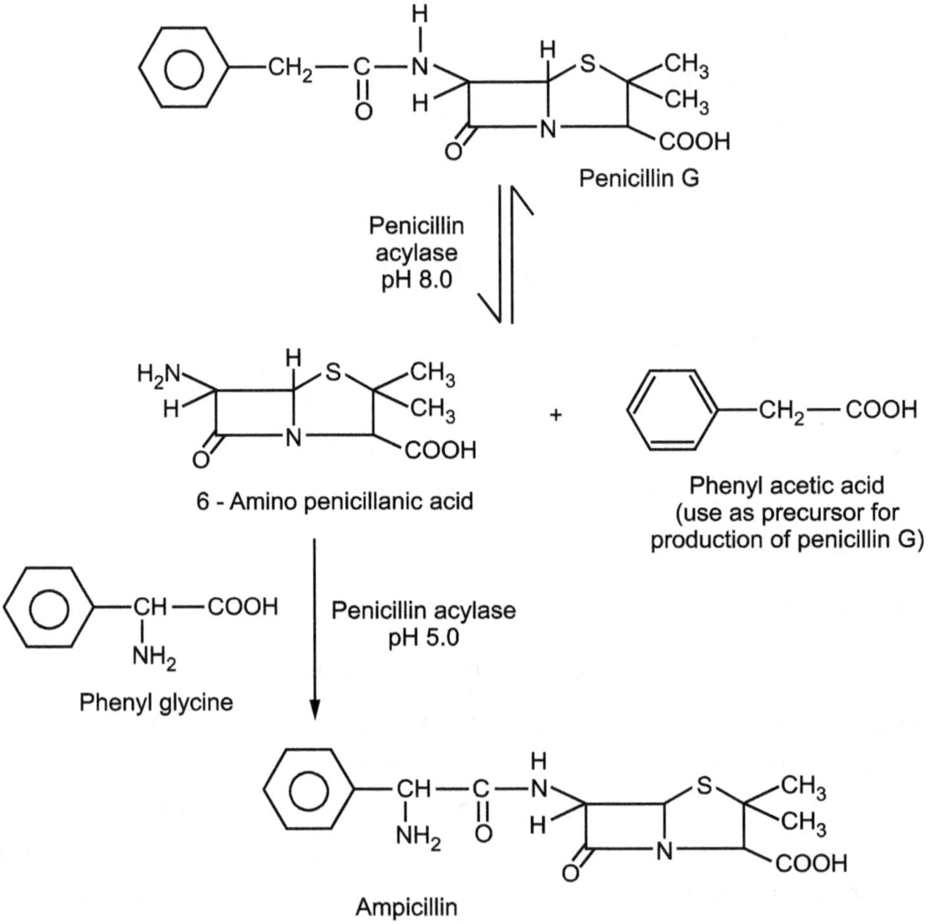

Penicillin G

Penicillin acylase
pH 8.0

6 - Amino penicillanic acid

\+

Phenyl acetic acid
(use as precursor for production of penicillin G)

Phenyl glycine

Penicillin acylase
pH 5.0

Ampicillin

Fig. 17.2: Preparation of semisynthetic penicillin (ampicillin) from 6-aminopenicillanic acid

Inoculum development:

The selected strain of *Penicillium chrysogenum* is maintained in the form of a master culture and preserved by lyophilization, or by mixing the spores in sterilized soils. For inoculum preparation, spores from working solid cultures are suspended in water. These spores are added in flasks containing nutrient solution and incubated for 4 to 6 days at 25°C. The resulting spores are used directly to inoculate inoculum tank. The inoculum tanks are incubated for 48 hours with agitation and aeration to grow more mycelium. The resulting inoculum is used for a production tank or it is added to a second or even third-stage inoculum tank to produce more inoculum for large-scale fementation.

Production media:

The exact composition of penicillin production media used in the industry for production of penicillin is unknown. These media are considered to be trade secrets of that particular fermentation industry. A typical medium described by **Jackson** (1958) contains fermentable carbohydrates, such as corn steep liquor solids (3.5%), lactose (3.5%) and glucose (1%); potassium dihydrogen phosphate (0.4%), calcium carbonate (1%), edible oil (0.4%), and penicillin precursor. The pH of this medium after sterilization is 5.5 to 6.0. Inoculum media are similar to production media except that lactose and precursors are not added in the inoculum media. These media compositions may be slightly changed to increase yields and meet economic changes.

Fermentation:

The media are placed in a fermentation vessel, sterilized and inoculated with a suspension of *Penicillium chrysogenum* (inoculum). A flow sheet for large scale production of penicillin is shown in Fig. 17.3. The fermentation vessel is equipped with devices which allow continuous addition of nutrients, acids/bases to maintain the pH (7 to 7.4) and cooling coils to maintain the temperature (24°C). Maximum antibiotics are produced within 4 to 5 days.

The growth of mycelium is occur in first 20 to 30 hours of fermentation. The mycelium grows rapidly by utilizing glucose, lactic acid and organic nitrogen compounds. Fungal growth becomes very thick and heavy. The growth occurs as disperse mycelial strands or clumps of mycelium, which are 0.5 to 2 mm in diameter. Initially pH may decrease with glucose utilization and production of acids. Ammonia is liberated by deamination of the amino acids of the corn steep liquor and pH becomes 7 to 7.5. Glucose and lactic acid are utilized first them lactose is available for the continuation of fermentation.

Lactose is slowly utilized, hence pH remains constant (Fig. 17.4). In stationary phase of culture, nutrients start depleting and adaptive enzymes are produced for addition of phenyl acetyl group side chain to penicillin nucleus. It is during the lactose utilization period, that the actual synthesis of penicillin. In penicillin synthesis period, pH of medium may be controlled by addition of calcium or magnesium carbonates and by the phosphate buffer. Lipids and fatty acids are utilized by the fungus during the production of penicillin. These ingredients increase both mycelium and yield of penicillin. The medium pH may rise to 8 to higher at the end of fermentation because of exhausting of lactose and autolysis of mycelium to release ammonia. Fermentation is stopped before this stage to avoid degradation of active compounds at higher pH. The yield of penicillin is dependent on composition of medium. Generally, the yield of penicillin is more than 60,000 units per ml in the fermentation broth.

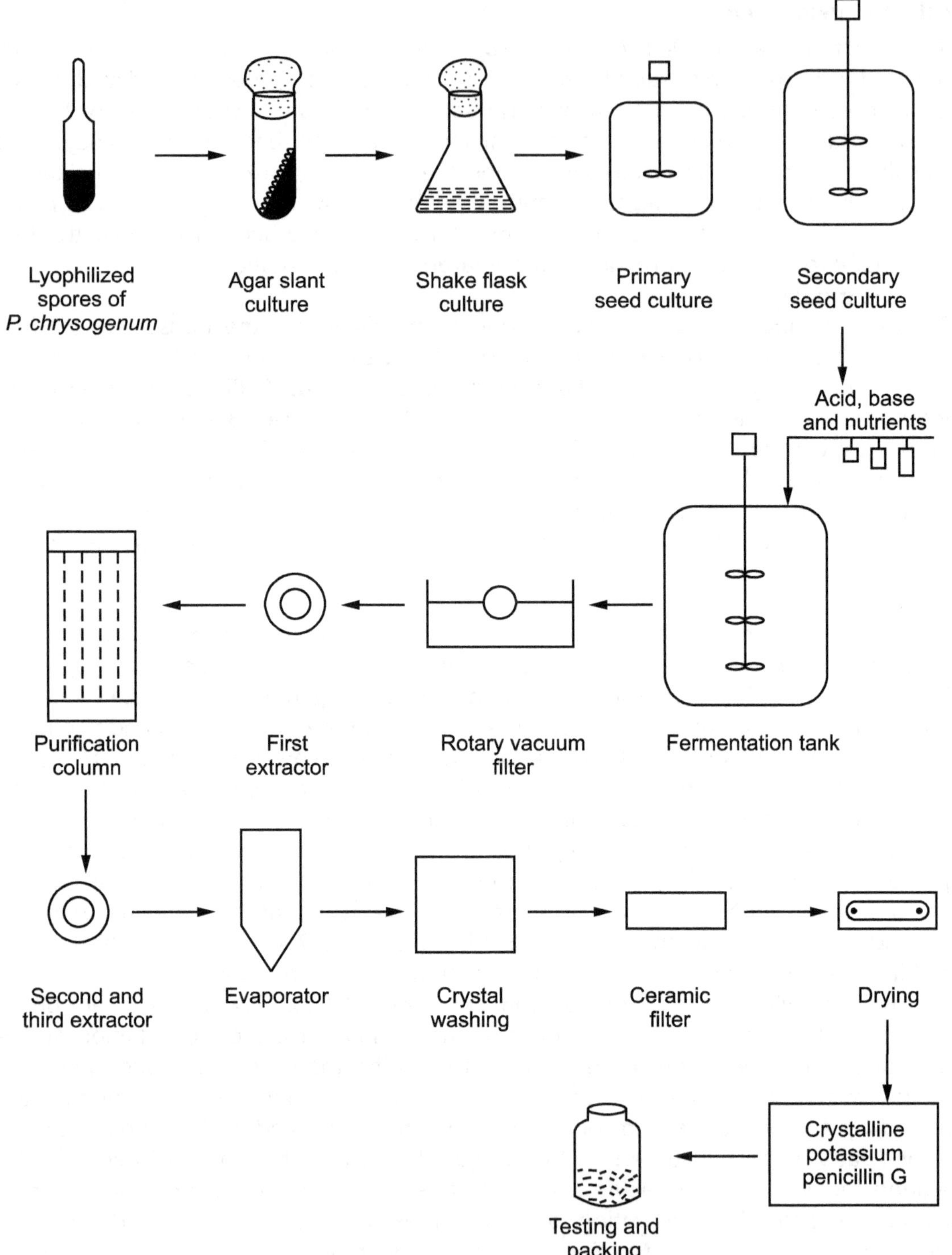

Fig. 17.3: Flow sheet for large scale production of penicillin

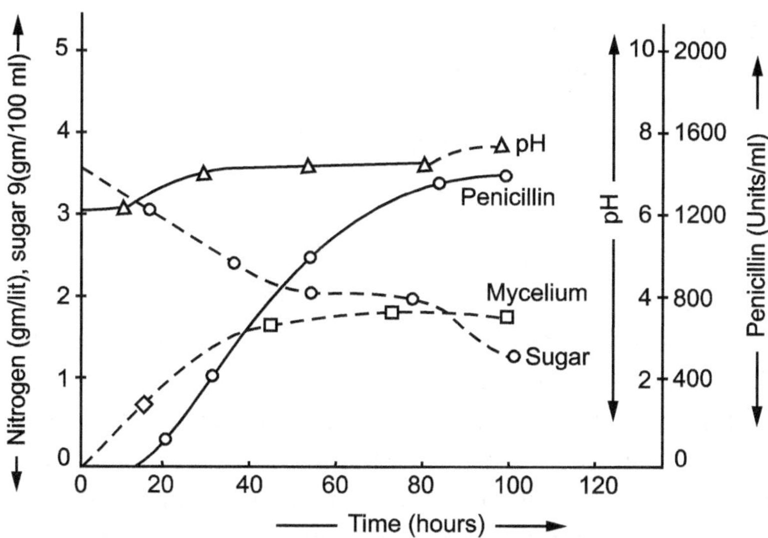

Fig. 17.4: Events in batch fermentation of penicillin

Recovery and purification:

A schematic flow diagram for the recovery of potassium penicillin G (down stream process) is incorporated in Fig. 17.3. The first step in the recovery process is the removal of mycelium or cells by filtration (rotary vacuum filter) or centrifugation. These stages are carried out under aseptic conditions, to avoid contamination of the filtrate with penicillinase producing microorganisms (*Bacillus* species) which may cause loss of antibiotics. Penicillin is extracted under controlled conditions of temperature, pH and sterility to minimize chemical and enzymatic degradation. It is extracted in the form of acid into amyl acetate, methyl isobutyl ketone or butyl acetate in a counter-current solvent extractor at pH 2.5 to 3.0. A penicillin containing solvent is treated with active charcoal to remove pigments and other impurities. The charcoal is separated from the extract on a precoated rotary vacuum filter and then washed with the solvent. Penicillin from the solvent is crystallized by the addition of sodium or potassium hydroxide to form its salt. The end product of penicillin is then crystallized into sodium or potassium penicillin.

Penicillin may be passed through gel filtration columns to separate and remove all contaminating proteins from medium. Procaine salt of penicillin may be prepared to modify release (slow release) of drug in the body.

17.3 CITRIC ACID

Citric acid is a natural constituent and common metabolite of plants and animals. It is the most versatile and widely used organic acid in the field of food and pharmaceuticals. Citric acid (Fig. 17.5) was isolated from lemons but today about 99% of the world's citric acid produced from microbial fermentation. Citric acid fermentation was first observed by

Wehmer (1893) the fungus species of *Penicillium glaucum*. Now, citric acid mainly produced by submerged fermentation using *Aspergillus niger* or *Candida* species from different sources of carbohydrates.

$$
\begin{array}{c}
H_2C\text{—}COOH \\
| \\
OH\text{—}C\text{—}COOH \\
| \\
H_2C\text{—}COOH
\end{array}
$$

Fig. 17.5: Structure of citric acid

Citric acid is mainly used in food industry because of its high solubility, pleasant taste and palatability. It is commonly used as a flavouring agent in food and beverages e.g. jams, jellies, candies, desserts, soft drinks, etc. Citric acid also acts as antioxidants and preservatives. It is used for pH adjustment in different beverages to provide uniform acidity. It is used in chemical industry (antifoam agent), pharmaceutical industry (preservative) and detergent industry (cleaning agent). It can be utilized as an stabilizing agent of fats, oils or ascorbic acid.

Strains and microbial biosynthesis for citric acid:

A large number of microorganisms are used for production of citric acid including bacteria, mould and yeasts (Table 17.1). *Aspergillus niger* and certain yeasts such as *Saccharomycopsis* sp are most commonly used for commercial production of citric acid. Mutant strains of *A. niger* have been developed for industrial production to tolerate high sugar concentration and low pH with suppression of undesirable byproducts (oxalic acid, gluconic acid and isocitric acid)

Table 17.1: Microorganisms used for production of citric acid

Microbial group	Species
Moulds	*Asperigillus niger, A. wentii, A. aculeatus, A. awamori, A. foetidus, A. carbonarius, Penicillium luteum, P. citrinum,*
Yeasts	*Saccharomycopsis lipolytica, Candida tropicals, C. oleophila, C. guilliermondii, C. parapsilosis, C. citroformans, Hansenula anamola.*
Bacteria	*Arthobacter paraffinens, Bacillius licheniformis, Corynebacterium* sp.

Citric acid is a primary metabolic product formed in the tricarboxylic acid (Krebs) cycle. Glucose is the main carbon source for production of citric acid. The biosynthetic pathway of citric acid production involves glycolysis where glucose is converted to two molecules of pyruvate. Pyruvate in turn forms acetyl CoA and oxaloacetate which condense to get citrate. The steps in biosynthesis of citric acid is given in Fig. 17.6.

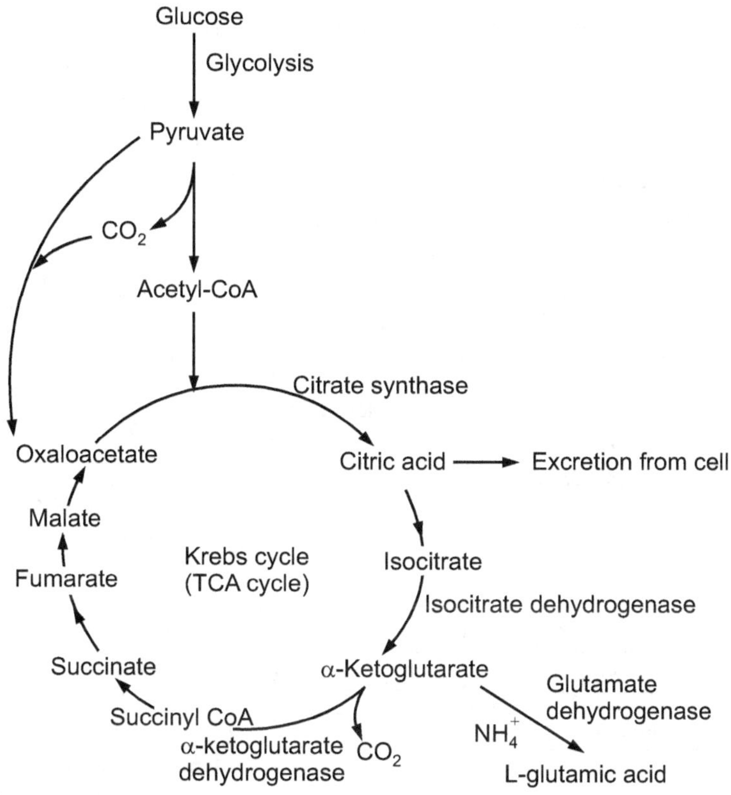

Fig. 17.6: Biosynthetic pathway of citric acid and glutamic acid

Preparation of inoculum:

Mutant species of *Aspergillus niger* is commonly used for production of citric acid for commercial use. Stock culture of species are mainited in culture tubes in form of lyophilized spores or storage in refrigerator. Spores are produced in glass bottles on solid substrates upto 12-14 days incubation at 25 to 27°C. A nutrient medium containing 15% sugar from molasses is used in seed fermentation to induce mycelium formation in the form of pellets. The spores germinate at 30 to 32°C within 20-24 hours to form pellets. These pellets are used as the incoulum for production medium.

Production processes of citric acid:

Citric acid is produced by both surface as well as submerged methods.

Surface fermentation: In this method, microorganisms can grow as a layer or a film on a surface of nutrient medium, which may be liquid (liquid surface fermentation) or solid (solid-state fermentation) in nature. Liquid surface fermentation is the oldest method for production of citric acid. This is more sophisticated and simple method requires less effort in operation and installation, less energy costs and higher reproducibility. The inoculum in the form of spores is sprayed over the medium and fungus develops as a mycelial mat on the surface of the medium. The trays are made of high purity aluminium or special grade steel.

The sterilized nutrient solution automatically flows over a distribution system onto the trays (Fig. 17.7). Microbial culture is inoculated in the incubation chamber at 30-40°C by blowing dry spores or by spraying spore suspensions. The fermentation chambers are provided with an effective air circulation to control temperature (30°C) and humidity. Within 24 hours after inoculation, the germinating spores form a thin cover of mycelium on the surface of medium. The fermentation is stopped after 7-14 days.

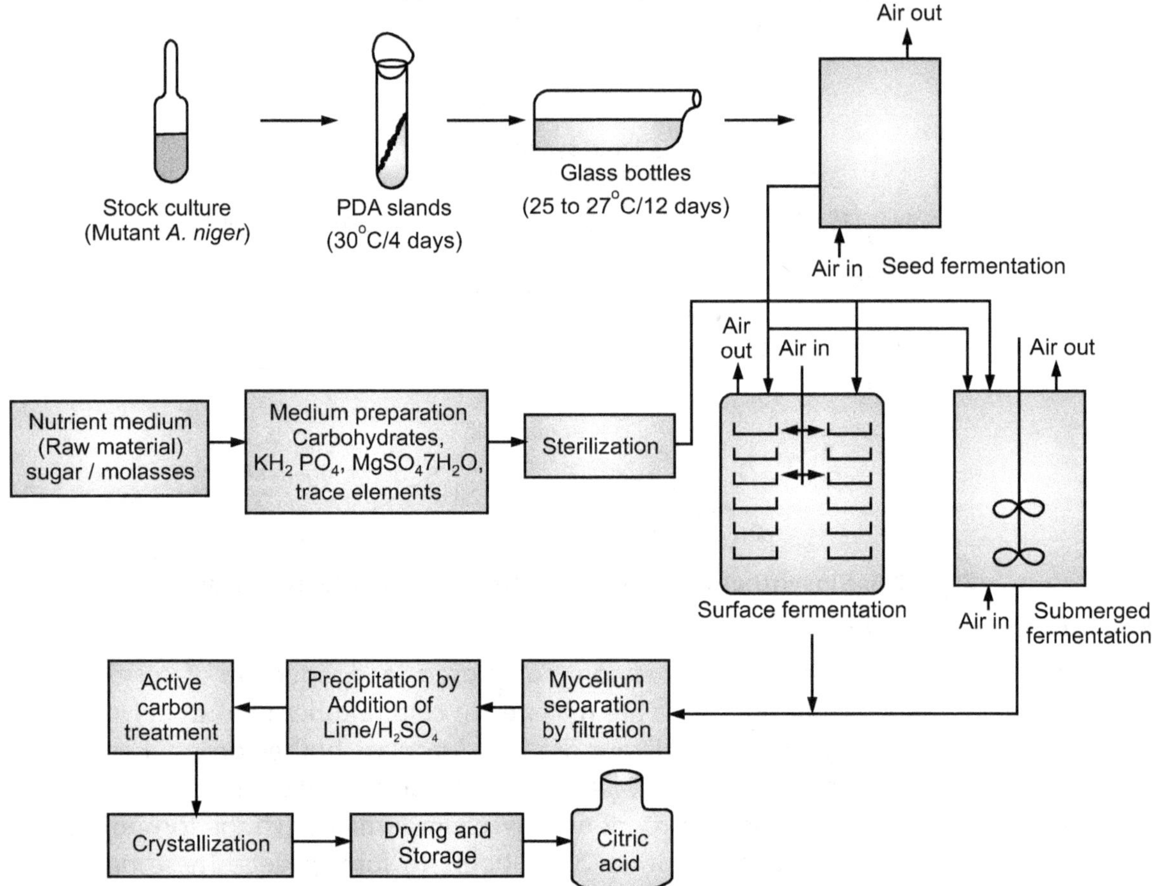

Fig. 17.7: Flow diagram for production of citric acid

Solid-state fermentation (SSF) is an alternative method to produce citric acid from agro-industrial residues. SSF (Koji processs) is an simplest method for production of citric acid and it was first developed in Japan. The solid substrate such as wheat bran or pulp from sweet potato starch are used in culture media. The pH of medium is adjusted to 4-5, then sterilized and inoculated the spores of *A. niger*. The spores can spread as a layers (3-5 cm thickness) and incubated at 28°C. The growth of the cells/mycelium can be accelerated by the addition of α-amylase. This fermentation process require 80-90 hours and at end, the entire solution is extracted with hot water to isolate the citric acid.

Submerged fermentation: Around 80% of the world's supply of citric acid is produced by submerged processes. This is most preferred method due to higher yield, easy automation and lower labour costs. The limitations or disadvantages of this methods are adverse effect of trace metals, other impurities and require highly trained personnel. Stirred bioreactor and airlift bioreactor are commonly used for submerged fermentation. The vessels of the bioreactors are made up of high quality stainless steel. After inoculation, the medium must be aerated by bubbling the air to allow maximum growth of fungal cells. The yield of citric acid is depends on the structure of mycelium. The mycelium with bulbous hyphae to form very small solid pellets is ideal for citric acid production. Supply of oxygen is required for good production of acid and ideal rate of aeration is 0.4-1.2 volume volume/minute (vvm).

Culture medium contains carbohydrates, KH_2PO_4, $MgSO_4$. $7H_2O$ and few trace elements. The carbohydrates (12 to 24%) most suitable for citric acid production are sucrose, glucose, maltose, molasses (sugar cane), starch (potatoes), cotton wastes, banana extract, pineapple waste water etc. Ammonium salts, urea, ammonium sulfate, peptone, malt extract and nitrates are the nitrogen sources used in the fermentation media. It is necessary to maintain pH because nitrogen consumption leads to reduce pH. Trace element such as Fe, Cu, Zn, Mn, Mg are essential for the growth of *Aspergillus* species and some of elements (Mn, Fe and Zn) increase the yield of citric acid.

The pH of a culture medium may change by secretion of organic acids such as citric, acetic or lactic acids. The pH for optimum production of citric acid is below 2.5. The lower pH is responsible for suppression of oxalic acid and gluconic acid production as well as minimize the contamination of other organisms. Antifoam agents (lard oil) and mechanical antifoam devices are used to prevent foam formation. Fermentation process is completed in about 5 to 7 days at 28-32°C°. Generally 90 to 110 gm/lit of citric acid is obtained from 140 gm/lit of sucrose.

Recovery of citric acid:

The steps for the recovery of citric acid from both processes (surface or submerged) are given in Fig. 17.7. The recovery starts with the filtration of the culture broth and washing of mycelium. Oxalic acid (unwanted byproduct) can be removed by precipitation by adding lime ($Ca(OH)_2$) at pH less than 3. Citric acid present in the solution (mono-calcium citrate) is separated by precipitation at pH 7.2 and temperature 70 to 90°C. Citric acid is dissolved in sulphuric acid and separates calcium sulfate in form of insoluble precipitate. The filtrate containing citric acid is purified by treating with active carbon and passing through cation and anion exchangers. The filtrate is concentrated in vacuum crystallizers at 22 to 25°C to form citric acid monohydrate. Citric acid crystallizers in an anhydrous form at above 40°C.

17.4 VITAMIN B_{12}

Vitamin B_{12} is a water-soluble vitamin, commonly known as cobalamin. It is an important dietary component for normal growth in human beings and animals. **Ricke E. L.** and **Smith L.** (1948) isolated small amount of active material from liver and crystallized it as vitamin B_{12} which was active in the treatment of pernicious anemia.

Vitamin B_{12} is one of the largest and the most complex molecules. The main part in the structure of vitamin B_{12} is porphyrin ring containing cobalt as the central element. The cyanide (CN) group, hydroxyl group (– OH) or nitrite group (– NO_2) attached to the cobalt is called cyanocobalamin (vitamin B_{12}), hydroxocobalamin and nitritocobalamin respectively.

Vitamin B_{12} is produced by bacteria and actinomycetes (Table 17.2). *Streptomyces olivaceus, Pseudomonas denitrificans, Propionibacterium shermanii* and *Propionibacterium freudenreichii* are mainly used for commercial production of vitamin B_{12}. Generally, vitamin B_{12} is prepared by the submerged culture process. Production of vitamin B_{12} from *Streptomyces olivaceus* have been discussed here.

Table 17.2: Vitamin B_{12} producing microbial species

Microbial group	Species
Actinomycetes	*Streptomyces olivaceus, Nocardia* species, *Streptomyces albidoflavus, S. antibioticus, S. aureofacieus, S. griseus, S. roseochromogenus.*
Bacteria	*Pseudomonas denitrificans, Aerobacter aerogenes, Bacillus subtilis, Bacillus megaterium, Propionibacterium shermanii, Propionibacterium freudenreichii, Clostridium butyricum, Flavobacterium acetylicum, Flavobacterium flavescens, Lactobacillus arabinosus, Mycobacterium smegmatis, Serratia marcescens, Proteus vulgaris, Streptococcus faecalis*

Preparation of inoculum:

Pure culture of *Streptomyces olivaceus* is inoculated in inoculum medium contained in Erlenmeyer flasks. Bennett's broth [yeast extract (0.1%), beef extract (0.1%), glucose (1%) and enzymatic hydrolysate of casein (0.25%)] is employed for development of inoculum. Flasks are kept on the mechanical shaker during incubation for the aeration. These flask cultures are used to inoculate the large amount of inoculum media. The required amount of inoculum (5% of the volume of production medium) is prepared by successive transfers.

Fermentation:

The culture of *Streptomyces olivaceus* is grown with aeration at 28°C in a nutritionally rich crude medium. Distiller's soluble (4%), dextrose (1%) and calcium carbonate (0.5%) are mainly present in typical production medium used in production of vitamin B_{12}. Cobalt chloride ($COCl_2 \cdot 6H_2O$) at approximately 2 to 10 ppm is added to this medium as a precursor. The flow diagram for the production of vitamin B_{12} by *Streptomyces olivaceus* is shown in Fig. 17.8. The pH of the medium is adjusted to 7 to 7.5 before sterilization and may

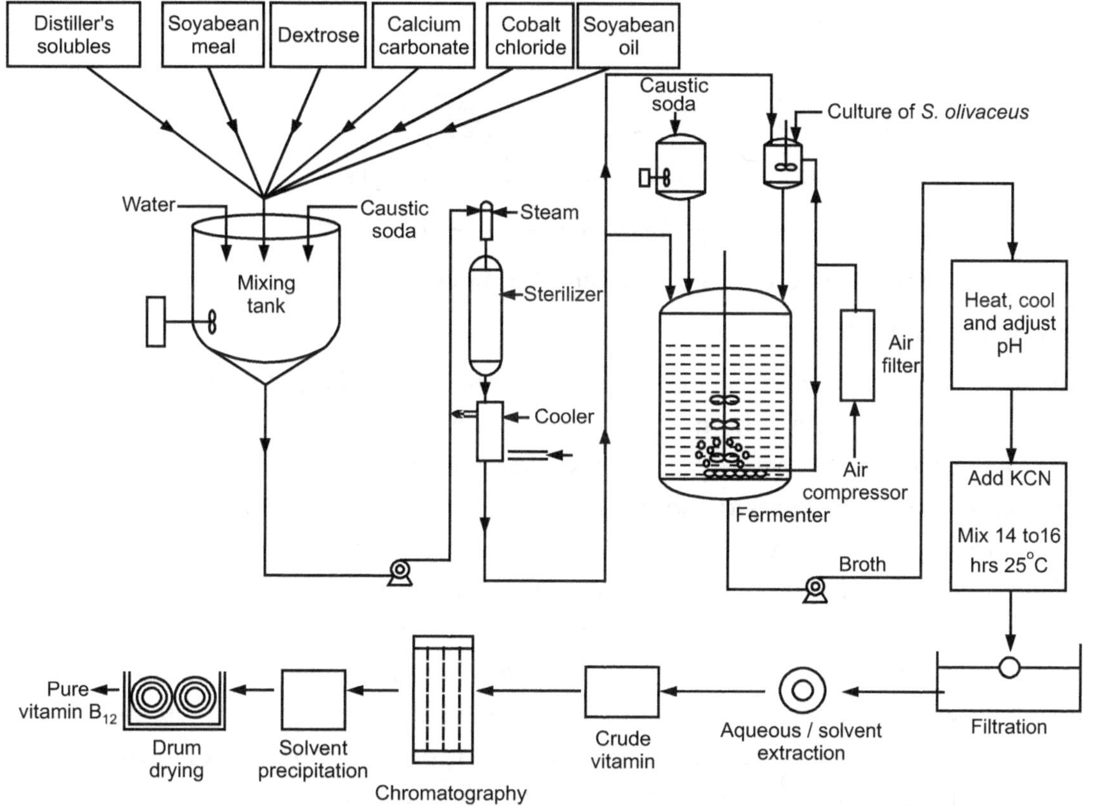

Fig. 17.8: Flow diagram for production of vitamin B_{12}

or may not be controlled during fermentation. In the first 24 hours, pH of fermentation is reduced due to rapid sugar consumption and again pH increases after 48 to 96 hours due to lysis of mycelium. The change in pH, sugar and production of vitamin B_{12} during a typical fermentation process is shown in Fig. 17.9. A correct rate of aeration and speed of agitation are required for proper growth of microbial strains. The optimium rate of aeration is about 0.5 volume air/volume medium/minute. Soyabean oil, corn oil, lard oil etc. are used as antifoaming agents to suppress the foam formation.

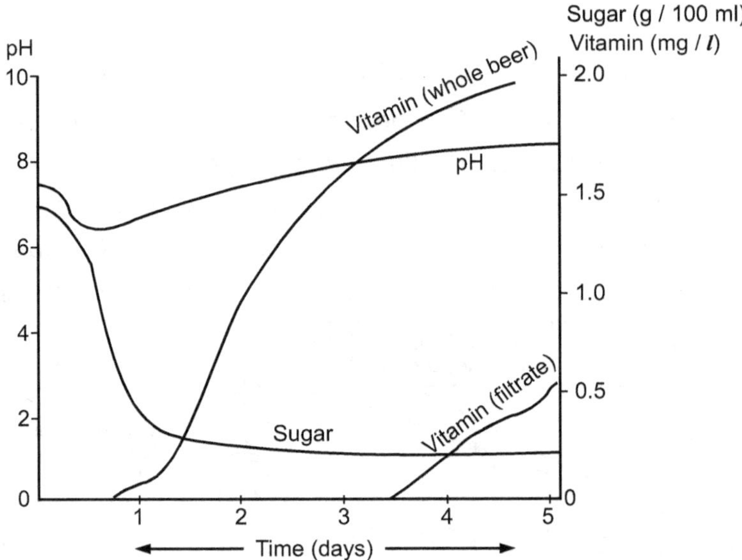

Fig. 17.9: Changes in medium during vitamin B_{12} production

Recovery of vitamin B_{12}:

Vitamin B_{12} is mainly associated with the mycelium of *Streptomyces* species. Most of cobalamin is recovered with the mycelium by centrifuging or filtering the whole beer after 3 to 4 days. Concentrated vitamin B_{12} is also obtained by reducing the pH of the beer to 5 with sulfuric acid and heating the mixture to boiling. Sodium sulfite (100 ppm) may be added in the mixture for the protection of vitamin. The medium is filtered to remove mycelium and then the filtrate broth is treated with cyanide to convert cobalamin to cyanocobalamin. The adsorption of the cyanocobalamin from the solution is done by using activated charcoal, fuller's earth, bentonite etc. Finally, elution of cyanocobalamin is performed by using an aqueous solution of materials ranging from organic bases to hydrochloric acid. Single step extraction into an organic solvent or counter-current extraction and product purification is carried out by the process of precipitation. Chromatography on alumina and final crystallization from ethanol-acetone is performed. The final product is drum-dried or spray-dried. The vitamin B_{12} content may vary from 10 to 30 mg/l in the final product.

17.5 GLUTAMIC ACID

L-glutamic acid was the first amino acid to be produced by microorganisms, *Corynebacterium glutamicum*. Glutamic acid is widely used in the production of monosodium glutamate which is commonly known as the 'seasoning salt'. Monosodium glutamate is condiment and flavour enhancing agent and it commonly used in convenient food-stuffs.

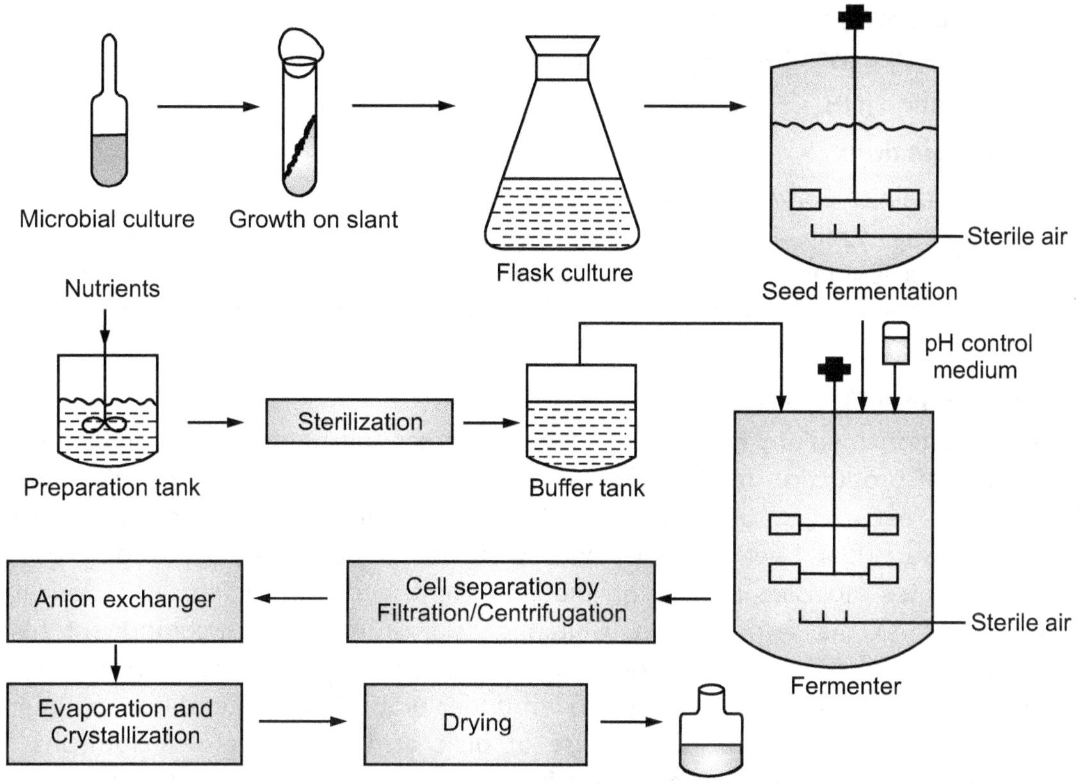

Fig. 17.10: Flow diagram of production of glutamic acid

This amino acid can be synthesized by number of techniques such as:

(i) Hydrolysis of wheat glutin, soyabean cake or by other protein rich food components.

(ii) Cleavage of pyrrolidone carboxylic acid found in stiffens molasses.

(iii) One step fermentation process using single microbes.

(iv) Two steps process involving α-ketoglutaric acid by fermentation and its conversion to glutamic acid by enzymatic process or use of another microbes.

Microbial strains and biosynthesis:

L-glutamic acid can be synthesized from a wide species of bacteria, actinomycetes and fungi. In addition of *Corynebacterium glutamicum*, the other different strains are used for production of acid such as *Escherichia coli, Bacillus subtilis, Cephalosporium salmosynnematum, Bacterium α-ketoglutaricum, Bacillus megatherium, Aerobacter cloacae, Pseudomonas fluoresences, Serratia marcescens, Microbacterium* species etc. *C. glutamicum* is a Gram-positive, non-sporulating, non-motile bacterial strain and its mutants are developed to produce high yield of acid.

The pathway for the synthesis of glutamic acid from glucose as the carbon source is given in Fig. 17.6. The glucose is broken down into fragments by microbes through the Embden Meyerhof-Parnas (EMP) pathway and the pentose-phsophate pathway. The key precursor of glutamic acid is α-ketoglutarate, which is formed in the tricarboxylic acid (TCA) cycle via citrate and isocitrate. α-Ketoglutarate is converted to L-glutamic acid through reductive amination (NH_4^+).

Inoculum Production:

A suitable strain of *Corynebacterium glutamicum* from stock culture is used for inoculum development. The strain is inoculated in sterilized medium and incubated at 35°C for 16 hours. Sufficient inoculum (6%) can be developed and then added in final production fermenter. The general flow diagram for the production of L-glutamic acid is given in Fig. 17.10.

Production of glutamic acid:

The production medium consists of carbon sources, nitrogen sources, minerals and vitamins. One of production medium for glutamic acid contains glucose, K_2HPO_4, KH_2PO_4, $MnSO_4$: $7H_2O$, $FeSO_4.7H_2O$, urea and biotin. Carbon sources such as glucose, sucrose fructose, maltose, sugar beet molasses and sugarcane molasses are commonly used in fermentation. Since molasses has a high biotin content, penicillin or fatty acid derivatives must be added to the fermentation. Glutamic acid is intracellular component hence, production and excretion is dependent upon cell permeability. Permeability of acid producing bacteria can be increased by growth under biotin limiting condition, addition of penicillin and saturated fatty acids and use of oleic acid and glycerol auxotrophs. The concentration of ammonia is very important for converting carbon source to glutamic acid. biotin is an important growth factor and an essential coenzyme in fatty acid synthesis. The addition of penicillin in the logarithmic growth phase enhance excretion of L-glutamic acid. Fig. 17.11 shows the process of typical fermentation with glucose as carbon source.

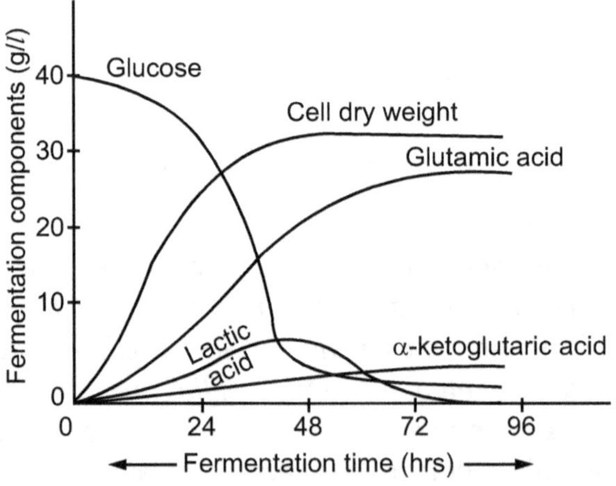

Fig. 17.11: Production of L-glutamic acid by *C. glutamicum* using glucose (carbon source)

The oxygen concentration should be optimum for production of acid. High oxygen concentration inhibits growth of the organisms while a low concentration responsible to produce lactic acid and succinic acid. The fermentation is carried out at 30-32°C for

40-48 hours. The pH of fermentation medium is adjusted to 7 to 8. In two stage fermentation process, α-ketoglutaric acid is converted to L-glutamic acid by another microbes or enzymes (Fig. 17.12).

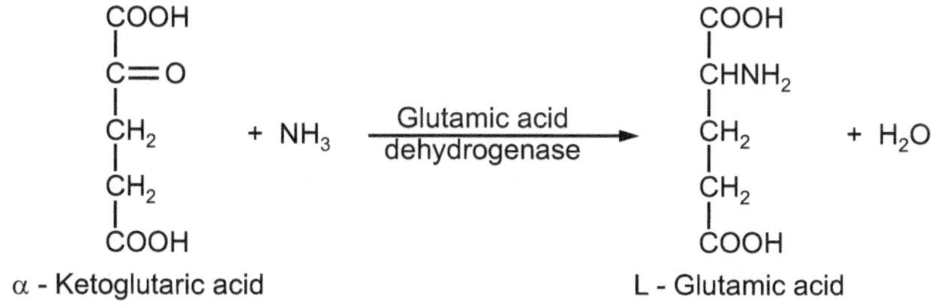

$$\underset{\alpha\text{ - Ketoglutaric acid}}{\begin{array}{c}COOH\\|\\C{=}O\\|\\CH_2\\|\\CH_2\\|\\COOH\end{array}} + NH_3 \xrightarrow[\text{dehydrogenase}]{\text{Glutamic acid}} \underset{\text{L - Glutamic acid}}{\begin{array}{c}COOH\\|\\CHNH_2\\|\\CH_2\\|\\CH_2\\|\\COOH\end{array}} + H_2O$$

Fig. 17.12: Conversion of α-ketoglutaric acid to L-glutamic acid

The culture broth contains glutamate in the form of ammonium salt. Glutamic acid forms monosodium glutamate (MSG) which can be purified by passing through anion exchanger. MSG can be subjected to evaporation and crystallization.

17.6 GRISEOFULVIN

Griseofulvin is an antifungal antibiotic first isolated from a *Penicillium* species in 1939. It is a benzofuran derivative (Fig. 17.13) produced by *Penicillium griseofulvum, P. nigricans, P. patulum* and other species of *Penicillium.* Commercial griseofulvin is produced by high yielding strain of *Penicillium patulum.* Different other strains of fungi are also used for production of griseofulvin such as *Penicillium janczewskit, P. urticae, P. albidum, Aspergillus versicolour, Khauskia oryzae, Nigrospora musae, N. splaerica*, etc.

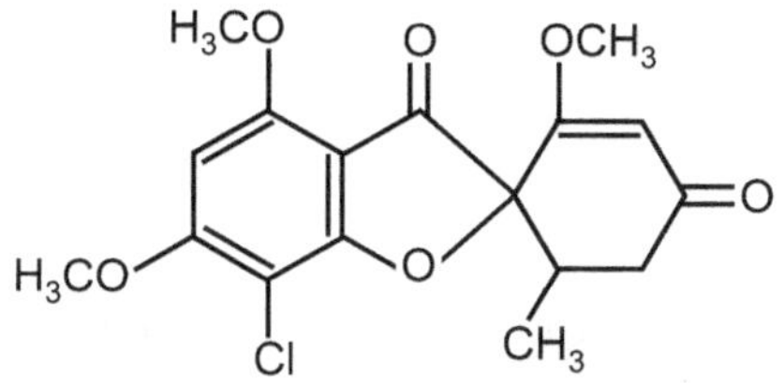

Fig. 17.13: Structure of griseofulvin

Griseofulvin is used in the treatment of various fungal skin infections. It is also employed in the treatment of plant diseases caused by *Biotrytis* and *Alternaria solani.*

Inoculum Development and Media:

Spore suspensions as well as vegetative cells are suitable to develop inoculum for laboratory scale fermentations. The media for inoculum development, fermentation and culture conditions are quite similar for all antibiotic producing fungal cells. Czapek - Dox agar medium is commonly used for growth and maintaining fungal cultures on agar plates.

P. griseofulvum may grown in different media such as sporulation medium (whey powder lactose, whey power nitrogen, KH_2PO_4, KCl, corn-steep liquor solids), germination medium (protopeptone, malted cereal extract, glucose, starch, $NaNO_3$, KH_2PO_4, $MgSO_4$,

$FeSO_4$) and seed stage medium (corn-steep liquor, brown sugar, chalk, corn oil, Hodag MF). Medium composition contains in production of antibiotic is corn steep liquor, $CaCO_3$, KH_2PO_4 and KCl. Carbon source (12%), phosphate (0.5%) and chlorine are most commonly used for better yield production.

Fermentation process:

The production is carried out by an submerged fermentation with a glucose rich medium. The optimal conditions for fermentation are: pH 6.8 - 7.2, temperature 24-26°C, aeration 0.8-1 vvm and the period is 6-8 days.

The wet mycelium is collected from a rotary string discharge filter and extracted three times with butyl acetate. The final ester extract is clarified by centrifugations and concentrated under reduced pressure at 50°C. The crude component is further purified by washing with chloroform, recrystallized from aqueous acetone and final product is washed with butyl acetate.

QUESTIONS

(A) Objective Type Questions:

1. Draw a flow sheet for production of penicillin.
2. How will you prepare inoculum for citric acid production?

(B) Short Answer Questions:

1. Write in short fermentation process of citric acid.
2. Write notes on:
   (a) Production of glutamic acid (b) Up-stream process of penicillin.

(C) Long Answer Questions:

1. Explain in detail about the down stream process for production of penicillin.
2. Explain the production of vitamin B_{12} by considering the following points:
   (a) Strains used (b) Inoculum development
   (c) Fermentation phases (d) Recovery of vitamin B_{12}
3. Explain the production of Griseofulvin by considering the following points:
   (a) Strains used (b) Inoculum development
   (c) Fermentation phases (d) Recovery of griseofulvin

(D) Multiple Choice Questions:

1. _______ is an extracellular enzyme produced by most of *Bacillus* species, which hydrolyzes penicillin to penicilloic acid.
   (a) Lipase (b) Streptokinase (c) Penicillinase (d) Amylase

2. Today, penicillin is produced from ______.
   (a) *Penicillium notatum* (b) *Penicillium chrysogenum*
   (c) *Penicillium griseofulvum* (d) All of the above
3. Raw material mainly used for commercial production of penicillin.
   (a) Peptone (b) Corn steep liquor (c) Soya meal (d) Glucose
4. In two stage fermentation process of glutamic acid, _____ is converted to L-glutamic acid by another microbes.
   (a) α-Ketoglutaric acid (b) Citric acid
   (c) Oxaloacetate (d) Succinate
5. ______ is a primary metabolic product formed in the tricarboxylic acid (TCA) cycle.
   (a) Glutamic acid (b) Citric acid
   (c) Succinate (d) Malate
6. ______ is used in industrial production of glutamic acid.
   (a) *Pseudomonas* (b) *Corynebacterium*
   (c) *Mycobacterium* (d) *Bacillus*

■■■

Chapter ... 18

BLOOD PRODUCTS AND PLASMA SUBSTITUTES

♦ LEARNING OBJECTIVES ♦

After completing this chapter, reader should be able to understand:

- *Introduction*
- *Collection and Storage of Blood and Blood Products*
- *Blood Products*
  - *Concentrated Human Red Blood Corpuscles*
  - *Dried Human Plasma*
  - *Human Plasma Protein Fraction*
  - *Dried Human Serum*
  - *Human Fibrinogen*
  - *Human Thrombin*
  - *Human Fibrin Foam*
  - *Human Normal Immunoglobulin*
  - *Human Albumin*
- *Quality Control of Blood Products*
- *Plasma Substitutes*

18.1 INTRODUCTION

Blood is composed of a clear, straw-coloured, watery fluid called plasma in which several different types of blood cells are suspended. It is an important regulator and a mirror of proper functioning of body cells. It circulates throughout the body by the circulatory system.

Blood transports oxygen from lungs to the tissues and carbon dioxide from the tissues to the lungs for excretion. It is also used to transport nutrients from the alimentary tract to the tissues and cell wastes to the excretory organs (kidney). Blood also plays an important role in transport of hormones to target tissues, protective substances to area of infection and clotting factors to part of ruptured blood vessels. Blood makes up about 7-8% of body weight consisting 5.6 litres in a 65 to 70 kg weight in adult. The temperature of blood is about 38°C and pH is 7.4. Blood volume and the concentration of its many constituents are kept within narrow limits by homeostatic mechanisms.

Hospital blood banks and blood centres provide a wide range of services to patient by prescription of doctor. It includes whole blood, platelets, granulocytes, single donar plasma, frozen plasma etc. The use of blood and its components is accompanied by some risk of accidental transmission of infectious agents e.g. Hepatitis, AIDS, herpes simplex, syphilis, malaria, infectious mononucleosis etc. The risk of microbial contamination is different depending on selection of donors and preparation techniques. The accidental pathogenic infection is prevented by careful screening of blood donors and finished products.

Whole blood is blood that has been aseptically withdrawn from humans who are certified by a physical as being free of transmissible disease and mixed with a suitable anticoagulant. Whole human blood is the final mixture of blood and anticoagulant solution contains not less than 9.7% w/v of haemoglobin. Whole blood is a mixture of a plasma and blood cells (Fig. 18.1).

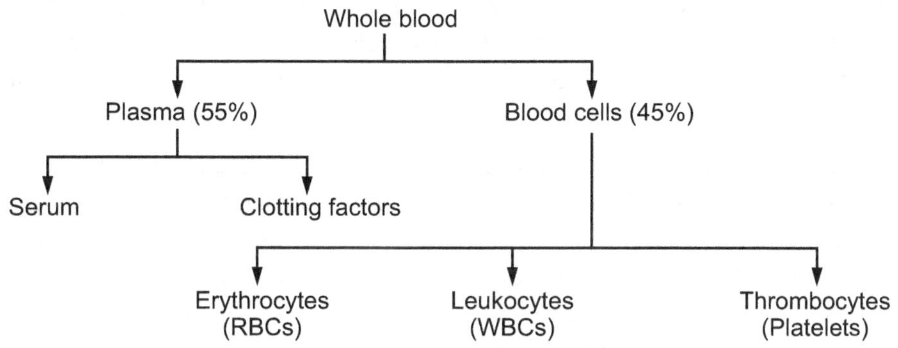

Fig. 18.1: Components of blood

The blood plasma is made up of water (92%), plasma proteins, inorganic salts, nutrients, waste materials, hormones and gases. Albumins are the most abundant plasma proteins. The main function of albumin is to maintain normal plasma osmotic pressure and it act as carrier molecules for free fatty acids, some drugs and hormones. Fibrinogen is responsible for coagulation of blood. Immunoglobulins are complex proteins produced by lymphocytes that plays an important part in immunity which interact with antigen to form antigen-antibody complex. Electrolytes are used for muscle contraction (calcium ions), transmission of nerve impulses (calcium and sodium ions) and maintenance of acid-base balance (phosphate ions). Nutrients such as glucose, amino acids, fatty acids, glycerol, vitamins and mineral salts are absorbed from the alimentary tract and are used by body cells for energy, heat repair and for synthesis of other blood components. Gases such as oxygen, carbon dioxide and nitrogen are transported round the body dissolved in plasma. Urea, creatinine and uric acid are the waste products of protein metabolism. They are formed in the liver and carried in blood to kidneys for excretion.

Blood cells contains erythrocytes, leukocytes and thrombocytes. Blood cells are synthesized mainly in red bone marrow. The active cellular bone marrow is called red bone marrow whereas the inactive marrow is called yellow bone marrow. The blood cells are derived from stem cell called Hemopoietic/Pluoripotent stem cell. The process of blood cell formation is called haemopoiesis.

18.2 COLLECTION AND STORAGE OF BLOOD AND BLOOD PRODUCTS

The blood is collected aseptically from the median cubital vein, in front of the elbow. Blood serves as a transport medium for carrying all its different components to and from the different organs of the body. Blood is collected in sterile plastic bags or medical research council blood bottles containing an anticoagulant solution. During collection the bottle is gently shaken to mix blood and anticoagulant solution. This collected blood is known as 'whole blood' transfusion. One unit of donated blood may be divided into components as red cell concentrates, fresh frozen plasma, platelet concentrates etc.

Transfusion medicine is a specialized branch of hematology that is concerned with the study of blood groups, along with the work of a blood bank to provide a transfusion service for blood and other blood products. Blood bank involves testing of blood from both donors and recipients to ensure that every individual recipient is given blood that is compatible and safe.

Blood is withdrawn, not more than 420 ml at once. This blood is transferred to plastic containers, sealed and cooled to 4 to 6°C. Refrigerators are commonly used for storage of blood components. The temperature in all areas of refrigerator must be maintained at between 2-6°C. The interior of refrigerator must be clean, insulated and there must be well organization of storage areas which are properly labeled and designated for cross matched blood, labelled blood and outdated blood. All blood storage refrigerators must contain recording thermometers and audible alarms. Temperature records are maintained for atleast 5 years as a part of blood blank records. A freezer that can achieve a storage temperature of – 20°C or lower is required for storing fresh frozen plasma and cryoprecipitate.

The whole blood or its components may be procured by the primary health centre or any hospital from the Government blood banks, Indian red cross society blood banks or regional blood transfusion centres.

18.3 BLOOD PRODUCTS

Blood centres and blood banks provide a wide way of services which reach the patient on prescription usually through a hospital blood bank or transfusion service. The major blood product includes whole blood, concentrated human R.B.C., dried human plasma, platelets, human thrombin etc. (Fig. 18.2). These are called as blood and blood products. They are distinguished by the fact that they are prepared locally in blood center and are dispensed in the form of individual units identified by donor.

18.3.1 Concentrated Human Red Blood Corpuscles

Concentrated Red Blood Cells (RBCs) are units of whole blood with most of the plasma removed. It is prepared by centrifugation or undisturbed sedimentation for the separation of plasma and anticoagulant solution. The quantity of fluid removed is not less than 40% of the total volume of whole human blood. A certain amount of plasma is left to ensure optimal cell preservation and maintain viscosity for administration. All surfaces that come in contact with the red cells and plasma must be sterile and free from pyrogen. The containers containing concentrated human red blood cells are stored at a temperature between 2° and 8°C. It may be stored for a period not longer than that for which the whole human blood from which it is prepared. However, if the seal is broken during processing, the product must be used within 24 hours.

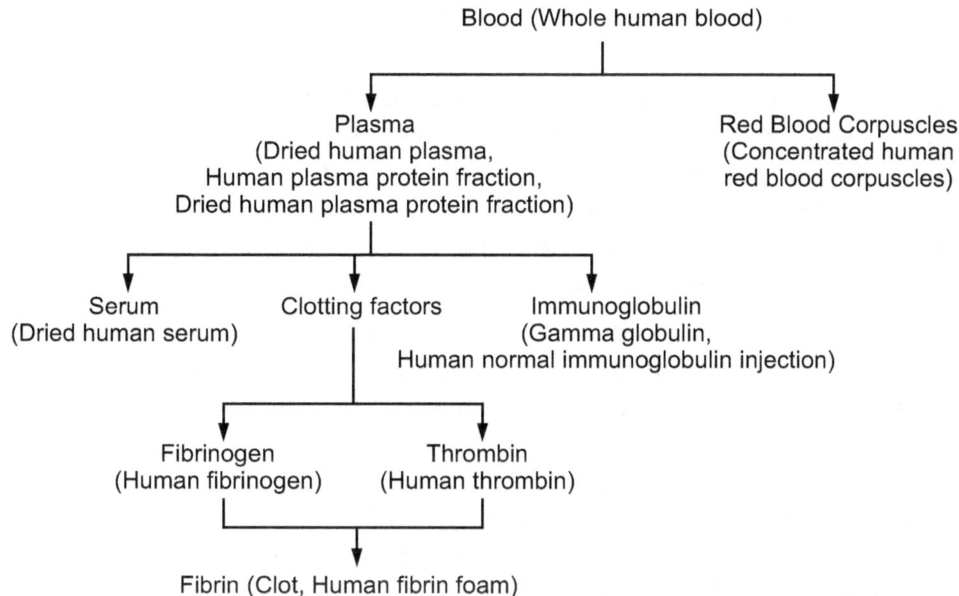

Fig. 18.2: Blood products

The haemoglobin concentration of the final preparation is not less than 15.5% w/v.

The final container must be labelled with the reference number of the whole human blood from which the preparation is made, the ABO and Rh groups of the whole human blood, the date of collection of the whole human blood from which the preparation is made, the date after which the preparation is not suitable for transfusion and the storage conditions. This product is used principally in the treatment of anaemia. Red blood cell fractions are also administered to patients with sickle cell anaemia and new born babies suffering from haemolytic disease.

18.3.2 Dried Human Plasma

Dried plasma has several advantages as compared with whole blood. It can be given to patients of any blood group and well stored plasma can be used for five years. Dried plasma can be stored at room temperature (below 20°C) if protected from light.

The plasma of same donors contains haemagglutinating antibodies of the ABO system which on transfusion into patients of certain blood groups may cause intravascular agglutination and haemolysis. This risk can be avoided by neutralization of the haemagglutinins with the soluble blood group substances present in the plasma of other donors of appropriate blood groups. The most satisfactory ratio for mixing is A (9 parts) : O (9 parts) : B or AB (2 Parts).

Viral jaundice (infective hepatitis and homologous serum jaundice) is one of the most serious ill effects of transfusion of plasma. Control of infection is partly effected by refusing to accept donors with a history of jaundice but not all cases are recognized. Attempts have been made to kill the infective viruses by treatment with ultraviolet irradiation or β-propiolactone or in combination of both. But treated plasma shows electrophoretic and other abnormalities.

Dried plasma is usually prepared from time-expired citrated blood. The supernatant fluid is separated by centrifugation or undisturbed sedimentation. Batches of not more than ten bottles are pooled, choosing the correct ratio of blood groups to neutralize powerful agglutinins. The pools are kept at 4 to 6°C while samples are tested for sterility. Pools which have passed the test for sterility are then redistributed in transfusion bottles in quantities suitable for freeze drying or sublimation drying.

In pre-freezing, the plasma bottles are sealed with bacteriologically efficient fabric pads covered by ring-type closures and then centrifuged at – 18°C. The content freezes in a shell round the walls of the bottle in a similar manner to formation of the roll tube used in microbiology. This process provides large area for sublimation and the maximum area for heat transfer (Fig. 18.3). In primary drying, then plasma bottles containing frozen material are mounted horizontally in the drying chamber and a high vacuum is applied. The ice sublimes onto a condensing coil (– 50°C) and a small heater provides the latent heat required for evaporation. The primary drying process leaves products with about 2% moisture and this is removed in the secondary drying process. Secondary drying is preformed in another chamber by vacuum desiccation over phosphorus pentoxide. The final product is left with about 0.5% of moisture. Each fabric seal is replaced by MRC type closure perforated by a plugged hypodermic needle. The bottles are returned to the secondary drying chamber, re-evacuated and then the vacuum is broken with dry sterile nitrogen. Finally, the needles are removed and the closure is protected with a sterile cap.

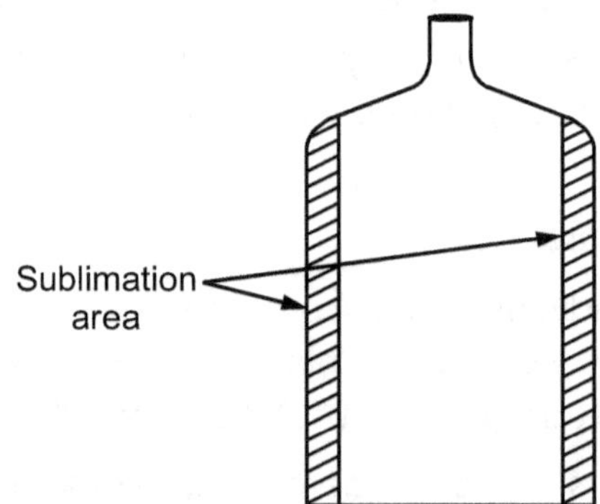

Fig. 18.3: Container showing large surface area of sublimation

The dried plasma is a cream-coloured powder, free from streaks of red or pink indicative of red cells or haemoglobin. It is reconstituted with water for injection equivalent to the original volume of plasma at room temperature. It must dissolve completely within ten minutes. The protein content is not less than 45 gm/lit. Dried plasma is stored in dry conditions, below 20°C and protected from moisture, light and oxygen. The containers must be labelled in addition to general requirements containing the names and percentages of anticoagulant and other contents, the quantity of water for injections required for reconstitution and the protein content. It must be used immediately (before 3 hr.) after reconstitution. Reconstituted plasma is an alternative to whole blood, in conditions where there is no loss of red cells. In emergencies, to restore blood volume when whole blood is not available or while awaiting the results of compatibility tests. It is also used in acute fibrinogen deficiency. Reconstituted plasma is used in patients suffering from severe burns, scalds or crush injury.

Fresh frozen plasma is prepared by centrifugation from whole human blood within a few hours of its collection from the donor. It is stored in frozen state (below – 30°C). Frozen plasma is used after by immersion in a water bath at a temperature not exceeding 37°C for 45 min. It is used as a source of factor VIII for treating minor hemorrhage in mildly affected haemophiliacs.

18.3.3 Human Plasma Protein Fraction

Human plasma protein fraction is a sterile aqueous solution by proteins of plasma or serum containing albumin and globulins. It is an isotonic solution containing 4.0 to 5.0% w/v of total protein and prepared by fractionating pooled citrated plasma. The plasma or serum is obtained from healthy human donors and free from detectable agents of infection transmissible by transfusion of blood or blood derivatives. Mainly, hepatitis B surface antigen and HIV antibodies are carried out by suitable sensitive methods.

The fractionation procedures is used to make use of following facts:

(i) Proteins are precipitated from solutions without denaturation by the addition of organic solvents such as diethyl ether or ethanol.

(ii) The different proteins are minimally soluble at different pH values.

(iii) Solubility in presence of organic solvents is differentially affected by variations in the salt concentration.

In a series of precipitation steps in which these factors are carefully controlled, various components are separated by centrifugation from a single pool of plasma. The final sedimented paste of proteins containing the desired component in concentrated form is dissolved in a suitable solvent, the composition of which is carefully controlled with respect to pH, ionic strength and temperature. The final product contain not less than 85% of the total protein in albumin. The solutions obtained are freeze-dried to remove residual organic solvent and gives stable product.

The product is dissolved in water and sufficient quantities of a suitable stabilizer, such as sodium caprylate or acetyl tryptophan is added to allow the preparation to be heated for several hours without denaturation of proteins. Sodium chloride is added to make the preparation isotonic but no antibiotic or antimicrobial preservative is added at any stage during preparation. The solution is sterilized by filtration and distributed aseptically into sterile containers. The solution in its final container is heated at 60 ± 0.5°C for ten hours to destroy the viruses of infective hepatitis and homologous serum jaundice. The containers are then incubated at 30 to 32°C for not less than 14 days or at 20 to 25°C for not less than 4 weeks and examined visually for evidence of microbial contamination. It must be stored between 2 and 25°C and protected from light.

Dried human plasma protein function is prepared by freeze drying human plasma protein fraction. Both are used for the same purposes as dried plasma.

18.3.4 Dried Human Serum

Dried human serum is prepared in the same way as dried plasma except that the blood is collected into dry bottles and allowed to clot. The supernatant serum is pooled, bottled and freeze-dried. Its storage and use are the same as for dried plasma except that it can not be used as a source of fibrinogen.

18.3.5 Human Fibrinogen

Fibrinogen is a soluble plasma protein with a molecular weight of 3,40,000. The fibrinogen molecules are elongated and in clotting process, they interact irreversibly to form a three-dimensional network of a semi-solid polymer (fibrin). The polymerization of fibrinogen is brought about by the action of an enzyme, thrombin, which is obtained from the activation of prothrombin.

After separation from plasma by fractionation, the precipitate is collected by centrifugation and dissolved in a citrate-saline solution. The citrate binds calcium ions and prevents spontaneous clotting of the product. The solution is freeze-dried to obtain dried human fribrinogen, yielding a white powder or friable solid. The dried powder is mixed with the stated volume of water for injection to reconstitute for use. The contents are mixed gently so as to avoid frothing. The cloudy solution obtained after 20 to 30 min. contains 10-15 gm./lit. of fibrinogen. The fibrinogen content is determined by adding thrombin to a known volume of solution and measuring the protein content of the separated and washed clot.

Dried human fibrinogen is stored in dry conditions, protected from light and temperature below 25°C. The solution is used immediately after preparation (before 3 hours). It is used for the treatment of fibrinogen deficiency. It is also used in conjunction with thrombin to repair severed nerves and to aid the adhesion of grafts.

18.3.6 Human Thrombin

Human thrombin is the enzyme that converts fibrinogen to fibrin. The prothrombin obtained from the fractionation of plasma is washed with distilled water and dissolved in citrate saline. Prothrombin is converted to thrombin by adjustment to pH 7 and adding thromboplastin in the presence of calcium ions. The solution is clarified, sterilized by filtration and freeze-dried. It is reconstituted with saline solution when required.

Dried human thrombin is stored in dry conditions, protected from light and temperature below 20°C. Thrombin is mixed with fibrinogen to produce fibrin clot and it is used in surgery to suture severed nerves and to assist adhesion of skin grafts. The clot also acts as haemostat.

18.3.7 Human Fibrin Foam

Human fibrin foam is prepared by adding thrombin into the solution of fibrinogen and mix immediately to form foam. The semi-solid foam of fibrin is poured into trays, freeze-dried and sterilized by dry heat at 130°C for three hours. It is issued in suitable size and shape pieces in sealed sterile containers. The fibrin foam is stored below 20°C temperature and protected from light.

Fibrin foam is used as absorbable surgical haemostatic agent. It is usually impregnated with human thrombin and applied locally.

18.3.8 Human Normal Immunoglobulin

Human normal immunoglobulin is a sterile solution or freeze-dried preparation containing immunoglobulins, mainly immunoglobulin G (I_gG), together with smaller amount of other plasma proteins. Human immunoglobulin is the name given to that fraction (IgG Immunoglobulin), separated from human plasma. This fraction was previously known as γ-globulin or immune serum globulin. When the fraction is prepared from random pools of human plasma it is called human normal immunoglobulin.

Human normal immunoglobulin is obtained from source materials such as blood, plasma, serum or placentae frozen immediately after collection from healthy donors. This preparation is a solution of IgG immunoglobulin separated from random pools of plasma. Each pool is derived from not less than 1500 individual donations of blood. The paste obtained by solvent precipitation is freeze-dried and then dissolved in a suitable solvent, usually sodium chloride (0.9% w/v) solution or glycine (2.25% w/v) solution. Thiomersal (0.01%) or other bactericide in suitable concentration is added and pH is adjusted to 6.8 ± 0.4. The solution is sterilized by filtration and distributed into previously sterilized containers and sealed. The liquid preparation is clear pale yellow or light brown in colour. A trace of flocculent protein may precipitate during storage. The freeze-dried preparation is a white to slightly yellow powder or solid, friable mass.

It is stored at temperature between 2-8°C with protection from light. Its use is based on the fact that adults have been exposed to a variety of virus infections. Plasma collected from large number of different donors contains useful levels of a number of important antiviral antibodies. Normal immunoglobulin is effective in preventing measles, rubella, chickenpox, infective hepatitis and bacterial infections.

18.3.9 Human Albumin

Human albumin is sterile, non-pyrogenic preparation of serum albumin obtained by fractionating blood, plasma, serum or placentas from healthy human donors. It is tested individually for the absence of hepatitis B surface antigen, HCV antibodies and HIV antibodies and complies with other tests and requirements prescribed by the appropriate national control authority.

Human albumin is prepared from pooled source materials by precipitation with organic solvents under controlled conditions of pH, ionic strength and temperature. Residual organic solvent is removed by freeze drying or other suitable treatment. The product is dissolved in sufficient water to obtain a suitable concentration. The preparation is free from antimicrobial agent but may contain sodium acetyltryptophanate with or without solution caprylate as a stabilizing agent. The solution is sterilized by filtration and transferred aseptically into final containers. The solution is heated at 60°C for 10 hours so as to prevent the transmission of infectious agent. It is then normally incubated at 30 to 32°C for a further 14 days and subsequently examined for any signs of microbial growth. Human albumin is stored at a temperature between 2 to 25°C and protected from light.

Human serum albumin (HSA) is the single most abundant protein in blood. Its normal concentration is approximately 42 g/lit., representing 60% of total plasma protein. HSA is responsible for over 80% of the colloidal osmotic pressure of human body, hence, it retain sufficient fluid within blood vessels. Human serum albumin preparations are given to patients suffering from kidney, liver diseases and as plasma volume expander in patients suffering from shock due to heavy loss of blood. Hyperoncotic albumin solutions may be used to cause transient diuresis in edematous patients or in those undergoing renal dialysis.

18.4 QUALITY CONTROL OF BLOOD PRODUCTS

All the blood products can save life but many products are dangerous as they can be heavily contaminated with microorganisms. Rigorous application of good manufacturing practice (GMP) with regard to the manufacture of blood products is required to minimize the risk of pathogen transmission. Most GMP or related guidelines contain sections that address issues particularly relevant to the production of blood products. The risk of contamination of blood during processing is minimized by using closed systems and strict aseptic technique. The official standards and labelling are designed to reduce the hazards and prepare quality blood products.

Identification: All blood products contain proteins, hence, standard methods are used in protein identification. Precipitation tests with specific antisera are used to show that only human serum proteins are present in dried serum, dried plasma, the plasma protein fractions, fibrinogen, thrombin and immunoglobulin. Different types of gamma globulin are identified by their sedimentation rate in an ultra-centrifuge. Fibrinogen and thrombin are identified by their clotting behaviour. Normal immunoglobulin is identified by a suitable immunoelectrophoresis technique. Whole blood is identified by determination of the blood group under the ABO and Rh system.

Assay: Whole blood and concentrated human red blood corpuscles assay is performed by determining haemoglobin content by photometric haemoglobinometry. Protein content of many blood products are detected by chemical method except thrombin and fibrin foam. For assay of thrombin, a clotting dose being the amount of thrombin required to clot 1 ml of fibrinogen (0.1%) is saline buffered at pH 7.2 in 15 seconds. Determination of K and Na ions in plasma protein fraction ensure the electrolyte balance of the recipient.

Solubility: All solid preparations are soluble in an appropriate volume of the usual solvent in a specified time. Solubility parameter helps in detection of deteriorated protein constituents. Normal immunoglobulin solubility is determined by adding the volume of the liquid stated on the label and allow it to stand at 20°C for 15 minutes, it dissolves completely.

Sterility and Pyrogens: All blood products must comply with the official tests for sterility and some preparations that are exposed to special risk of contamination with pyrogen due to lengthy processing must also pass the pyrogen test. Pyrogen test for normal immunoglobulin is performed by injecting per kg of the rabbit's mass a volume equivalent to 0.5 g of immunoglobulin but not more than 10 ml per kg of body mass.

Blood products are routinely tested for sterility, identity, pyrogenicity, solubility, stability, assay, abnormal toxicity, loss on drying, protein and moisture contents etc. The quality of the plasma protein fractions is also controlled by electrophoretic, immunoelectrophoretic, ultracentrifugal and chromatographic analysis; assay of specific activities such as coagulation factor or antibody activity; and tests of heat stability. All blood products are properly labelled with all official specifications, storage conditions, contents, expiry date, dose etc.

18.5 PLASMA SUBSTITUTES

The limited supplies of blood, risk of transmitting serum hepatitis and the cost involved in storing, cross matching, processing and dispensing blood and blood products stimulates to find substitutes of non-human origin that could be used to restore the blood volume. The majority of blood substitutes are used as plasma expanders. These blood substitutes are used to maintain blood pressure by providing vascular fluid volume after haemorrhage, burns or shock. Standard electrolyte solutions or physiological saline have been shown to be effective but relatively inefficient plasma volume expanders. The electrolyte solutions (crystalloid fluids) diffuse out of the vascular system or distribute over the entire extra cellular fluid space. Hence, large volume of crystalloid fluids are required to result in effective plasma volume expansion. Colloidal fluids contain larger molecules that diffuse slowly across the semipermeable capillary membranes. These fluids such as dextran, gelatin, starch derivates are used as effective plasma expanders. The major drawbacks of colloidal therapy are high cost and the risk of prompting a hypersensitivity reactions. The ideal properties of plasma substitutes are as follows:

- Low cost, ease of preparation and ready availability.
- Isotonic, equal to blood plasma.
- Same colloidal osmotic pressure as whole blood.
- Viscosity similar to plasma.
- Freedom from toxicity, antigenicity, pyrogenicity and confusing effects on important tests.
- High stability in liquid form at normal and sterilizing temperatures and storage.
- Low rate of excretion or destruction by the body and complete elimination from the body.
- A high molecular weight such that the molecules do not easily diffuse through the capillary walls.

Polyvinylpyrrolidone:

Polyvinylpyrrolidone, a synthetic colloid was introduced by Germany in the Second World War for the treatment of shock. It was marketed in this county in the 1950s but it was not used further because of suspected carcinogenicity.

Gelatin:

Gelatin is produced by partial acid or partial alkaline hydrolysis of animal collagen. It has a wide variety of therapeutic and pharmaceutical uses. Gelatin solution (4%) or succinylated gelatin is also used as a plasma expander. Rapid infusion of the gelatin solution has been known to initiate hypersensitivity reactions. Gelatin is excreted quickly and mostly via the urine.

Hydroxyethyl Starch:

Starch is the energy storage polysaccharide of plants and is analogous functionally and structurally to glycogen, the energy storage polysaccharide molecule of animals. Starch is composed of two types of glucose polymers such as amylose (linear molecule) and amylopectin (branched molecule). Amylopectin is well tolerated when infused intravascularly into animals but is rapidly hydrolyse by amylase. Amylopectin molecule is modified and make it more stable within the plasma by substituting hydroxyethyl groups to create hydroxyethyl starch (HES).

HES solutions contain a heterogeneous solution of HES molecules with an average molecular weight of 69,000, similar to albumin. Hydroxyethyl starch appears to be an extremely well-tolerated plasma expander. Allergic reactions to HES are distinctly uncommon. The incidence of allergic reactions to HES was 0.085% compared with 0.011% for albumin infusion. The important adverse effect of HES infusion appears to be some impairment of coagulation after moderate (20 ml/kg) doses.

Hydroxyethyl starch has been well studied for its efficacy as a plasma volume expander. HES solution (6%) in saline increases plasma volume from 71% to 230% of the volume infused. The colloid osmotic pressure is increased significantly following HES infusion. HES infusion has good hemodynamic effect. In comparative studies of fluid therapy patients, in fusing, HES solutions (6%) has increased central venous pressure, cardiac output and ventricular strike work, with efficacy equivalent to that of 5% albumin infusion. HES and dextran both effectively raise colloid osmotic pressure and plasma volume, though the plasma volume increase may be greater and more sustained following infusion of higher molecular weight dextrans.

Perfluorochemicals:

Perfluorochemicals (PFCs) are 8 to 10 carbon fluorinated hydrocarbons and used as an oxygen carrying blood substitute. Fluosol (Fluosol - DA 20%) is a fluorocarbon emulsion of perfluorodecalin and perfluorotripropylamine. This emulsion is prepared by using poloxamer 188 (Pluronic F-68) or egg yolk phospholipid as a emulsifying agent and hydroxyethyl starch is added to increase oncotic pressure. Fluosol emulsion can absorb, transport and release both oxygen and carbon dioxide. It is used as an effective oxygen carrier during coronary angioplasty. Fluorocarbon emulsions (20%) can be administered regardless of blood type. It is free from blood borne pathogens and is stable for years at room temperature.

Perfluorochemical emulsions are eliminated unchanged through the airways. The particle size of the fluosol emulsion is small (0.1 μ), which contributes to elimination through the alveolar membrane. There is some uptake of PFC emulsions by the reticuloendothelial cells. The plasma half-life of fluosol is about 17 hours after infusion of 20 ml/kg.

Stroma-free Hemoglobin:

Hemoglobin is principal protein found in erythrocytes. Human hemoglobin is a tetramer of molecular mass 64 kDa consisting of two α-chains (141 amino acids) and two β-chains (146 amino acids). Each of the four polypeptide chains has heme as prosthetic group and it is responsible for oxygen binding of hemoglobin.

Human hemoglobin solutions has number of advantages, including the potential to develop a stable, oxygen-binding, colloid volume expander with no antigenicity. Renal toxicity is the main problem with hemoglobin solutions which has led to the development of stroma-free hemoglobin solutions. There are highly purified hemoglobin solutions, free from erythrocytic membrane fragments, which are responsible for renal toxicity.

Stroma-free hemoglobin solutions are prepared from the hemolysis of washed, outdated, banked, human packed erythrocytes. Pure crystalline hemoglobin is produced by sequentially crystallization and washing of hemolysate. This protein is stored in dry form or it may be reconstituted into a solution. These preparations are relatively stable and shelf-life is greatly prolonged if stored in frozen state.

Stroma-free hemoglobin has high ability to bind oxygen. The oxygen half-saturation pressure (P-50) of stroma-free hemoglobin solutions varies from 12 to 16 torr compared with a value of 26 to 27 torr for fresh blood. This increased oxygen affinity is due to the loss of tetrameric hemoglobin, the lack of 2, 3-diphosphoglycerate (2, 3-DPG) and a higher pH compared with the intracellular erythrocyte pH. The increased affinity for oxygen by stroma-free hemoglobin solutions could lead to inadequate release of oxygen to the tissues. The major problem with stroma-free hemoglobin is their rapid clearance from the vascular space due to renal excretion and reticuloendothelial cell uptake.

Hemoglobin is conjugated to additional high molecular weight substances (dextran, polyethylene glycol) to prolong vascular retention, reduce antigenicity and potent plasma volume expansion properties. Polymerized hemoglobins are prepared by cross-linking with gluteraldehyde to prolong product half-life by preventing disassociation into dimmers or manomers. Hemoglobin has been successfully produced by recombinant DNA technology is *Escherichia coli* and *Saccharomyces cerevisiae*. Human hemoglobin α and β genes have been expressed in a wide variety of prokaryotic and eukaryotic systems, including transgenic plants and animals.

Dextran:

Dextrans are polysaccharides produced by the conversion of sucrose into long glucose polymers (Fig. 18.4) by the bacterial enzyme dextransucrase isolated from *Leuconostoc mesenteroides*.

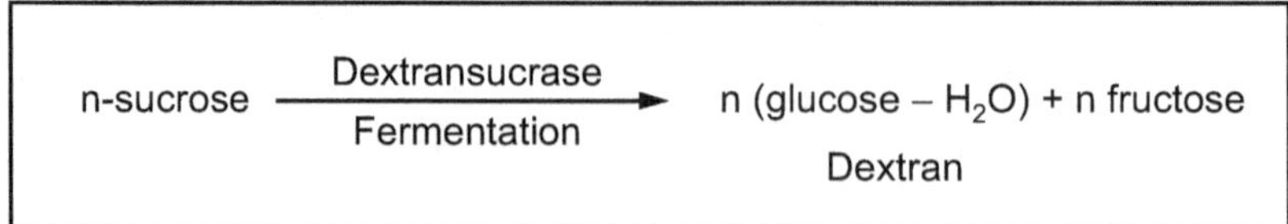

Fig. 18.4: Production of dextran

Dextrans of various molecular masses usually 1, 40, 60, 70 or 110 kDa are often used as plasma expanders. Two dextran solutions are now most widely used, a 6% solution with an average molecular weight of 70,000 (dextran 70) and a 10% solution with an average weight of 40,000 (dextran 40)).

Production of dextran by fermentation is similar in many respects to the antibiotic production. Growth of the dextran producing strain is carried out in large fermenters in media containing high percentage of carbohydrates. The dextran produced by the fermentation have molecular weight 2 to 2.5 lakhs. For clinical use, dextran have the molecular weight upto 1 to 1.1 lakhs. Less molecular weight dextrans are produced by the process of acid hydrolysis, thermal degradation, ultrasonic disintegration and seeding the fermenter with low molecular weight dextran (Refer Chapter 5, Page 5.18). The final dextran molecule is purified by solvent precipitation, adsorption or membrane filtration.

Higher molecular weight dextrans (mainly dextran 70, 75 and 110) are used to promote short-term expansion of plasma volume thus preventing shock due to blood loss. A solution of these dextrans (6% w/v) exerts an osmotic pressure similar to that of plasma proteins. The initial dose of 500 to 1000 ml is administered by intravenous infusion but not more than 20 ml/kg of body weight. In addition to plasma volume expansion, dextran solutions are also used as antithrombotic effects, probably mediated by inhibition of platelet aggregation and to improve blood flow. The low molecular weight dextrans are mainly responsible for improvement of microcirculatory flow by decreasing the viscosity of blood and inhibiting erythrocytic aggregation. The low molecular weight dextran (40 kDa) shows similar therapeutic effects to the high molecular weight dextrans, although it must be used at higher concentrations (10% w/v) in order to achieve the same osmotic pressure.

The rate of renal excretion of dextran depends on molecular size and it mainly excreted unchanged in the urine. Large molecules not excreted in the urine slowly diffuse into the interstitium where uptake into the retriculoendothelial cells. Dextran molecules has severe side effects such as renal failure, coagulation disorders, congestive heart failure, hypervolemia, hypersensitivity, severe dehydration and allergic reactions. Dextrans may interfere with cross-matching of blood if unsuitable dilutions of erythrocytes and serum are used.

QUESTIONS

(A) Objective Type Questions:

1. What is blood? Write the importance of blood donation.
2. Write the ideal properties of plasma substitutes.
3. Explain in short quality control of blood products.

(B) Short Answer Questions:

1. Write in short production and applications of dextran.
2. Write short notes on:
   (a) Human fibrinogen
   (b) Dried human plasma
   (c) Human normal immunoglobulin

(C) Long Answer Questions:

1. Explain in detail collection, processing and storage of blood and blood products.
2. Write in detail the production and importance of different plasma substitutes.

(D) Multiple Choice Questions:

1. Dextrans are produced by the bacterial enzyme _______ isolated from *Leucohostoc mesenteroides*.
   (a) Dextransucrase (b) Amylase
   (c) Lipase (d) Protease
2. _______ is a naturally occurring anticoagulant made by the mast cells.
   (a) Disodium edetate (b) Heparin
   (c) Citrates (d) None of above
3. The breakdown of fibrin is catalyzed by _______ .
   (a) Urokinase (b) Protease
   (c) Renin (d) Plasmin
4. Freezing point of normal human plasma is_______.
   (a) 4°C (b) -4°C
   (c) 0.54°C (d) -0.54°C

■■■

APPENDICES

APPENDIX I - ANSWER KEY

Chapter 1: Introduction to Biotechnology

(D) 1 – (a), 2 – (d), 3 – (d), 4 – (b), 5 – (d), 6 – (b)

Chapter 2: Enzyme Biotechnology

(D) 1 – (d), 2 – (b), 3 – (d), 4 – (a), 5 – (b), 6 – (c)

Chapter 3: Biosensors

(D) 1 – (a), 2 – (c)

Chapter 4: Protein Engineering

(D) 1 – (a), 2 – (c)

Chapter 5: Cloning Vectors and Enzymes

(D) 1 – (c), 2 – (b), 3 – (a), 4 – (b), 5 – (c)

Chapter 6: Recombinant DNA Technology

(D) 1 – (b), 2 – (d), 3 – (a)

Chapter 7: Polymerae Chain Reaction

(D) 1 – (a), 2 – (a), 3 – (c), 4 – (d), 5 – (d)

Chapter 8: Immunity

(D) 1 – (b), 2 – (a), 3 – (a), 4 – (c)

Chapter 9: Hypersensitivity Reactions

(D) 1 – (a), 2 – (b), 3 – (a), 4 – (b), 5 – (b)

Chapter 10: Vaccines and Sera

(D) 1 – (c), 2 – (b), 3 – (d), 4 – (b), 5 – (d), 6 – (d), 7 – (d),

Chapter 11: Hybridoma Technology

(D) 1 – (c), 2 – (d), 3 – (d)

Chapter 12: Immunoblotting Techniques

(D) 1 – (d), 2 – (a), 3 – (c)

Chapter 13: Eukaryotes and Prokaryotes

(D) 1 – (b), 2 – (b), 3 – (d), 4 – (c), 5 – (b), 6 – (c), 7 – (b), 8 – (b), 9 – (c)

Chapter 14: Microbial Genetics

(D) 1 – (b), 2 – (d), 3 – (d), 4 – (a), 5 – (d), 6 – (a), 7 – (a), 8 – (d)

Chapter 15: Microbial Biotransformation

(D) 1 – (d), 2 – (b), 3 – (a), 4 – (a)

Chapter 16: Fermentation

(D) 1 – (c), 2 – (a), 3 – (d), 4 – (b), 5 – (c), 6 – (d)

Chapter 17: Production of Pharmaceuticals

(D) 1 – (c), 2 – (b), 3 – (b), 4 – (a), 5 – (b), 6 – (b)

Chapter 18: Blood Products and Plasma Substitutes

(D) 1 – (a), 2 –(b), 3 – (d), 4 – (d)

■■■

APPENDIX II - QUESTION PAPER FORMAT

Third Year B. Pharmacy : Semester - VI

PHARMACEUTICAL BIOTECHNOLOGY

(PCI SYLLABUS)

Time : 3 Hours] ***[Maximum Marks : 75***

Instructions to the Candidates:

1. *Figures to the right indicate full marks.*
2. *All questions are compulsory.*

SECTION - I

Q.1 Multiple Choice Questions (MCQs) = 20 × 1 = 20

1. Pencillin was discovered by ______
   (a) Paul Ehrlich (b) Louis Pasteur
   (c) Milstein and Kohler (d) A. Fleming
2. ______ is the method of covalent bonding.
   (a) Adsorption (b) Diazotation
   (c) Phase separation (d) Polymerization
3. The pBR 322 is the first artificial vector developed from ______
   (a) *B. subtilis* (b) *Saccharomyces cerevisiae*
   (c) *Escherichia coli* (d) Hepatitis B virus
4. Insulin is made up of ______ amino acids.
   (a) 119 (b) 51
   (c) 86 (d) 35
5. The polymerase chain reaction is ______
   (a) A method of gene amplification (b) A type of DNA repair
   (c) Require for ligation of DNA ends (d) Essential for chromosome replication
6. B-lymphocytes are processed in ______
   (a) Bone marrow (b) Liver
   (c) Lung (d) Brain
7. The immunoglobulin most often associated with immediate type (type 1) allergic reactions ______
   (a) I_gA (b) I_gE
   (c) I_gM (d) I_gD
8. Delayed hypersensitivity reaction is mediated by ______
   (a) T-lymphocytes (b) B-lymphocytes
   (c) Killer cells (d) Natural killer cells

9. Which of the following are live viral vaccines?
   (a) Rabies (b) Cholera
   (c) Influenza (d) Small pox
10. Killed bacterial vaccine is _____
   (a) MMR (b) Small pox
   (c) Rabies (d) Pertussis
11. Hybridoma cell technology is widely used for producing _____
   (a) Organ culture (b) Tissue culture
   (c) Recombinant vaccines (d) Monoclonal antibodies
12. Southern blotting technique is commonly used for the specific identification of _____
   (a) DNA (b) RNA
   (c) Protein (d) DNA and RNA
13. Where does energy production occur in prokaryotes?
   (a) Mitochondria (b) Endoplasmic reticulum
   (c) Cytoplasmic membrane (d) Golgi apparatus
14. Drug resistance in tuberculosis is due to _____
   (a) Transformation (b) Transduction
   (c) Conjugation (d) Mutation
15. The highest rate of conjugation and recombination is associated with the _____
   (a) F-plasmid (b) R-plasmid
   (c) C-plasmid (d) M-plasmid
16. Steroidal transformation mainly occurs at _____
   (a) Growth phase (b) Transformation phase
   (c) Death phase (d) None of the above
17. Sparger is used in fermenter for a addition of _____
   (a) Antifoaming agent (b) Antimicrobial agent
   (c) Sterile medium (d) Sterile air
18. _____ is an extracellular enzyme produced by most of *Bacillus* species, which hydrolyzes penicillin to penicilloic acid.
   (a) Lipase (b) Streptokinase
   (c) Penicillinase (d) Amylase
19. Dextrans are produced by the bacterial enzyme _____ isolated from *Leucohostoc mesenteroides*.
   (a) Dextransucrase (b) Amylase
   (c) Lipase (d) Protease
20. Freezing point of normal human plasma is _____
   (a) 4°C (b) -4°C
   (c) 0.54°C (d) -0.54°C

OR

Q.1 Answer the following (10 × 2) = 10 × 2 = 20.

1. Explain the applications of Lipase.
2. Define vector. Write the features of a good vector.
3. Write the functions of MHC.
4. Differentiate between monoclonal antibodies and polyclonal antibodies.
5. Differentiate between induced mutation and spontaneous mutation.
6. Write the applications of moist heat sterilization in fermentation.
7. What is microbial transformation? Explain microbial transformation by reduction.
8. How will you prepare inoculum for citric acid production?
9. Draw a flow sheet for production of streptomycin.
10. Explain in short quality control of blood products.

Q.2 Answer the following (Answer 2 out of 3) = 2 × 10 = 20.

1. Explain in detail methods for enzyme immobilization.
2. Explain different types of biosensors used in diagnostics with applications.
3. Explain different hypersensitivity reactions with suitable examples.

Q.3 Answer the following (Answer 7 out of 9) = 7 × 5 = 35.

1. Explain in detail importance of Biotechnology with reference to Pharmaceutical Sciences.
2. What is Protein engineering? Write its applications.
3. Write in detail applications of genetic engineering in medicine.
4. How will you prepare Hepatitis-B vaccine by recombinant technology?
5. Explain the applications of polymerase-chain reaction.
6. Explain the general method for preparation of bacterial vaccines.
7. Explain in detail principle and applications of Southern blotting.
8. Explain in detail genetic organization of Prokaryotes.
9. How will you monitor and control different parameters in large scale fermentation?

■■■

APPENDIX III - BIBLIOGRAPHY

- Balasubramanian D. et. al. (eds); (2004). Concepts in Biotechnology, First edition, Universities Press (India) Private Limited.
- Casida L. E., (2000). Industrial Microbiology, New Age International, Delhi.
- Crueger W. and Cruegar A. (2005). Biotechnology, Second Edition, Panima Publishing Corporation, New Delhi.
- Cruickshank R. (ed.), (1965). Medical Microbiology, Eleventh Edition, E. and S. Livingstone Ltd.
- Debnath M. (2005). Tools and Techniques of Biotechnology. First Edition, Pointer Publishers, Jaipur.
- Demain A. L. and Davies J. E. (eds), (1999) Manual of Industrial Microbiology and Biotechnology, Second Edition, ASM Press, Washington, D.C.
- Dubey R. C., (2006). A Text book of Biotechnology, Fourth Edition, S. Chand and Company Ltd.
- Gangal S., (2007). Principles and Practice of Animal Tissue Culture. Universities Press (India) Private Limited, Hyderabad.
- Gupta P. K., (2007). Elements of Biotechnology, First Edition, Rastogi Publications, Meerut.
- Hugo W. B. and Russell A. D., (1998). Pharmaceutical Microbiology, Sixth Edition, Backwell Science.
- Ian Freshney R., (2000). Culture of Animal Cells – A manual of basic technique, Fourth Edition, Wiley-Liss Publication.
- Ketchum P. A., (1988). Microbiology- Concepts and Applications, John Wiley and Sons, New York.
- Kokare C., (2013), Pharmaceutical Microbiology – Experiments and Techniques, Fourth Edition, Career Publications, Nashik, India.
- Kokare C., (2018), Pharmaceutical Microbiology – Principles and Applications, Fifteenth Edition, Nirali Prakashan, Pune.
- Kokare C., (2017), Pharmaceutical Biotechnology- Fundamentals and Applications. Fifth Edition, Nirali Prakashan, Pune
- Kokare C., (2017), Pharmaceutical Biotechnology- Experiments and Techniques. Fourth Edition, Nirali Prakashan, Pune.
- Kokare C. and Kokare S., (2016), Research Methodology, Third Edition, Nirali Prakashan, Pune.

- Lachman L. et al., (1987). The Theory and Practice of Industrial Pharmacy, Third Edition, Varghese Publishing House.
- Nelson D. L. and Cox M. M., (2005), Lehninger Principles of Biochemistry, Fourth Edition, W. H. Freeman and Company, New York.
- Patel A. H. (2005). Industrial Microbiology. First Edition, Macmillan India Ltd.
- Pelczar M. J. et al., (1986). Microbiology, Fifth Edition, MaGraw Hill, New York.
- Philopose P. M. (2004). A Textbook of Biotechnology, First Edition, Dominant Pubishers and Distributors, New Delhi.
- Rehm H. J. and Reed G. (eds.), (1989), Biotechnology, Volume 7b, VCH Publishers.
- Salle A. J., (1974). Fundamental Principles of Bacteriology, Seventh Edition, Tata McGraw-Hill Publishing Company Ltd., New Delhi.
- Sambrook J., Russel D. W., (2001), Molecular Cloning, A laboratory manual, Vol. – I, Third Edition, Cold Spring Harbor Laboratory Press, New York.
- Satyanarayana U (2005). Biotechnology, First Edition , Books and Allied (P) Ltd. Kolkatta.
- Singh B.D. (2005). Biotechnology, Second Edition, Kalyani Publishers, Ludhiana.
- Stanbury P. F. et. al., (1995). Principles of Fermentation Technology, Second Edition. Butterworth-Heinemann.
- Swarbrick J. and Boylan J. C., (1994). Encyclopedia of Pharmaceutical Technology, Vol.9, Marcel Dekker, Inc., New York.
- Talaro K. and Talaro A., (1996). Foundations in Microbiology, Second Edition, Wm C. Brown Publishers, U. S. A.
- Tortora G. J. et al., (1998). Microbiology: An Introduction, Third Edition, Benjamin/ Cummings Publishing, California.
- Vyas S. P. and Dixit V. K. (2003), Pharmaceutical Biotechnology, First Edition, CBS Publishers and Distributors.
- Vyas S. P. and Kohli D.V. (2004), Methods in Biotechnology and Bioengineering. First Edition, CBS Publishers and Distributors, New Delhi.
- Walsh G., (2003), Biopharmaceuticals, Biochemistry and Biotechnology, Second Edition, Antony Rowe Ltd., Great Britain.
- Winfield A. J. and Richards R. M. E. (eds.), (1998). Pharmaceutical Practice, Second Edition, Varghese Publishing House.

■■■

www.ingramcontent.com/pod-product-compliance
Lightning Source LLC
LaVergne TN
LVHW061937220826
846092LV00004B/1024

* 9 7 8 9 3 8 9 6 8 6 3 4 0 *